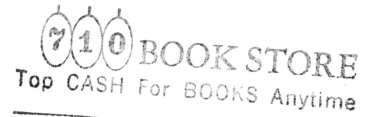

Textbook of
Head and Neck Anatomy

Second Edition

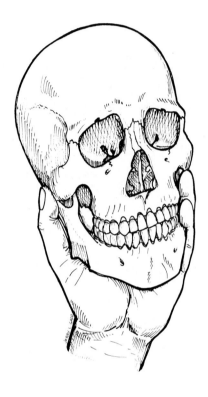

Alas, poor Yorick! I knew him well Horatio, a
fellow of infinite jest, of most excellent fancy. He
hath borne me on his back a thousand times.
Shakespeare, Hamlet.

Textbook of
HEAD AND NECK ANATOMY

Second Edition

James L. Hiatt, Ph.D.
Associate Professor of Anatomy

Leslie P. Gartner, Ph.D.
Associate Professor of Anatomy

Department of Anatomy
Baltimore College of Dental Surgery
Dental School, University of Maryland
Baltimore, Maryland

Illustrated by Jerry L. Gadd

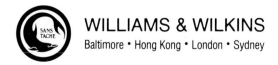

WILLIAMS & WILKINS
Baltimore • Hong Kong • London • Sydney

Editor: John Gardner
Associate Editor: Victoria M. Vaughn
Copy Editors: Deborah Tourtlotte, Shelley Potler
Design: JoAnne Janowiak
Illustration Planning: Lorraine Wrzosek
Production: Raymond E. Reter

Copyright © 1987
Williams & Wilkins
428 East Preston Street
Baltimore, MD 21202, U.S.A.

Printed in the United States of America

First Edition, 1982

Library of Congress Cataloging in Publication Data

Hiatt, James L., 1934–
    Textbook of head and neck anatomy.

    Bibliography: p.
    Includes index.
    1. Head—Anatomy. 2. Neck—Anatomy. I. Gartner,
Leslie P., 1943—   II. Title. [DNLM: 1. Head—
anatomy & histology. 2. Neck—anatomy & histology.
WE 705 H623t]
QM535.H48 1987   611'.91   86-22434
ISBN 0-683-03975-X

    88 89 90 91   10 9 8 7 6 5 4 3

Dedicated to our wives,
Nancy and *Roseann,*
and to our children,
Drew, Beth, Kurt, and *Jennifer.*

Preface to the Second Edition

It is always gratifying to learn that your efforts have been well received, and thus it has been with the first edition. Many of our colleagues expressed an endorsement of this text and from students we learned how well it had served them.

Since this book was not intended to be a scholarly treatise, but a textbook designed to enhance and facilitate learning for the student, we were pleased to learn that students found it especially helpful in their study of head and neck anatomy and in their preparations for boards examinations.

This second edition has not undergone drastic changes; however, we have made every effort to correct errors including those pointed out by colleagues and students. We believe the style and format utilized in the first edition are optimal for student learning, and they have been retained in this edition. In addition to correcting errors, we have rewritten Chapter 20, Lymphatics of the Head and Neck, and added two new chapters.

Chapter 20 was totally revised in an attempt to make it more understandable from the standpoint of lymph node involvement in lymphatic drainage of the head and neck. This information was summarized in tabular form to assist the student in assimilating this subject matter. While the format of the text is presented in a regional manner, a few of the chapters naturally lend themselves to being presented systemically, for example, Chapter 18, Cranial Nerves. One of the new chapters (Chapter 21, Vascular Supply of the Head and Neck) presents this subject in this fashion, to assist the student in comprehending the continuity of the system.

The remaining new chapter (Chapter 22, Fascia of the Head and Neck) details a necessary but difficult subject that the dental professional must understand. We have strived to present this material in a manner that is not overly simplified nor intensely complex, but sufficiently complete for student understanding.

Finally, we have revised the Index in an effort to make it more useful through cross-referencing. Particular attention was given to the sections referencing muscles, nerves, arteries and veins, as these items are the ones most frequently searched.

We wish to express our sincere thanks to all of those colleagues and students who offered constructive criticisms which we have attempted to incorporate in this edition. We especially thank the faculty of the Department of Anatomy for their continued interest, comments, and discussions which helped us in evaluating the needs for this edition. We are also grateful to JoAnn Walker for her expert typing of the manuscript on a very tight schedule.

Working with our friends at Williams & Wilkins has been a pleasure. So many there have helped and their efforts are greatly appreciated. We especially wish to mention Debbie Tourtlotte, our copy editor, Lorraine Wrzosek, layout, JoAnne Janowiak, design; to you we offer our thanks. A special thank you also to Ray Reter, our Production Sponsor, who kept everything straight, Pamela Caras, Domestic Marketing Manager, for her guidance, and of course our Associate Editor, Vicki Vaughn, who was there at every request. Finally, a warm thanks to John Gardner, Vice President and Editor-in-Chief, for having the faith once again.

Although we have made every effort to ensure care and accuracy, we realize that some mistakes, errors, and omissions may have escaped our attention. Therefore, criticisms, suggestions, and comments that could help to improve this textbook will be appreciated.

Preface to the First Edition

This book was written for students, remembering that they enter the study of head and neck anatomy with varying backgrounds and much apprehension. We have attempted to circumvent many of the problems that students face by making the book complete, concise, yet easily read. It is profusely illustrated to aid the student who does not always have access to anatomical specimens. Additionally, this text contains numerous tables in order to make the student's formidable task somewhat easier. New words, when first introduced, are printed in italics, some of which are redefined in the Glossary. Although this is not an elementary textbook, it is not meant to be a reference text. Anatomical variations, except for those most common, are usually not discussed. This textbook was conceived and written from a regional approach; yet certain aspects, such as osteology, the nervous system and lymphatics, which are easier to comprehend from a systemic point of view, are detailed in both manners.

In the first three chapters we have included introductory information which is not normally found in specialized textbooks of head and neck anatomy, such as generalized anatomical concepts, a rather complete but concise summary of cogent materials on body systems and a brief history of anatomy. The fourth chapter examines the oral cavity so that students become involved with the subject of their profession relatively early in their study of anatomy. This and most subsequent chapters contain a treatment of pertinent clinical considerations, correlating anatomical material with clinical practice. Chapter 5 presents an overview of the development of the head and neck with particular attention devoted to the embryology of the face and palate. Osteology of the skull and neck follows development, thus providing an orderly sequence and foundation for the remaining chapters which detail regional presentations of the head and neck. The brain and spinal cord and cranial nerves are considered in separate chapters and are presented as overviews with information being detailed where applicable to the study of the head and neck. The autonomic nervous system is discussed with the functional relationships of its components to the nerves transmitting taste and secretomotor functions. Oral anesthesia is presented as related to the components of the trigeminal nerve and pertinent anatomical landmarks. Lymphatics of the head and neck conclude the chapter presentations. The last two subjects are often omitted from textbooks and anatomy curricula, yet are important to students whose future practice will entail the region of the head and neck. Following the Glossary is a short list of Selected References for students professing interest or requiring additional information. The final segment of the text provides a fully cross-referenced index for expedient use by the student.

We would like to thank our artist Jerry Gadd for his excellent illustrations and the time that he so freely gave; our typists Mary Eccleston and Carolyn Jones for their cheerful and efficient attention to detail; the Department of Oral Diagnosis of the Dental School, University of Maryland at Baltimore for permitting us to use their intra-oral photography equipment; Donna Muir, one of our students, for permitting us to photograph her eyes; members of the Anatomy Department for their support during our writing of this text; and our many friends at Appleton-Century-Crofts, including Marcia Kipnees, who demonstrated an interest in our project from the beginning, Judith Warm-Steinig, Associate Managing Editor and Text Designer, for seeing it through and especially Elizabeth Stueck, Acquisitions Editor, for her devoted help, interest and support in guiding us through the amazing complexities of preparing and publishing a textbook.

While we appreciate all the assistance we received, we acknowledge that the responsibility for shortcomings, errors and omissions is ours. And in view of that fact, we welcome criticisms and suggestions for improvement of this text.

Contents

PREFACE TO THE SECOND EDITION .... *vii*

PREFACE TO THE FIRST EDITION .... *ix*

LIST OF TABLES .... *xv*

1. INTRODUCTION *1*

2. ANATOMICAL CONCEPTS *5*
  Anatomical Variation/7

3. BODY SYSTEMS *9*
  Integumentary System/9
  Muscular System/12
  Skeletal System/16
  Circulatory System/21
  Nervous System/24

4. THE ORAL CAVITY, PALATE, AND PHARYNX *31*
  Lips/31
  Vestibule/33
  Oral Cavity Proper/36
  Pharynx/48
  Clinical Considerations/51

5. EMBRYOLOGY OF THE HEAD AND NECK *57*
  Pharyngeal Arch, Groove and Pouch Development/58
  Floor of the Pharynx/63
  Face, Nose and Palate Development/65
  Clinical Considerations/68

6. OSTEOLOGY *73*
  Skull and Cervical Vertebrae/73
  The Skull/73
  Mandible/103
  Hyoid Bone/109
  Cervical Vertebrae/109

7. NECK *113*
  Surface Anatomy/113
  Superficial Structures of the Neck/114
  Deep Fascia/117
  Posterior Aspects of the Neck/121
  Triangles of the Neck/128
  Deep Prevertebral Muscles of the Neck/149
  Clinical Considerations/149

8. SUPERFICIAL FACE   *153*
   Surface Anatomy/153
   Scalp/153
   Face/155
   Clinical Considerations/164

9. CRANIAL FOSSA   *167*
   Dura Mater/167
   Diploic and Emissary Veins/172
   Cranial Nerves/173

10. ORBIT AND EAR   *175*
   Orbit/175
   Clinical Considerations/185
   Ear/185
   Clinical Considerations/189

11. PAROTID BED   *191*
   Superficial Anatomy and Boundaries/191
   Parotid Gland/191
   Carotid Arteries/195
   Facial Nerve/197
   Structures Deep to the Parotid Bed/197
   Clinical Considerations/199

12. DEEP FACE   *201*
   Descriptions and Boundaries/201
   Muscles and Fascia/202
   Vascular Supply/211
   Innervation/213
   Mastication/215

13. TEMPOROMANDIBULAR JOINT   *217*
   Joint Anatomy/217
   Types of Movement/221
   Clinical Considerations/223

14. PTERYGOPALATINE FOSSA, NASAL CAVITY, AND
    PARANASAL SINUSES   *225*
   Pterygopalatine Fossa/225
   External Nose/227
   Internal Nose/228
   Clinical Considerations/233

15. SUBMANDIBULAR REGION AND FLOOR OF MOUTH   *235*
   Contents and Boundaries/235
   Muscles and Fascia/236
   Salivary Glands/240
   Innervation/241
   Vascular Supply/242
   Lymphatics/243
   Clinical Considerations/244

16. PALATE, PHARYNX, AND LARYNX   *245*
    Palate/245
    Pharynx/250
    Esophagus/255
    Larynx/255
    Trachea/261
    Deglutition/261
    Clinical Considerations/262

17. BRAIN AND SPINAL CORD   *265*
    Meninges/265
    Brain/266
    Spinal Cord/277

18. CRANIAL NERVES   *279*
    Cranial Nerves/280

19. ANATOMICAL BASIS FOR LOCAL ANESTHESIA   *307*
    Plexus Anesthesia/307
    Trunk Anesthesia/308

20. LYMPHATICS OF THE HEAD AND NECK   *311*
    Lymph Nodes of the Head and Neck/311
    Lymphatic Drainage of the Head and Neck/313
    Clinical Considerations/317

21. VASCULAR SUPPLY OF THE HEAD AND NECK   *319*
    Common Carotid Artery/319
    Subclavian Artery/330
    Veins of the Head and Neck/332

22. FASCIAE OF THE HEAD AND NECK   *337*
    Cervical Fascia/337
    Cervical Fascial Spaces/341
    Fasciae of the Face and Deep Face/342

    GLOSSARY   *347*

    SUGGESTED READINGS   *361*

    INDEX   *363*

List of Tables

Table 5.1.	Pharyngeal Arch Derivatives and Their Innervation	59
Table 5.2.	Derivatives of the Pharynx and the Pharyngeal Pouches	65
Table 5.3.	Derivatives of Facial Components	68
Table 6.1.	Bones of the Skull	74
Table 6.2.	Foramina of the Skull and Their Contents	106
Table 7.1.	Muscles of the Back of the Neck	122
Table 7.2.	Boundaries and Contents of the Suboccipital Triangle	128
Table 7.3.	Boundaries of the Cervical Triangles	130
Table 7.4.	Muscles Associated with the Posterior Triangle	132
Table 7.5.	Branches of the Cervical Plexus	135
Table 7.6.	The Infrahyoid Muscles	140
Table 7.7.	Deep Prevertebral Muscles of the Neck	150
Table 8.1.	Muscles of the Face and Scalp	156
Table 8.2.	Branches of the Facial Nerve in the Superficial Face	163
Table 10.1.	Bones of the Orbit	176
Table 10.2.	Communications of the Orbit	177
Table 10.3.	Muscles of the Eye	183
Table 10.4.	Bony Ossicles and Their Associations	187
Table 12.1.	Boundaries, Communications and Contents of Infratemporal Fossa	203
Table 12.2.	Muscles of Mastication	204
Table 13.1.	Muscles Acting on the Temporomandibular Joint	223
Table 14.1.	Openings of the Paranasal Sinuses	231

Table 14.2.　Vascular and Sensory Nerve Supply of the Paranasal Sinuses　233

Table 16.1.　Muscles of the Palate and Pharynx　248

Table 16.2.　Intrinsic Muscles of the Larynx　259

Table 18.1.　Cranial Nerves　281

Table 18.2.　Parasympathetic Ganglia of the Head　286

Table 20.1.　Lymph Nodes of the Head and Neck　314

Introduction

Anatomy has always fascinated man not only because of his interest in the delivery of children but also due to the importance of understanding anatomy in healing wounds and caring for the sick. Although anatomical representations and the study of anatomy have been noted in almost every culture, Occidental medicine traces its origin to philosophers in the Golden Age of Greece and the Arabic physicians, who studied, instructed, and wrote about anatomy and attempted to relate it to function and disease. They also named observed structures, while their students expanded this knowledge by discovering and naming yet other structures. Students of anatomy during the Middle Ages— even as late as the 18th century—utilized Greek and Latin, the *lingua franca* of learned men. Hence, most of the structures named during those centuries of discoveries were named in those languages, a practice continued into modern times.

The earliest written treatise on anatomical studies was set down by the Greek philosopher Alcmaeon about 2500 years ago. He discovered and dissected the optic nerves, traced them back to the optic chiasma, and deduced their role in binocular vision. He also discovered and described the auditory tube, suggested that the brain is responsible for intelligence, and studied the ramifications of blood vessels.

Writing at about the same time, the philosopher Pythagoras also suggested that the brain was the center of intelligence. He believed that the physical and emotional well-being of an individual was related to the ratio of the four humors: phlegm, yellow bile, black bile, and blood. These four humors were related to the four elements: water, fire, earth, and air, respectively, whose properties were moist, dry, cold, and hot. A healthy individual would possess a proper combination of these fluids, while a disproportionate ratio would be responsible for a diseased state of the body and/or mind. This belief in humors became a basic tenet of Hippocratic Medicine. Unfortunately, Aristotle's writings lent credence to this line of thinking; thus it persisted well into the Middle Ages. Aristotle, however, did make major contributions to the study of anatomy by correctly describing many organs and structures of the human body. He may also have been the first anatomist to illustrate his descriptions with drawings.

Shortly after the decline of Athens, the Greek scholars of Alexandria, especially Herophilus, pioneered in the teaching of anatomy by the use of human dissections. For his work in this field, Herophilus is considered the Founder of Anatomy, and his dissertations (all lost) encompassed many areas of the subject. The next four centuries saw a decline in anatomical studies until the advent of Galen, possibly the greatest physician of his age. His writings on anatomical structures were so precise and well researched that they constituted the solid bases of medicine for well over a millenium. He believed that structure and function were closely interrelated, and his painstaking studies of the spinal cord illuminated his theories, which survived into the early 19th century. Soon after Galen, the Roman Empire collapsed and Europe entered its Dark Ages. During this period, it was the Arabic physicians, chiefly Avicenna writing around 1000 A.D., who were responsible for keeping the scientific perspectives of Medicine and Anatomy alive.

A major landmark of anatomical history occurred in 1224, when Frederick II proclaimed that in order to be permitted to perform surgery one must have studied anatomy by dissecting a human body. Although this edict established Anatomy as a discipline unto itself, no major advance occurred for another 350 years. The next important achievement came with Leonardo da Vinci, whose brilliant anatomical illustrations added new emphasis to the functional appreciation of structure. He, more than anyone before him, was able to display the results of his dissections and simplify the complexities of the human body. Hence, the study of human anatomy returned to Europe, flourishing in the Age of Renaissance. This enlightened period of humanistically oriented culture permitted questioning of secular dogma. The teachings of the ancients were at last openly opposed by the Belgian physician Andreas Vesalius, who applied strict scientific discipline to his anatomical observations. He single-handedly revised the discipline of Anatomy and wrote a treatise that was the forerunner of modern anatomy textbooks. Within a generation or so of Vesalius, another great anatomist, William Harvey, wrote about the blood vessels and the heart. His work, the cornerstone of the study of the structure and function of the circulatory system, revolutionized Medicine, Physiology, and Anatomy.

The invention of the microscope around this time opened new vistas in anatomy, permitting the marvelous discoveries of Wirsung, Malpighi, Purkinje, Golgi, Cajal, and Ehrlich. Discussion of these anatomists is outside the scope of this brief historical survey, but interested readers are encouraged to refer to one of several books dealing with the history of Medicine or Anatomy.

Modern anatomy textbooks approach the subject from a systemic, regional, or surgical point of view. A systemic anatomy textbook, as the name implies, treats the body as if it were organized into neat, self-contained systems, such as the skeletal, muscular, nervous, and circulatory systems, each of which is detailed in the text. Such an approach is valuable, especially in a reference textbook, for it describes each structure in a continuous fashion.

Textbooks that treat the subject in a regional manner divide the body into specific areas—such as upper extremity, lower extremity, thorax, head and neck—and discuss each region as to its contents—that is, osteology, myology, nervous, and vascular elements. Descriptions do not exceed the boundaries of the region, regardless of the fact that many structures (vessels, nerves, and muscles, for example) are not wholly contained within that specified area. Textbooks of surgical anatomy are based on such a regional approach, with emphasis on surgical techniques, approaches, and normal anatomic variations.

The head and neck comprise a highly specialized region of the body. The structures contained within this region are closely interrelated, since they are compacted into a small, complicated area. Other regions of the body, where interrelationships are less complex, lend themselves to a systemic approach. The head and neck does not. Consequently, the present textbook is written from a regional point of view, since the authors believe this approach will be more likely to promote student understanding. The regional method synthesizes morphology for the reader by correlating relationships as the reader progresses through the various anatomical divisions of the head and neck. Furthermore, this approach aids not only those who have constant access to a laboratory situation but also those who do not. And, finally, this approach eliminates the need to synthesize the final product from its component parts, thus assisting the student in mastering the intricacies of this fascinating region of the body.

Anatomical Concepts

The word *anatomy,* which has been derived from the Greek words *ana* and *tomē,* literally means to "cut up" or dissect. The human body, therefore, is described in an anatomy text as if it were dissected layer by layer. Since the study of anatomy is a descriptive science and since the descriptions are related spatially, it is evident that a student of anatomy must become familiar with the language an anatomist utilizes in describing these spatial relationships. Without understanding the basic vocabulary, the student would be unable to learn the subject effectively or to communicate with peer professionals.

The science of human anatomy is generally divided into four major categories of study. *Developmental anatomy* deals with the study of how the mature body is formed from a fertilized ovum. *Neuroanatomy* is the specialized study of the nervous system. *Microscopic anatomy* is the division of anatomy which studies the fine details of the human body utilizing the microscope. This division is often referred to as *Histology,* the study of tissues. *Macroscopic* or *Gross anatomy,* on the other hand, is that division of anatomy which studies the human body with the unaided eye.

Gross anatomy of the human body may be studied from one of two approaches. *Systematic anatomy* is the approach which discusses each system separately and in its entirety, for example, studying all of the muscles of the body which comprise the muscular system before discussing the components of any other system. The other study approach, *regional anatomy,* details a region of the body, such as the head and neck, studying all systems in that area as a complete, integrated unit.

The regional approach employed in this text provides the student with a more comprehensive understanding of an anatomical region thus enhancing an understanding of interrelationships between the various systems of the body.

Human anatomical structures are described spatially relative to the anatomic position, defined for the human as an erect position with the palms of the hands facing forward (Fig. 2.1). Structures located on the "front" side of the body are described as being *anterior,* while those located on the "back" of the body are termed *posterior.* Occasionally, other terms may be used for anterior and posterior, such as *ventral* in place of anterior and *dorsal* in place of posterior (Fig. 2.2).

Similarly, alternate terms may be utilized in referring to directions aimed at the head or tail. *Cranial* or *superior* means "toward the head," while *caudal* or *inferior* refers to "tailward." The terms *superficial* and *deep* are employed to describe positions relative to the surface of the body from any aspect. The ribs

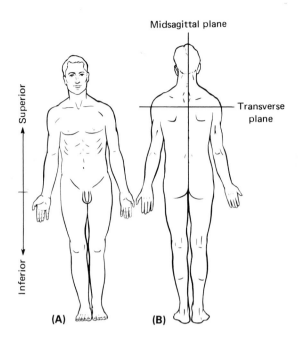

Figure 2.1. Human figure in the anatomical position illustrating planes and directional references. **A.** Anterior view. **B.** Posterior view.

are superficial to lungs yet deep to the skin. Alternate terms for superficial and deep are *external* and *internal* respectively. *Proximal* and *distal* are terms generally applied to positions close to or away from the body. For example, the wrist is proximal to the finger but distal to the elbow. The teeth are described as being either *mesial* or *distal* to each other in the dental arch from the median plane of the face. For example, the canine tooth is mesial to the first

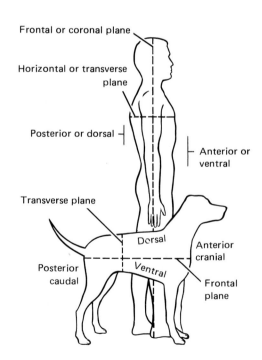

Figure 2.2. Comparative planes and directional references with alternate terminology.

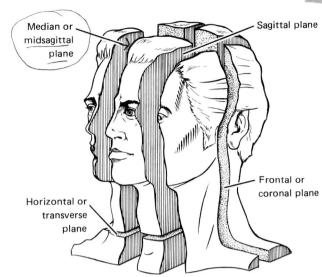

Figure 2.3. Planes of reference and alternate terminology.

premolar and distal to the lateral incisor. *Medial* and *lateral* are terms applied in relationship to the midline of the body. A structure, A, located closer to the midline than another structure, B, is therefore medial to structure B.

An anatomy student must also learn to visualize several imaginary planes passing through the body serving to divide it in one way or another. The *median plane* passes vertically through the body from anterior to posterior at the midline. This plane serves to divide the body in symmetrical right and left halves except for certain of the viscera. This plane may also be referred to as the *midsagittal plane.* Any plane parallel to this plane is simply a *sagittal plane.* A plane through the body at right angles to the midsagittal plane is the *horizontal plane* or *transverse plane*, providing a cross section with superior and inferior parts. Another plane passes at right angles to the midsagittal plane again in a vertical direction and is the *frontal* or *coronal plane*, dividing the body into anterior and posterior sections (Fig. 2.3).

Although the previously described terms are applied to the entire body, they are also appropriately employed in describing the structures in head and neck anatomy.

ANATOMICAL VARIATION

A student of anatomy must learn early that anatomical variation is sometimes the rule rather than the exception. Structures observed in the cadaver often do not conform to the descriptions found in anatomy textbooks. The major structures may not vary so much, but as the finer details are studied, variations clearly emerge. For example, a student would not expect great variation in the number of bones present in a cadaver, and there is not a great variation. However, the individual processes on the bones and their relationships are not at all constant from one individual to another. Similarly, muscles may display slightly different origins, insertions, and tendons. Nerves may not arise from the segment as described. Variations in blood supply are very common; a particular region may be supplied from an entirely different source than that described.

It is important that the student learn to recognize anatomical variations as they exist, whether they are described or not. Further, the student must learn to interpret logically the significance of these variations and perhaps to extrapolate their effects upon the living individual. Mastering this diagnostic technique helps in enabling the professional to make rational decisions regarding anatomical variations observed in clinical practice.

Body Systems

Human beings, like all other animals, are composed of a complex aggregate of specialized *cells*. These cells, the building blocks of all living things, have become specialized to perform certain functions, a "division of labor."

Since structure and function are interrelated, it is possible to group cells into functional classifications based on morphology. Thus the cell classifications of epithelium, connective tissue, muscle, and nerve represent all of the specializations relative to structure and function. Similar specialized cells organized to perform a specific role are grouped into *tissues.*

Tissues fabricated together and performing in unison to accomplish a particular function make up an *organ.* Organs acting together to accomplish specific functionary roles are referred to as *systems.* Thus, the body possesses a myriad of cells organized into tissues and organs performing together as the integumentary, skeletal, muscular, circulatory, endocrine, digestive, respiratory, excretory, reproductive, and nervous systems.

It is not the purpose of this text to detail the systems of the body. It is essential, however, that the student possess a satisfactory knowledge of the systems encountered in the head and neck. By learning a brief overview of these systems, students will reach a common starting point for studying the anatomy of the head and neck.

INTEGUMENTARY SYSTEM

The integument, or skin, includes its derivatives—the hair, nails, and glands. It functions to protect the underlying structures against intrusion from the outside as well as loss from within. Furthermore, it serves as a sensory receptor, regulates body temperature, and functions as an organ of secretion and excretion.

The skin forms a pliable covering over the body and becomes continuous with mucous membranes at the orifices of the body, as at the nares and the oral cavity. The skin is thickest over the back, palm of the hand, and sole of the foot where it is about 6 mm thick. The thinnest skin is about 0.5 mm in thickness where it overlies the tympanic membrane and the eyelid. In most areas of the body the skin is loosely attached to the underlying structures, thus permitting it to be easily displaced. It is, however, firmly attached to the periosteum of the tibia, to cartilage of the ear, and over joints of the fingers and the palm of the hand.

Skin color is primarily controlled by three factors: blood, carotene, and melanin. Variation in color is related to degree of vascularity, oxygen content of blood, skin thickness, and profuseness of pigmentation. Under certain conditions, physiological changes may produce a transient increase in pigmentation, as evidenced in the tanning process from exposure to sunlight. The external genital areas, the axilla, and the areola of the mammary gland display constantly deeper pigmentation.

Skin possesses fine furrows or creases extending in various directions across the surface. These furrows tend to divide the surface into polygonal areas. Some of these are large, while others—for example, on the back of the hand—are small. Epidermal ridges and sulci (furrows) on the fingers, palms, and soles are organized in a specialized fashion of whorls and curves peculiar to each individual. This individual uniqueness provides the basis for fingerprint identification. Epidermal ridges provide friction against slippage in walking and in grasping. Ducts of sweat glands open on the summits of the ridges, while in areas covered with hair, the shafts emerge at points of intersection of the furrows. Typically, the secretions of the sebaceous glands empty in the furrows also.

Structure

Skin is composed of two layers: the *epidermis,* or surface layer, and the underlying *dermis.* The epidermis is without blood vessels but is penetrated by sensory nerve endings. In general, the epidermis is only about 1 mm in thickness and is composed of several layers of stratified squamous epithelial cells. Histologists have subdivided these layers into five distinct groups based on morphology and function. The deepest layer, *stratum germinativum,* overlies the dermis and is primarily responsible for producing all of the epidermal cells above it, which are being constantly shed. As these cells mature, they produce *keratohyalin* which is eventually transformed into keratin in the superficial layers. The most superficial layer, *stratum corneum,* composed of dead cells and keratin, forms a horny layer whose thickness is related to the trauma it experiences.

The dermis underlying the epidermis possesses the blood supply, lymphatic channels, and nerve endings. It also contains sebaceous and sweat glands, hair follicles, and the smooth muscles of the skin. The interface of the epidermis and dermis is thrown into interdigitations of *epidermal pegs* and *dermal papillae* which serve to secure the two layers (Fig. 3.1).

The dermis is composed of two basic layers, a superficial papillary layer and the deeper reticular layer, containing collagenous and elastic fibers which account for its strength and elasticity. The deepest layer of the dermis sits upon a subcutaneous connective tissue layer. The interface of these two layers is somewhat interdigitated so that, when the layers are separated from each other, the dermal side appears to exhibit a dimpled appearance similar to an orange peel. These dimples are sites of entry for nerves and blood vessels into the skin from the subcutaneous connective tissue.

The *subcutaneous connective tissue* (hypodermis) is a loose, fibrous connective tissue containing fat and some elastic fibers. It may be termed *loose areolar tissue* or *superficial fascia.* Some areas of the body possess large deposits of fat in this layer and are designated *panniculus adiposus.* Certain other

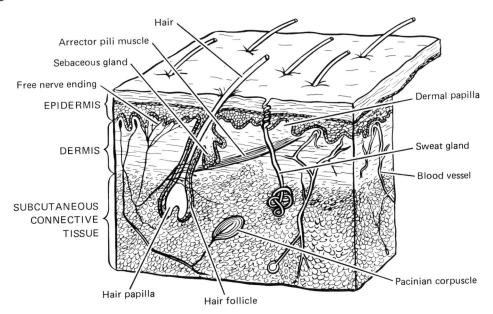

Hair

Arrector pili muscle

Sebaceous gland

Free nerve ending

EPIDERMIS

DERMIS

SUBCUTANEOUS
CONNECTIVE
TISSUE

Dermal papilla

Sweat gland

Blood vessel

Pacinian corpuscle

Hair papilla

Hair follicle

Figure 3.1. Skin structure.

areas—notably the eyelids, penis, scrotum, as well as the nipple and areola of the mammary gland—are devoid of subcutaneous fat. Embedded in this layer are the roots of the hair follicles, blood vessels, secretory portions of the sweat glands, and nerves with special sensory endings for pressure. Overlying some joints, the hypodermis contains *bursae,* which are fluid-filled sacs providing lubrication for movement of the skin as the joint is flexed. Many mammals, such as the horse, possess voluntary muscles located in this layer which permit flinching of the skin. Muscles of this nature, originating in the hypodermis and inserting in the dermis, are found in the scalp, face, and neck. Here they are grouped in man as the *muscles of facial expression.* Involuntary (smooth) muscles are also represented in this layer, muscles such as the dartos muscle of the scrotum and the muscles of the nipple and areola of the mammary gland.

Hair

Hair is found on nearly all parts of the body with the exception of the palms, soles, dorsum of the terminal digits, nipples, umbilicus, and the skin portion of the genitalia. Hair is also absent in areas of skin transitional to mucous membrane, such as the lips and nares. Hair varies in shape: it may be round causing it to be straight, or it may be flattened producing curly hair. The eyelashes, hair of the pubic region, and hair in the beard are very thick, while that in other areas of the body may be so thin that it may go unnoticed. Hair on the scalp may remain for up to four years, while the eyelashes may only survive for a few months.

Hair is a product of the epidermis, whose deeper cells invade the dermis forming a hair follicle from which the nonliving hair develops. The dermis responds by forming a papilla to nourish the germinative cells of the follicle. Thereafter, the hair grows surfaceward, finally exiting the skin. The free part of the hair is called the *shaft*, while that within the follicle is the *root*. Color is imparted to the hair by melanin and red pigment in the hair cells.

Each hair has in association with it one or more sebaceous glands whose ducts open into the neck of the hair follicle. Involuntary muscle fibers *(arrector pili)* arise in the dermis and attach to the hair follicle, serving to erect the hair, squeezing out the secretions of the sebaceous glands and producing "goose bumps" on the flesh (Fig. 3.1).

Nails

The nails, which grow approximately 1 mm per week, are modifications of epidermal-cell layers on the terminal digits. The vascular nail bed, formed by the lower germinal layer of the epidermis and the dermis, upon which lies the translucent nail plate, imparts a pinkish hue to the nail. The visible part of the nail is the body and the hidden portion behind the nail wall is the root. The nail is formed in the proximal part near the whitened lunula which may be covered by eponychium (cuticle). The epidermis is thickened under the distal portion of the nail, forming the hyponychium.

Glands

Glands of the skin include the sebaceous, sweat, and mammary glands (the last will not be discussed in this text since they are remote to the head and neck). The sebaceous glands have been described in their association with hair follicles, but they are found in other places in the body devoid of hair, namely the lips, corners of the mouth, and sometimes within the oral cavity. Additionally, these glands may be found in most areas of the genitalia as well as the areola and nipple. The secretory cells are constantly destroyed and become part of the oily secretion *sebum* which protects the skin from undue drying.

Sweat glands are widely distributed, being absent only on the lips, parts of the ear, skin of the nipple, and some skin areas of the genitalia. They are most dense over the palms and soles. The clear noncellular fluid produced by the sweat glands regulates body temperature as it evaporates from the surface of the skin, cooling it (Fig. 3.1).

MUSCULAR SYSTEM

Cells specialized to function in contraction upon stimulation comprise the muscles of the body. Muscles are usually attached from bone to bone, across a joint. Upon contraction, these muscles change the angle of the joint, producing motion. In this way, muscles acting in concert effect movement. Such motion may be under conscious control, *voluntary,* or not under conscious control, *involuntary.* Muscles which effect smiling, walking, writing, and so on are voluntary muscles, while those utilized in altering the diameter of blood vessels or controlling the bowel are in the involuntary category.

There are three types of muscles in the body: skeletal, cardiac, and smooth. The first two are striated while the last one is not. Skeletal muscle is under voluntary control, while cardiac and smooth muscles are involuntary.

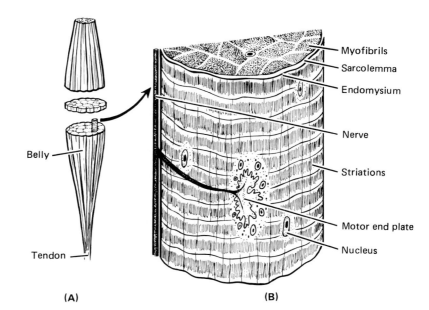

Labels: Myofibrils, Sarcolemma, Endomysium, Nerve, Striations, Motor end plate, Nucleus, Belly, Tendon

Figure 3.2. Skeletal muscle. **A.** Belly of muscle shown with fascicles in cross section. **B.** A detailed section of a single muscle fiber.

(A)   **(B)**

Structure

Microscopically, the muscle cell is referred to as a *muscle fiber.* The cytoplasm in a muscle cell contains many contractile elements called *myofibrils* which are composed of actin and myosin. The fibril arrangement in skeletal and cardiac muscles is such that the muscle fiber appears to be cross-banded in alternate light and dark striations. This appearance is responsible for the name *striated muscle.* Skeletal muscle fibers are long, cylindrical, multinucleated cells whose nuclei are located peripherally (Fig. 3.2).

Smooth muscle cells, in contrast, each possess only one centrally located nucleus. Microscopic evaluation reveals no striations within the cytoplasm.

Cardiac muscle is found mostly in the muscular pump, the heart. The cardiac muscle fibers are striated in a fashion similar to skeletal muscle cells, but each cell possesses only one centrally located nucleus. Features unique to cardiac muscle are the branching and anastomosing, or joining together, of the cells and transversely oriented *intercalated discs,* located at the junction of any two fibers. This muscle type is unique in that it possesses an ability to modify its contractive actions by altering the wave of impulses received from the nervous system.

Skeletal muscle is by far the most abundant muscle in the body. In fact, it comprises about 40 percent of the total body weight. Skeletal muscle size varies from the large muscles of the leg, to the very small stapedius muscle (about 2 mm in length) which is attached to the tiny stapes bone of the middle ear cavity.

Each skeletal muscle fiber is encased in a thin connective tissue covering, the *endomysium.* A *muscle fascicle,* composed of a group of muscle fibers, is bundled into a separate connective tissue sheath, the *perimysium.* The entire muscle, composed of many fasciculi, is wrapped in yet another connective tissue sheath, termed the *epimysium* or *deep fascia.*

Attachment

At the attachment to bone, the muscle fiber membrane (especially the endomysium), along with the epimysium, blends into the tendon, a white, dense regular collagenous connective tissue. The tendon is extremely strong and is continuous with the periosteum of the bone at the attachment site where the two interlace. In certain regions of the body—for example, in the muscles of the scalp—attachment is by an *aponeurosis,* a broad, flat sheet-like structure, instead of a tendon.

Some attachments are provided with *bursae* which lubricate the tendon as it passes over bone. Often a *synovial sheath* encloses a tendon, forming a tubular sac that is capable of secreting a *synovial fluid,* constantly bathing the tendon in a fluid environment to reduce friction. Friction is also reduced by the epimysium, the deep fascia of the body. Since the deep fascia encloses muscles and bone in a continuous manner, it also serves to contain the spread of infection.

Tendinous attachments to bone are usually described as the *origin* and *insertion* of the muscle. Generally, the muscle is described as arising from the origin, possessing a fleshy belly (the contractive portion), and inserting at the insertion site. Usually the origin is the more proximal and/or fixed area, with the insertion being the more distal or movable area. It must be stressed that these are not hard and fast rules, but they are rather arbitrarily employed by anatomists as aids in describing function.

Though the above description of bone-to-bone origin and insertion is the usual occurrence, the muscles of facial expression do not follow this rule. Generally, these muscles arise from bone or fascia and insert into the skin of the face. Upon contraction, they produce movements of the skin which we recognize as expressions in the face.

Form

Examining a muscle's size, form, and fiber arrangement in relation to its insertion into the tendon will indicate the relative strength of the muscle as well as the direction of its force. Those muscle fibers which approach the tendon in an oblique fashion afford more power. Muscles whose anatomy takes this form are *pennate.* Fibers entering a tendon at two oblique angles, as do the veins of a feather, are said to be *bipennate.* Multiples of this architectural arrangement produce *multipennate* muscles, which exhibit the greatest strength.

Action

Muscle action is described according to the movement effected in the part in motion from the anatomical position (this basic reference position was shown in Fig. 2.1). Though individual actions are often difficult to separate given the complexities of a variable motion—as, for example, in mandibular movement—they are expressed in a few anatomical terms. *Flexion* is described as motion which reduces the angle of a joint, while *extension* increases the joint angle. Making a fist utilizes the flexor muscles. Opening a closed fist utilizes the extensor muscles. *Adduction* and *abduction* are terms employed to describe motion toward the body centerline or away from it, respectively. Terms describing movements of the head and neck—*protrusion, retraction, elevation, rotation,* and *depression*—are self-explanatory.

There are several other terms used to describe various other motions created by the action of a muscle; however, since these are of no concern to the study of the head and neck, their discussion will be omitted. Often, names assigned to muscles reflect the architecture of the muscle, its form or shape, attachments and action, or in some cases, a combination of these features. However, seldom does a muscle function independently and alone. Indeed, movements are so complex that muscles must function in a cooperative and integrated manner to accomplish a total desired movement. To recognize this complexity, anatomists have created additional terms which indicate how a muscle functions in producing a total movement. Muscles may be *prime movers* or *synergists* which assist a prime mover. Certain other muscles, such as the strap muscles attached to the hyoid bone, serve as *fixators,* so that other actions may be initiated by yet other muscles. *Antagonists* function in such a manner that the action they develop is in opposition to the desired function of yet other muscles *(agonists).* In addition to aiding in the production of smooth movement, antagonists protect the musculoskeletal system from damaging itself, as might occur through a violent movement.

Nerve Control

Voluntary muscles must receive nerve stimulation in order to contract. The number of nerve fibers in a muscle is dependent on the muscle's size and the degree of control required of the muscle. The extrinsic muscles of the eye, for instance, are well endowed with nerve fibers, while the muscles of the back possess fewer nerve endings. As the nerve fiber approaches the muscle, it branches to innervate many muscle fibers. The *motor end-plate* is the zone of interaction between the nerve fiber and the sarcolemma of the muscle where the impulse is transmitted (Fig. 3.2). In addition to this nerve fiber which serves a motor function, other fibers enter the muscle which will conduct sensations of pain and proprioception from the muscle and surrounding connective tissue back to the central nervous system (CNS). These nerves provide sensory data to the CNS so that the motor function may be reprogrammed either voluntarily or involuntarily, as might be necessary for the individual to take protective measures.

When a muscle fiber is stimulated, it contracts maximally according to the "law of all or none." It holds, then, that fine movements are accomplished by stimulating fewer nerve fibers resulting in activation of only a portion of the total muscle fibers at a given time.

Energy requirements necessary for the work performed by the muscles demand a rich vascular supply. It is a general rule throughout the entire body that nerves and blood vessels travel together as *neurovascular bundles*, are named alike, and enter the muscle together. Larger muscles, requiring additional vascularization, may have additional arteries entering their surfaces without associated nerves. In such cases, the artery usually arises from a nearby vascular trunk. While nerve supply to a muscle is specific, vascular supply may not be; therefore, vascular supply is provided by region.

SKELETAL SYSTEM

The elements of the skeletal system—bone, cartilage, and the joints—are composed of intercellular materials and cells specialized in performing certain functions for the body. Functions unique to this system include support, protection, providing attachment for muscles, leverage, mineral storage, and blood formation.

Support is derived from the mineral salts that are deposited in the matrix and fibers secreted by the cells of the system. Through this process, the skeletal system provides form and a framework upon which all of the remaining systems of the body are supported and held together.

Protection is afforded to the soft tissues of the body, including the viscera, lungs, and brain, by encasing them in partially enclosed structures, such as the rib cage and pelvis, or in an enclosed chamber, the skull.

The skeletal system also provides sites of attachment for skeletal muscles along the bones and across the joints. The various parts of the skeletal system then can be utilized as levers for the production of motion as a result of muscle contraction. In addition to their function in providing leverage, bones become calcified by mineral deposits during development and growth and, therefore, serve as reservoirs for mineral storage. The predominant minerals stored are calcium, magnesium, and phosphate.

A final major function of the skeletal system is blood cell formation. The centers of several bones contain *bone marrow* whose specialized cells have the capacity of differentiating into blood cells.

Skeleton

The skeletal system, composed of 206 bones, is divided into the *axial skeleton* and the *appendicular skeleton* according to the following distribution:

Axial skeleton		
Skull	28	
Hyoid	1	
Vertebral Column	26	
Ribs and Sternum	25	
		80
Appendicular Skeleton		
Upper Limbs	64	
Lower Limbs	62	
		126
Total		206

This number is not constant, since there may be slight variations among individuals. Many of the bones do not fuse together until after infancy; therefore, infants possess more bones than do adults. Occasionally, some of the skull bones which develop as bilateral halves do not fuse in the midline, thus remaining doubled. The frontal bone is one example of this phenomenon, in some cases remaining divided into two separate bones at the *metopic suture* instead of fusing at the midline.

Additionally, *accessory bones* may develop in bones possessing multiple ossification centers that fail to unite. This condition gives rise to *wormian bones* often observed in the larger flat bones of the skull. *Sesamoid bones* develop within tendons either for additional leverage, as in the patella (knee cap), or as a means of reducing friction at the joint. There may be several of these bones, but again the number varies among individuals.

The *axial skeleton* is composed of the bones making up the longitudinal axis and serves to protect the spinal cord, brain, and vital organs. It also supports the head and neck, along with the trunk and its appendages. A major part of this portion of the skeleton is the *skull,* composed of many bones more or less tightly sutured together forming the cranial vault to protect the brain as well as bones forming the face. The mandible and bony ossicles of the ear are bones separate from the skull proper, but they are still considered part of it. Although the hyoid bone does not articulate with the skull, it is occasionally listed as part of the skull because of its functional association.

The *vertebral column* acts as the major foundation of the skeleton and protects the spinal cord. Attached to the vertebral column are the ribs, which enclose and protect the lungs and heart and attach anteriorly to the medial anteriorly-placed sternum. The five fused sacral vertebrae and four coccyx form part of the pelvis serving to protect the pelvic viscera. These last nine constitute the remaining components of the axial skeleton.

The *appendicular skeleton,* composed of some 126 bones, makes up the remaining skeletal system. The bones of the *superior extremity* include those of the hand, arm, and the pectoral girdle. The pectoral girdle attaches the bones of the superior extremity to the axial skeleton. The *inferior extremity* includes the bones forming the foot and leg and the pelvic girdle. Here the pelvic girdle attaches the extremity to the axial skeleton.

Classification

Bones may be classified on the basis of their general shape. These shapes include *long bones,* as found in the arms and legs, *short bones,* as in the wrist and ankle, *flat bones,* like those forming the skull, and *irregular bones,* such as the vertebrae. *Sesamoid bones* are also described as a separate category.

Bone is a composite of cells and organic matrix secreted by bone cells with deposited inorganic salts crystallized within the matrix. This complex organization produces a structure with a great tensile strength and the ability to withstand compression. The tubular design of the long bones, consisting of a thin layer of compact bone external to spongy bone with its trabeculae, increases the structural strength of the bone. The articular ends of bones usually covered by the articular cartilage are designated either a *condyle* or *head.* The shaft of the bone may possess several characteristic landmarks indicating much information. Terms employed to describe these features include: *smooth areas,* indicating a periosteum cover only; elevations, in the form of *lines, crests, ridges, processes, tubercles, tuberosities,* and *spines,* indicating points of attachments; depressions, such as *pits, foveae,* and *fossae,* indicating intervals between elevations or sites where a structure may be housed; *grooves* and *sulci,* indicating linear depressions housing particular structures; *foramina* and *notches* indicating openings or holes; and *canals* or *meatuses,* indicating passageways or tunnels.

Joints

Two or more bones coming together form a joint. Sometimes the unison is such that movement is prevented, while in other instances movement is the function of the joint. Joints can be classified as *fibrous, cartilaginous,* or *synovial,* depending upon the structural articulations of the opposing bones (Fig. 3.3).

Fibrous joints include two types: *syndesmoses* and *sutures.* The syndesmosis joint permits only slight movement between the two bones which are separated by a layer of fibrous connective tissue. The interosseous membrane between the radius and ulna is an example. Sutures are joints like those between the flat bones of the skull. Here the individual bones interdigitate tightly along serrated edges, rendering them almost immovable. The fibrous tissue between these bones is continuous with the periosteum.

Cartilaginous joints are represented by *synchondroses* and *symphyses.* Opposing bony surfaces of this group are united by cartilage. A synchrondrosis is a temporary joint that will eventually be ossified into a bony component. The epiphyseal plate on the ends of the growing long bones is an example of this type of joint. A symphysis is a cartilage joint between two bones. It is located in the midline and is interposed between the fusion of the bones, as in the mandibular symphysis and the pubic symphysis.

Synovial joints, the most abundant type in the body, afford the greatest degree of joint movement. The articular surfaces of the bones are covered by hyaline cartilage. The entire joint is in turn covered by ligaments forming an articular capsule which is lined by synovial membrane. Occasionally, the joint is separated by an articular disk. This meniscus is continuous with the capsule

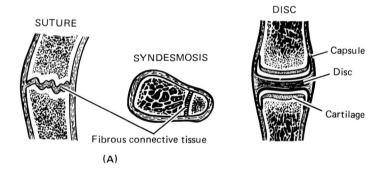

Figure 3.3. Joint types. **A.** Fibrous joints. **B.** Cartilaginous joints. **C.** Synovial joints. (Modified from R. C. Crafts, *A Textbook of Human Anatomy,* 2nd ed. New York, John Wiley & Sons, 1979, p. 14.)

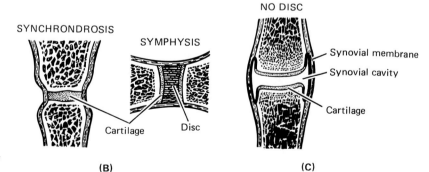

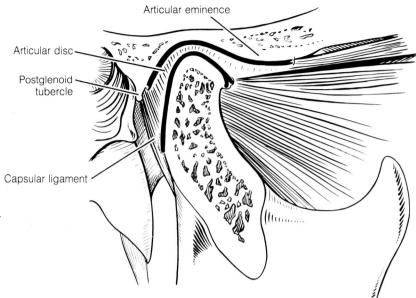

Articular eminence

Articular disc

Postglenoid
tubercle

Capsular ligament

Figure 3.4. Temporomandibular joint. A portion of the condyle has been cut away revealing the disc and joint cavity.

peripherally, but its articular surfaces are not covered with synovial membrane. A variety of synovial joints exist in the body, each permitting only a particular type of movement. These movements are categorized in six different terms. Since most of these terms are not associated with the joints of the head and neck, terms will be defined as discussion of individual joints requires.

Articulations of the synovial joint are usually of a gliding or sliding character. The joint contains synovial fluid which acts as a lubricant and also supplies nutrients to the avascular articular cartilage. The synovial joints are richly supplied with sensory nerve endings, principally of the proprioceptive variety, as well as with pain and stretch receptors. Articular capsules and ligaments are highly vascularized, forming capillary networks over the synovial membranes (Fig. 3.4).

Bone Development

During embryogenesis and postnatal growth, bone may develop in one of two ways. It may be formed directly in mesenchyme, in which case the mode is intramembranous. Most of the flat bones of the skull are formed in this manner. The other method of bone formation involves bone being elaborated on and replacing a cartilage template. This is endochondral bone formation and represents the manner in which the long bones and most of the other bones of the body are formed.

Intramembranous bone formation begins as the area destined to become bone becomes highly vascularized and the mesenchymal cells develop into *osteoblasts.* These bone-forming cells then begin secreting collagen and a matrix composed of mucoproteins, constituting the *osteoid.* These osteoblasts possess long cell processes that communicate with other osteoblasts and nearby blood vessels. At this stage, the osteoid is a rubbery, tough but elastic material yet uncalcified.

Mineral ions of calcium carbonate and calcium phosphate, circulating in the blood, begin to diffuse into osteoid tissue and are deposited on the surfaces of the collagen fibers as fine crystals. This imparts a hardness and rigidity to the osteoid in the process of becoming bone. Those cells that were responsible for secreting the matrix become trapped in *lacunae* and are now *osteocytes.*

Endochondral bone formation begins after a cartilage template has been formed in an area destined to become bone. The hyaline cartilage miniaturized model, which continues to grow while at the same time being replaced by bone, originally develops in mesenchyme in a fashion similar to that of intramembraneous bone. Condensation of mesenchymal cells is followed by differentiation into *chondroblasts* which secrete a viscous polysaccharide matrix interspersed with collagen and some elastic fibers. The chondroblasts eventually become entrapped in a lacuna within the matrix. Since the matrix may not become calcified soon after formation, if at all, chondroblasts may continue to divide within the lacuna producing *interstitial growth.* Later the entrapped cells become quiescent, ceasing to produce matrix, and are now termed *chondrocytes.* Once these cells stop secretion, the only method of enlarging the cartilage model is by *appositional growth* at the periphery by cells differentiated from the perichondrium.

Because of the nature of the cartilage matrix, it does not become infiltrated by blood vessels. Nutrients reach the cells by diffusion only; therefore, cartilage metabolism is low compared to that of the very vascular bone. This accounts for the slow repair of cartilage upon damage.

During endochondral bone formation, the perichondrium of the cartilage model becomes vascularized at mid-diaphysis, causing the chondrogenic cells to become osteogenic and begin to elaborate bone in this region. Eventually a *periosteal bud* of mesenchymal cells, and blood vessels invade the model, and the cartilage begins to calcify. Simultaneously, mesenchymal cells differentiate into *chondroclasts* (phagocytic cells) and begin to destroy the cartilage while other cells differentiate into osteoblasts and start elaborating bony tissue on the calcified cartilage as its remnants are removed, thus developing a *primary ossification center.* This process spreads outward from the center and, in the case of a long bone, for example, it may take many years to complete.

The ''bone'' continues to elongate at its *epiphyses* (ends) by cartilaginous growth. The center of the *diaphysis* (shaft) of the long bone is composed of *cancellous bone* which is finally remodeled to withstand stresses upon it. Later, much of it is replaced with *red bone marrow* composed of specialized stem cells with give rise to blood cells. The walls of the shaft are composed of very hard and strong *compact bone* to which are attached muscles via tendons (Fig. 3.5). The architecture of the bone is in a constant state of change in response to the mechanical stresses placed upon it. The mandible and maxillae, for example, are constantly being restructured to meet the changing stresses imposed by growth as well as by tooth eruption, movement, wear, and loss. This constant simultaneous growth and remodeling process is achieved by resorbing bone from certain areas and depositing new bone in other areas. The cells associated with the process of resorption are the *osteoclasts,* while the osteoblasts responsible for depositing new bone are derived from the osteogenic cells of the *periosteum* covering the bone or the *endosteum* lining the medullary cavity. This is the process which permits the orthodontist to move teeth, since tension stimulates new bone formation while pressure activates resorption *(Wolff's Law).*

Spongy bone   Pulp cavity

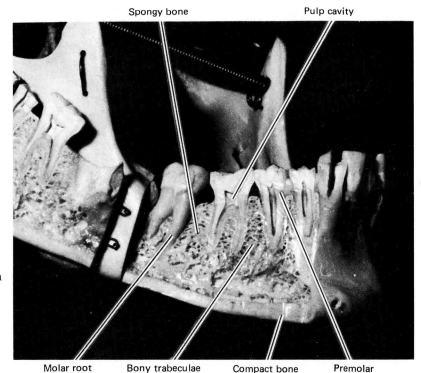

Figure 3.5. Bone structure. A section of the mandible reveals the cancellous bone located interior to the very hard compact bone located on the surface.

Molar root   Bony trabeculae   Compact bone   Premolar

Cartilage

Bones cannot be discussed without mention of the articulating cartilages which serve as connective tissue at the joints. Cartilage is a supporting tissue which possesses a firm but somewhat pliable anatomy permitting it to withstand great stresses at the joints.

Cartilage also serves as the template for endochondral bone formation and functions in long bone growth as previously discussed. Though it is formed in a fashion similar to bone, it is poorly vascularized and innervated. Three types are recognized: *hyaline, fibrous,* and *elastic.* Hyaline cartilage is the type found in the cartilage template of long bones and at their growing ends. Hyaline cartilage is located also at the joints as articulating cartilage and may be found also in the tracheal rings and larynx. Fibrocartilage is present in the intervertebral discs, in the pubic symphysis, and in the mandibular symphysis. In addition, the articulating parts of the temporomandibular joint are covered by fibrocartilage rather than by hyaline cartilage (Fig. 3.4). Elastic cartilage occurs in the external ear, auditory tube, epiglottis, and some components of the larynx.

CIRCULATORY SYSTEM

The circulatory system is composed of two parts working in unison to maintain the internal environment. The heart, arteries, veins, capillaries, and blood comprise the cardiovascular system, while lymph nodes, spleen, tonsils, thymus, lymph, and lymphatic vessels make up the lymphatic system.

Cardiovascular System

The cardiovascular system functions to provide transportation of oxygen, water, nutritive materials, and hormones to the tissues of the body in exchange for carbon dioxide and wastes that will be further transported to excretory organs for elimination from the body.

Blood, the fluid tissue of the cardiovascular system is composed of cells and plasma. The cells are *erythrocytes* (red blood cells) and *leucocytes* (white blood cells). Erythrocytes, which are manufactured in red bone marrow, transport oxygen and carbon dioxide gases to and from the body tissues, respectively. Leucocytes are diverse in origin and function. Non-granular leucocytes, which include *lymphocytes* and *monocytes*, originate in red bone marrow and lymphatic tissues and function in the defense system. The granular leucocytes include *eosinophils, neutrophils,* and *basophils.* These cells are generally assigned the functions of protecting from outside invasion and combating infection. *Blood platelets,* also found in the blood, assist in coagulating the blood. The *plasma* (liquid portion of the blood) is composed of water, proteins, enzymes, and salts as well as the products of digestion and excretion. This fluid leaks out of the capillary walls becoming tissue fluid bathing the cells with its contents and picking up wastes prior to its return to the circulatory system via either the venous capillaries or the lymph capillaries.

The heart, arteries, veins, and capillaries comprise the closed system for the transportation function of the cardiovascular system. The heart is a double pump in that it serves two circuits for blood flow that are completely separated from each other in a normal healthy adult heart. The *pulmonary circuit,* located in the right side of the heart, receives venous (deoxygenated) blood in the right atrium from the body via the *superior* and *inferior venae cavae* and from the heart itself via the *coronary sinus.* During muscular contraction, the pooled blood is pumped from the right atrium through the *right atrioventricular (tricuspid) valve* into the *right ventricle.* Blood in the ventricle is then pumped out the *pulmonary trunk* which divides into *right* and *left pulmonary arteries* transporting the blood to the lungs for oxygenation and some excretion (Fig. 3.6).

Oxygenated blood returns from the lungs in the *pulmonary veins* to enter the left side of the heart in the *left atrium.* The blood is now in the *systemic circuit* where it is pumped through the *left atrioventricular (bicuspid) valve* into the enlarged, very muscular *left ventricle.* From here, the blood will be pumped out the *aorta* to be distributed by arteries throughout the entire body (Fig. 3.6).

The *arteries* branch like a tree, becoming smaller and smaller with each branching leading away from the heart. The blood flows away from the heart from large arteries to small arteries to *arterioles* and finally to *capillaries* with a bore only large enough to permit blood cells to traverse one or two at a time (Fig. 3.7).

In the *capillary bed,* gases and nutrients are exchanged for wastes while hormones and enzymes are delivered for body maintenance. Muscles in the walls of the vessels control the blood flow to the periphery, thus aiding in the control and management of body temperature.

The cardiovascular system is under control of the nervous system. The rate and force of the heartbeat is modulated by the autonomic nervous system

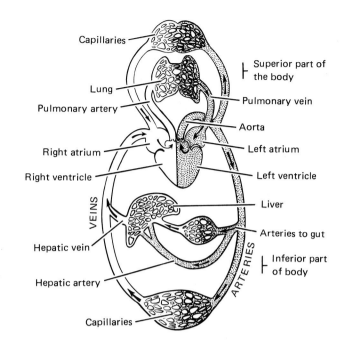

Figure 3.6. Schematic representation of the cardiovascular system. Note the darkened area is transporting oxygenated blood while the light regions transport deoxygenated blood. (Adapted from J. E. Crouch, *Functional Human Anatomy*, 2nd ed. Philadelphia, Lea & Febiger, 1972, p. 279.)

through the specialized cells within the heart musculature which have the capacity to perpetuate the beat determined by the nerve impulses. The blood vessels, particularly the arteries, are also under control of the autonomic nervous system. Nerve impulses to the muscular walls of the arteries will elicit either dilation or contraction of the vessel lumen thereby increasing or decreasing the rate of flow.

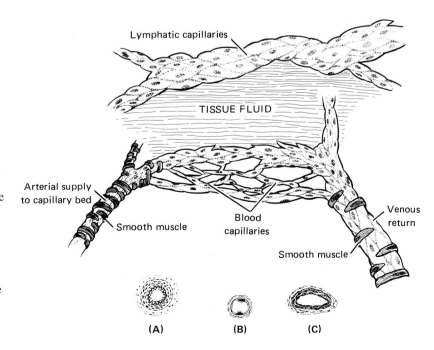

Figure 3.7. Diagram illustrating the capillary bed where tissue fluids leave the blood vessels to bathe the tissues prior to being taken into the lymphatic capillary. Cross-sectional drawings of an artery, capillary, and a vein are shown in **(A)**, **(B)**, and **(C)** respectively.

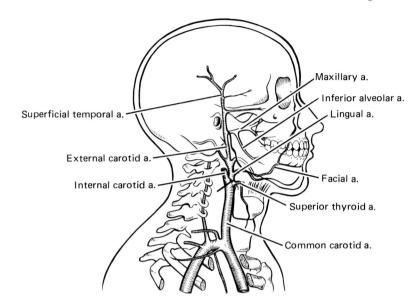

Figure 3.8. Schematic diagram of the carotid artery and the distribution of its vessels in the neck and head. The arrow indicates the approximate location of the carotid body and carotid sinus.

Labels: Superficial temporal a.; External carotid a.; Internal carotid a.; Maxillary a.; Inferior alveolar a.; Lingual a.; Facial a.; Superior thyroid a.; Common carotid a.

Specialized sensory mechanisms to monitor blood pressure and oxygen tension within the bloodstream are located in the carotid arteries within the neck. The *carotid sinus* located at the beginning of the internal carotid artery responds to changes in blood pressure. The *carotid body* located at the bifurcation of the common carotid artery is a chemoreceptor sensitive to changes in oxygen tension within the blood. When stimulated, both of these specialized receptors, served by cranial nerves, evoke an autonomic response aimed at returning the system to a homeostatic state (Fig. 3.8).

Lymphatic System

The lymphatic system begins as an extensive system of capillary beds collecting the lymph (tissue fluid) from the tissues (Fig. 3.7). The capillaries empty into larger lymphatic vessels and eventually the lymphatic vessels empty their contents into the bloodstream in the large veins at the base of the neck. Between the capillary beds and the point of entry into the bloodstream, the lymph passes through one to several *lymph nodes* which act as filters. Here lymphocytes reside in *lymph nodules* and are propagated for circulation in the bloodstream to sites for combatting foreign intrusion. Lymph capillaries within the gut, called *lacteals,* absorb fatty products of digestion and eventually transport it to the bloodstream via the *thoracic duct.*

In addition to the lymph nodes, the lymphatic system also includes the spleen, thymus, and tonsils, which are responsible for other lymphatic functions such as the maintenance of immunocompetence.

NERVOUS SYSTEM

The nervous system is a complex organization of tissue, ramifying throughout the body, functioning to collect information from within and from outside the environment of the body. The nervous system sorts this information, then activates, coordinates, reorders, and integrates body functions to meet these perceived challenges imposed upon it. Included within the functions of this system is the process of conceptual thought taking place in the highest centers of the system in the brain.

The system is divided morphologically, for descriptive purposes, into two divisions: the peripheral nervous system and the central nervous system. The *peripheral nervous system (PNS)* is comprised of twelve pairs of cranial nerves emanating from the brain and thirty-one pairs of spinal nerves originating from the spinal cord. The *central nervous system (CNS)* is composed of the brain and spinal cord (Fig. 3.9).

Structure

The tissue of this system is made up of specialized cells, *neurons,* which conduct impulses and *neuroglial* cells which serve in supporting capacity.

A neuron, the basic structural unit of the system, possesses the ability to perceive stimuli *(irritability)* and to transmit physiochemical impulses along its processes *(conduction)* to effector organs and/or other neurons. The neuron is composed of a *cell body* and its processes. The cell body contains the nucleus and cytoplasm with *Nissl bodies* which may be made visible through the use of special stains. Neuron cell bodies are located either in a *ganglion,* if outside the CNS, or in *nuclei,* if within the CNS. Radiating from the cell body are freely branching processes called *dendrites,* which transmit impulses toward the cell body, and a singular *axon,* which transmits impulses away from the perikaryon. The axon often emanates at the opposite side of the cell body from a bulge called the *axon hillock.* The arrangement of processes around the cell body may vary from that described here and are thus supplied with descriptive terms (Fig. 3.10).

Axons may or may not possess a fatty *myelin sheath* covering of variable thickness which completely surrounds the *axis cylinder* except at regular intervals along the axon. These intervals, called the *nodes of Ranvier,* impart a linked-sausage appearance to the axon. Myelinated or unmyelinated axons are covered by a *neurilemma sheath* composed of Schwann cells. The speed of conduction of an impulse along a nerve fiber is related to the absence or presence and thickness of the myelin sheath (Fig. 3.10).

Functional Components

Neurons are categorized functionally as: sensory, intercalary (connecting), or motor. Sensory (afferent) and motor (efferent) functions are each further subcategorized to facilitate description of a neuron's specific function. *General somatic afferent* refers to sensory function (modality) perceived from the body and transmitted to the spinal cord or brain. Sensations such as pain, temperature, and touch to the skin are perceived by neurons in this category. Also in this category is sensation from muscles, tendons, and joints, referred to as "proprioception." *General visceral afferent* is the sensory modality received from within the viscera (glands, organs, and membranes). *General somatic efferent,* a motor component, serves to provide innervation to all of the skeletal muscles of somatic origin, while *general visceral efferent* stimulation provides motor innervation to smooth muscles, cardiac muscles, and glands.

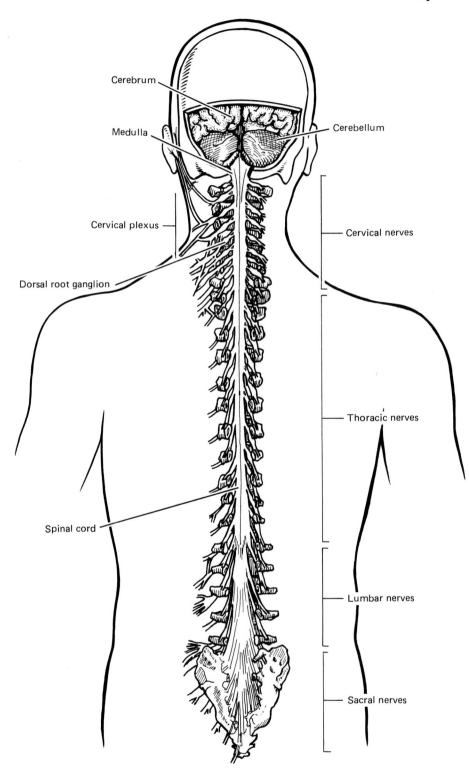

Figure 3.9. The brain, spinal cord, and the proximal portions of the spinal nerves. Observe the nerve plexus in the neck.

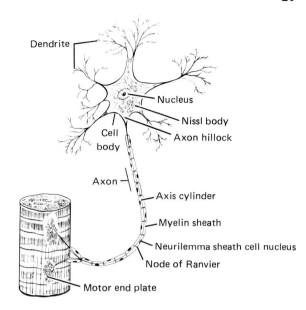

Dendrite

Nucleus

Nissl body

Cell body

Axon hillock

Axon

Axis cylinder

Myelin sheath

Neurilemma sheath cell nucleus

Node of Ranvier

Motor end plate

Figure 3.10. Motor neuron. Observe the axon synapsing with the muscle at the motor end-plate.

Sensory and motor functions within the head are carried on by the cranial nerves. Certain muscle groups and the sense organs for hearing, smell, taste, and sight make this group "special." The senses of sight and hearing are transmitted by *special somatic afferent* sensory neurons, while taste and smell are transmitted by *special visceral afferent* sensory fibers. Similarly, the motor component to the "special" muscles (branchiomeric origin) is the *special visceral efferent.* Since there is no "special" category for glandular secretomotor function in the head, the *general visceral efferent* component remains for the glands, smooth muscles, and mucous membranes of this region. It should be noted that certain of the cranial nerves carry *general visceral afferent* sensory components from the viscera of the head as well.

Peripheral Nervous System

Sensory neurons originating peripherally (in skin, for example) may possess nerve endings specialized for receiving various stimuli, such as cold, hot, touch, and pressure. Nerve endings transmitting pain, on the other hand, are free and without specializations. Dendrites of the spinal nerves are connected to their cell bodies located in the *dorsal root ganglion* which is just outside the spinal cord. The axons pass from the ganglion via the *dorsal root* into the *dorsal horn* (sensory) of the spinal cord. Here they may terminate, they may enter the white matter of the cord to ascend or descend before synapsing on connecting neurons in the spinal cord, or they may ascend to conscious levels in the brain (Fig. 3.11).

Cell bodies of spinal motor neurons are located in the *ventral horn* (motor) of the spinal cord. Their axons traverse the *ventral root* upon leaving the spinal cord. Just beyond the dorsal root ganglion area, the sensory and motor roots unite forming a spinal nerve which thus carries both sensory and motor components. Motor fibers destined for muscle will continue on to *synapse* at the *motor end-plate,* a specialized ending between the nerve and the muscle (Fig. 3.10).

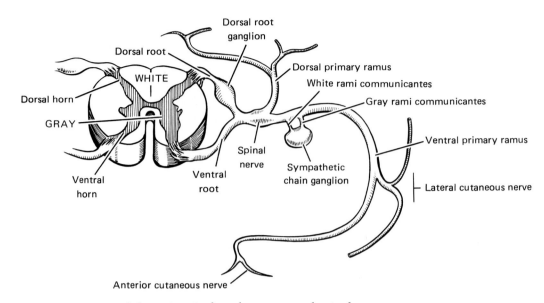

Figure 3.11. Typical thoracic spinal cord segment and spinal nerve.

Sensory nerve endings located, for example, in the patellar ligament of the knee, do not have their terminals in the dorsal horn but rather terminate directly on motor neurons in the ventral horn of the spinal cord, thus effecting a *reflex arc* bypassing the connecting neurons. Rapid opening of the mouth as a result of painful stimuli from biting down on a piece of bone while chewing is an example of a reflex arc in the fifth cranial nerve.

Coverings

The *central nervous system* (CNS) is composed of the brain and spinal cord. Each is delicately covered by several layers of meninges and protected by bone—either the skull around the brain or the bony vertebral column which surrounds the spinal cord.

The meninges covering the brain and spinal cord are continuous and completely enclose the CNS. Three separate layers make up the meninges: a tough outer layer, the *dura mater,* an inner delicate layer closely applied to the brain, spinal cord, and their vessels, the *pia mater,* and an intermediate layer, the *arachnoid,* which is closely applied to the dura. Only a potential space exists between the dura and arachnoid known as the *subdural space.* The *subarachnoid space,* located between the arachnoid and pia layers contains the cerebrospinal fluid bathing and further protecting the CNS.

Autonomic System

The *autonomic* (involuntary, visceral) *nervous system* exerts control over the viscera of the body, serving cardiac muscle, smooth muscle, and/or glands. By definition it is a system which is purely motor in function. Its manner of functioning is different from that previously described in that innervation is accomplished via a two-neuron chain between the central nervous system and

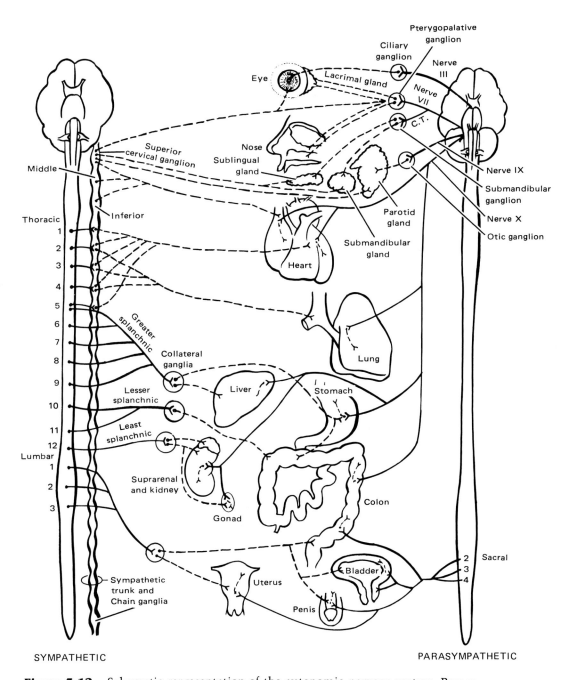

Figure 3.12. Schematic representation of the autonomic nervous system. Preganglionic fibers are represented by solid lines. Broken lines represent postganglionic fibers (adapted from several sources.)

the effector organ. The cell body of the first neuron in the chain is located in the central nervous system, while the cell body of the second neuron is located in one of the autonomic ganglia, all of which lie outside the central nervous system (Fig. 3.12).

The autonomic system is subdivided into two divisions, the sympathetic and parasympathetic systems. The *sympathetic system* generally prepares the body for action—as in the "fight or flight" response—by increasing heart rate, respiration, blood pressure, and blood flow to the skeletal muscles, dilating the pupils, and generally "shutting down" visceral activity. *Parasympathetic* innervation, conversely, functions to calm the body by decreasing heart rate, respiration, blood pressure, constricting the pupils, and increasing visceral activity. Both systems innervate many organs of the body where their antagonistic actions serve to balance functioning to maintain homeostasis.

Neurons of the sympathetic system originate in the lateral horns of the spinal cord in the thoracic and upper lumbar segments. Thus they are often referred to as the *thoracolumbar outflow* of visceral efferent fibers. Neurons of the parasympathetic system originate either in the brain *(cranial outflow)* or in the sacral spinal cord *(sacral outflow).* Together this system is known as the *craniosacral outflow* (Fig. 3.12).

The cell body of the first neuron within the two-neuron chain of the autonomic system is located within the visceral efferent column of the central nervous system. The axon of this neuron will synapse on the cell body of the second neuron located in one of the autonomic ganglia; thus, this axon is *preganglionic.* The axon of the second neuron is *postganglionic* and extends to the effector organ. The sympathetic system is served by the autonomic ganglia located along most of the spinal segments. These ganglia are known as the *chain ganglia* and are connected together by the *sympathetic trunk,* and the several *collateral ganglia* along the major abdominal blood vessels (Figs. 3.11, 3.12). Ganglia of the parasympathetic system are found close to the structures innervated and are called *terminal ganglia,* four of which are located in the head while others are located within the muscular coats of the viscera (Fig. 3.12).

Preganglionic sympathetic fibers reach the chain ganglia via the *white rami communicantes,* a connection between the spinal nerve and the ganglion transmitting the myelinated fibers. The postganglionic fiber may enter the spinal nerve via the *gray rami communicantes* directly or after ascending or descending in the sympathetic trunk. Preganglionic fibers synapse only one time; therefore, those destined to synapse in the collateral ganglia do not synapse in the chain ganglia (Figs. 3.11, 3.12).

Preganglionic parasympathetic neurons of the cranial outflow originate in cranial nerves III, VII, IX, and X only and may be distributed to the terminal ganglion via the cranial nerve of origin or by the named preganglionic fiber. Postganglionic fibers are distributed by other nerves serving the organ (Fig. 3.12).

The Oral Cavity, Palate, and Pharynx

This chapter provides an overview of the anatomy of the oral cavity as it would be observed in an oral examination. In addition, some pertinent clinical aspects of the variations in normal anatomy of the oral cavity are addressed at the end of the chapter. Subsequent chapters detail regional dissections pertinent to a thorough understanding of the anatomical structures of the head and neck.

The oral cavity (mouth) is the entry portal of the digestive system. It is bounded anteriorly by the *lips* and posteriorly by the *oropharyngeal isthmus (isthmus faucium)*, a more or less circular aperture which guards the entrance to the pharynx. The oral cavity is lined with mucous membrane composed of stratified squamous epithelial cells and connective tissue and contains accessory salivary glands. For purposes of description, it is subdivided into two major portions, the *vestibule* and the *oral cavity proper*.

LIPS

The lips are two fleshy mobile structures guarding the entrance to the mouth. They are covered externally with skin which overlies muscle, glands, and connective tissue. Internally they are lined with a mucous membrane. The red portion of the lips, whose coloration is caused by a rich vascular bed visible through the thin epithelium, is termed the *vermilion zone*. Since it is not a wet membrane, it must be kept moistened with the tongue to prevent drying. The skin and vermilion zone join at the *vermilion border*.

The superior lip is bounded laterally by the *nasolabial groove* extending from the *ala* (wing) of the nose to a short distance lateral to the corner of the mouth. A slight shallow vertical depression in the midline from the nose to the vermilion border is the *philtrum* (Cupid's bow). Just inferior to this depression is the *labial tubercle*, a fleshy bump of varying size in the vermilion zone (Fig. 4.1). The inferior lip is separated from the chin by the *labiomental groove*.

The two lips are connected laterally by the *labial commissures*, which are thin folds of tissue that are easily viewed when the mouth is slightly opened. Occasionally a slight depression is noted in the center of the labial commissure, known as the *commissural lip pit*. The *oral fissure* (rima of the mouth) is the zone between the superior and inferior lips which may be opened or contacted (Fig. 4.2).

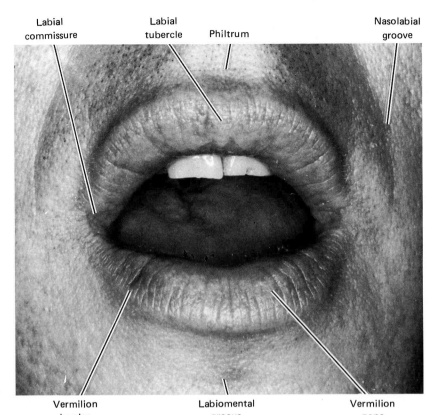

Labial commissure   Labial tubercle   Philtrum   Nasolabial groove

Vermilion border   Labiomental groove   Vermilion zone

Figure 4.1. Anatomy of the lips and adjacent area.

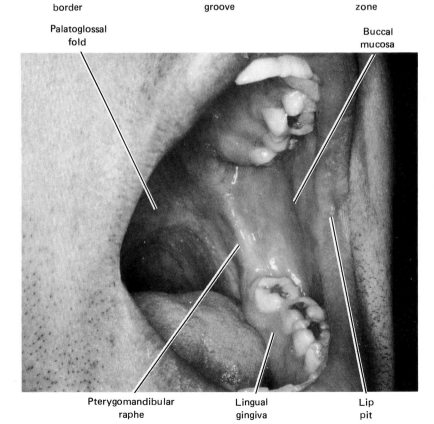

Palatoglossal fold   Buccal mucosa

Pterygomandibular raphe   Lingual gingiva   Lip pit

Figure 4.2. Lips and buccal vestibule illustrating lip pit and pterygomandibular raphe.

The lips develop from several sources, including the median nasal, maxillary, and mandibular processes. Many of the structures just described are fusion remnants of these embryological origins and often become more pronounced with advancing age. A more detailed description of the development and congenital deformities of the lip is presented in Chapter 5.

VESTIBULE

The vestibule is the cleft or space between the lips and cheeks externally and the teeth and gingiva of the dental arches internally when the teeth are in occlusion. The vestibule communicates with the exterior through the oral fissure of the lips, and with the oral cavity proper via the interdental spaces and the interval posterior to the last molar teeth in each dental arch. Laterally, the vestibule is referred to as the *buccal vestibule,* while anteriorly, in the region of the lips, it is termed the *labial vestibule.* The *mucobuccal* and/or *mucolabial folds* (fornix) represent the point at which regionally named vestibular mucosa turns to become the gingival mucosa. Located in the superior labial vestibule is the *incisive fossa* represented by a shallow depression superior to the incisor teeth. The bulge extending into the labial vestibule from the alveolar ridge over the root of the superior canine tooth is the *canine eminence,* while the shallow depression just lateral to it is the *canine fossa* (Fig. 4.3). Protruding into the roof of the buccal vestibule in the vicinity of the first molar

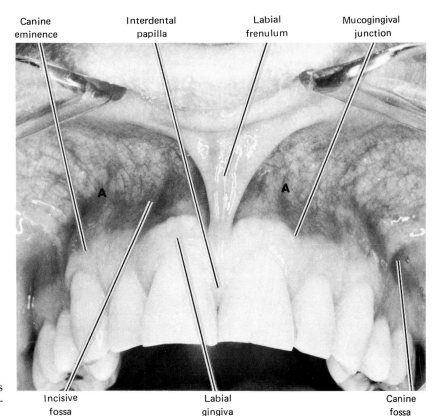

Canine eminence   Interdental papilla   Labial frenulum   Mucogingival junction

Incisive fossa   Labial gingiva   Canine fossa

Figure 4.3. Superior labial vestibule indicating regionally named gingiva covering anatomical regions of maxillae. Mucolabial folds (**A**).

is the zygomatic process of the maxilla which may be palpated. The nearly vertical anterior border of the masseter muscle may also be palpated in the posterior buccal vestibule, since it extends from the angle of the mandible to the zygomatic arch. The region of the maxilla posterior to the zygomatic process and superior to the last molar is the *maxillary tuberosity.* This is an important area anatomically, since it serves as an injection site for posterior superior alveolar anesthesia.

The parotid gland empties its salivary secretions into the buccal vestibule at a small orifice opposite the second maxillary molar. This opening which appears elevated in the mucosa is the *parotid papilla (Stenson's duct).* Several other small minor accessory glands which are regionally named—for example, the *buccal glands* and *labial glands*—also open into the vestibule at microscopic openings (Figs. 4.2, 4.4).

In some individuals, small yellow spots may be observed in the buccal mucosa lateral to the corner of the lips. These are *Fordyce's granules,* made up of isolated sebaceous glands that became incorporated into the mucosa during development (Fig. 4.5).

Extra reflections of labial mucosa appearing as folds of tissue attaching the superior and inferior lips to the gingiva are the *labial frenula* (sing. *frenulum*), the superior being the most prominent (Fig. 4.3). Often additional frenula may be observed in the labial and buccal vestibules. Occasionally the superior labial frenulum is so broadly attached that it interferes with normal eruption of the

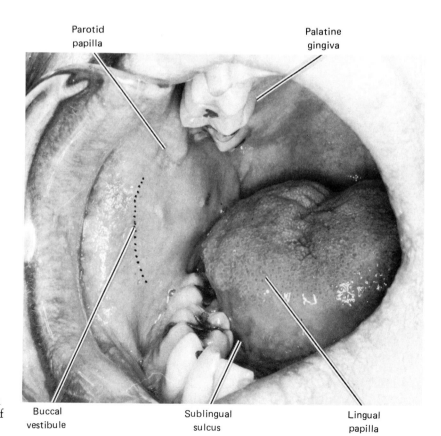

Parotid papilla

Palatine gingiva

Buccal vestibule

Sublingual sulcus

Lingual papilla

Figure 4.4. Buccal vestibule with opening of parotid duct opposite the second maxillary molar. Accessory buccal glands open onto the mucosa of the vestibule.

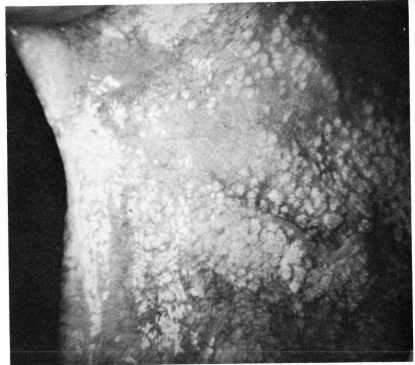

Figure 4.5. Ectopic sebaceous glands termed *Fordyce's granules* may be observed as white spots on the buccal mucosa and less frequently on the lips. (Courtesy of Dr. Mark Kutcher, Department Of Oral Diagnosis, Dental School, University of Maryland, Baltimore.)

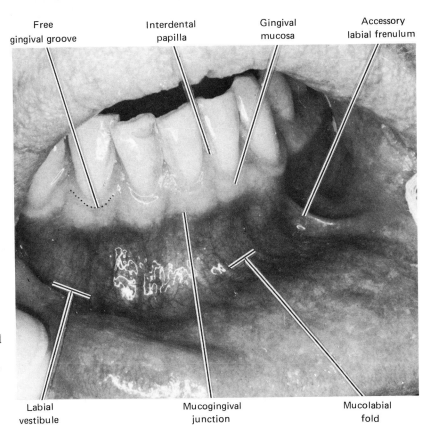

Free
gingival groove

Interdental
papilla

Gingival
mucosa

Accessory
labial frenulum

Labial
vestibule

Mucogingival
junction

Mucolabial
fold

Figure 4.6. Labial vestibule with labial frenulum and regionally named gingival reflections. The free gingival groove represents the area above dotted line.

central incisors thereby producing a diastema. Correction of this condition usually requires surgical removal of the frenulum between the central incisors to permit the teeth to return to the normal position.

The *gingiva* (gum) is covered by the *gingival mucosa*, which possesses a free edge surrounding the inferior margin of the clinical crowns of the teeth. The vestibular gingiva in this region becomes continuous with the gingiva of the oral cavity proper. The *interdental papilla* lies between the teeth in the interdental spaces and the *retromolar papilla* is that specialized area of the gingiva distal to the last molars in both dental arches. It should be noted that, in both of these areas, the gingiva is elevated on the vestibular and oral surfaces and usually possesses a concavity in the interface forming a col. The gingival mucosa is pale pink in color and stippled in good oral health. The *alveolar mucosa* overlies the alveolar processes of both the maxillary and mandibular arches. Its bright red hue is due to its vascularity. Where it blends into the remaining vestibular mucosa is not easily noticed. However, a rather sharp, scalloped line, the *mucogingival junction,* separates the gingival mucosa from the alveolar mucosa (Figs. 4.3, 4.6).

ORAL CAVITY PROPER

The oral cavity proper lies internal to the dental arches and their contained dentition and gingiva. It is bounded by the palate superiorly and inferiorly by the muscular tongue and reflections of the mucous membrane extending from the mandibular gingiva in the *sublingual sulcus (groove)* to the base of the tongue. Anterolaterally it is bounded by the lingual surfaces of the teeth, lingual gingiva, and lingual alveolar mucosa.

The posterior boundary is formed by the vertical portion of the soft palate superiorly and by the *anterior pillar of the fauces,* which is the *palatoglossal arch.* This arch which includes the palatoglossus muscle and overlying oral mucosa, extends from the soft palate to the sides of the base of the tongue (Fig. 4.7).

Communication of the oral cavity proper with the vestibule has been discussed previously, now its communication with the pharynx will be described.

The oral cavity communicates with the oral pharynx via the *oropharyngeal isthmus,* the *fauces.* This aperture is bounded by the soft palate superiorly, by the surface of the posterior one-third of the tongue inferiorly, and by the palatoglossal arch laterally. Anything posterior to these named structures lies in the pharynx. For example, the palatine tonsil lies in a tonsillar crypt between the palatoglossal and palatopharyngeal arches. Thus the tonsil is considered to be in the pharynx, since its position is posterior to the palatoglossal arch (Fig. 4.7).

Tongue

The tongue, a muscular organ, is divided for descriptive purposes into the body, which lies relatively free in the oral cavity, and a base that is fixed to the hyoid bone. It should be noted that the base spans the oral cavity and pharynx. The dorsum of the body possesses the *median sulcus,* a shallow groove superficially dividing the tongue longitudinally in the midline.

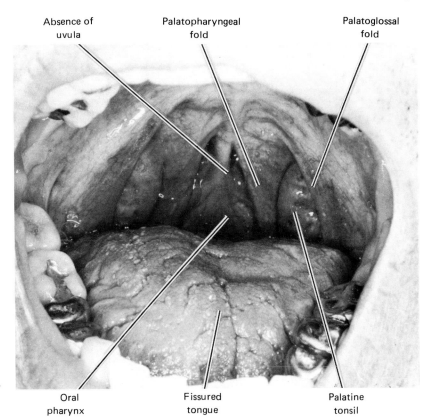

Absence of uvula   Palatopharyngeal fold   Palatoglossal fold

Oral pharynx   Fissured tongue   Palatine tonsil

Figure 4.7. Surgically repaired cleft palate. Oral vestibule and oral cavity displaying anterior and posterior pillars of the fauces. Note large palatine tonsils and the absence of a uvula.

The surface mucosa exhibits specialized zones demarcating the remnants of embryological origin. The *sulcus terminalis* may be observed as a posteriorly directed V-shaped shallow groove separating the anterior two-thirds (or body) from the posterior third (base) of the tongue. It should be noted that the terminal sulcus is the developmental dividing line. That is, anything anterior to it is in the oral cavity, while anything posterior to it is in the pharynx. The posterior third and base will be described here since they may be observed when the tongue is protruded, as in an oral examination (Fig. 4.8).

Lying alongside the terminal sulcus but anterior to it, is a row of eight to ten mushroom-shaped *vallate papillae,* often termed *circumvallate papillae.* These structures possess taste buds and receive the ducts of the serous *glands of von Ebner,* one of the few named groups of minor accessory salivary glands. The remaining anterior mucosal surface of the dorsum of the tongue possesses specialized projections which are the variously named papillae presenting a rough surface. Taste buds are present and associated with certain of these papillae. Located in the midline, just posterior to the apex of the sulcus, is the *foramen cecum,* a shallow pit-like depression which is a remnant of the developmental *thyroglossal duct* (Fig. 4.8). The remaining dorsal surface of the base of the tongue exhibits irregular bulges in the mucosa representing the *lingual tonsils.*

The mucosa of the ventral surface of the tongue is smooth and without surface papillae. The medially placed *lingual frenulum* attaches the anterior

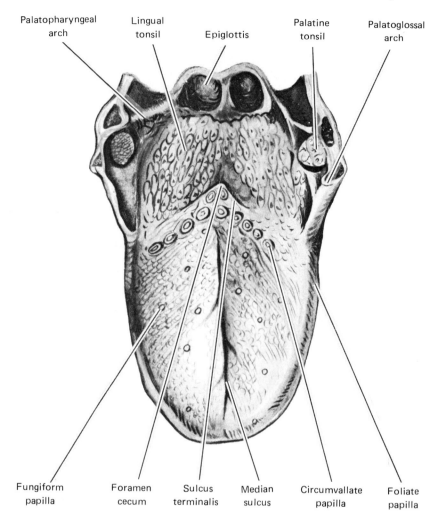

Palatopharyngeal arch · Lingual tonsil · Epiglottis · Palatine tonsil · Palatoglossal arch

Fungiform papilla · Foramen cecum · Sulcus terminalis · Median sulcus · Circumvallate papilla · Foliate papilla

Figure 4.8. Dorsum of the tongue.

two-thirds of the tongue to the floor of the mouth. On either side of the frenulum, extending almost to the tip of the tongue, surface bulges may be observed representing the underlying *glands of Blandin-Nuhn,* another group of the named, minor accessory salivary glands. These glands are mixed, producing both serous and mucous fluids which empty into the oral cavity via several minute pores. The *deep lingual vein* may be observed through the nearly transparent mucosa on either side of the frenulum coursing just deep to the mucosa along the tongue's inferior surface from the tip to the deep regions in the floor of the mouth, where the vein disappears from view. Lateral to the vein is a fringed fold of mucous membrane, the *plica fimbriata* (Fig. 4.9), which often exhibits tissue tags from its free edge. Just above the floor of the mouth on either side of the lingual frenulum is an elevation of the mucous membrane *(plica sublingualis)* overlying the bulging *sublingual gland* (Fig. 4.10).

Upon closer examination one may observe several small openings along the surface of the plica sublingualis representing the *small sublingual ducts (ducts of Rivinus).* In addition, a large *sublingual duct (duct of Bartholin)* from the sublingual gland joins the *submandibular duct (Wharton's duct)* just prior

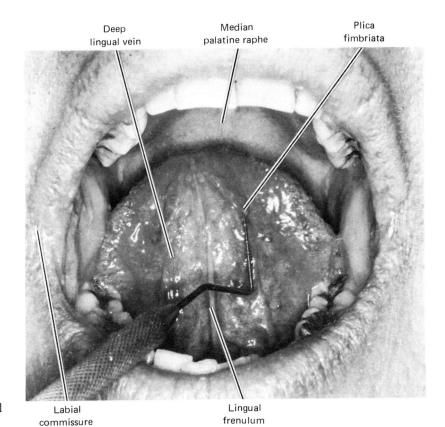

Deep
lingual vein

Median
palatine raphe

Plica
fimbriata

Labial
commissure

Lingual
frenulum

Figure 4.9. Ventral surface of the tongue illustrating plica fimbriata and lingual frenulum.

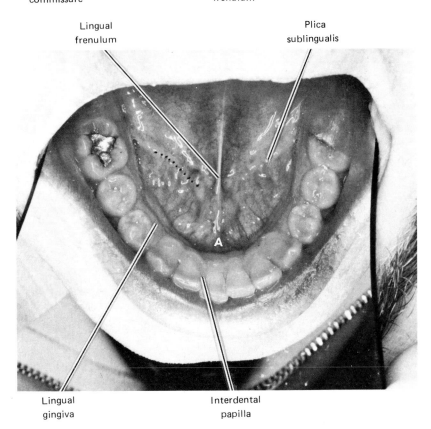

Lingual
frenulum

Plica
sublingualis

A

Lingual
gingiva

Interdental
papilla

Figure 4.10. Anterior floor of the mouth. Observe the plica sublingualis overlying the sublingual gland. Dots represent area where sublingual ducts open into the floor. Region of incisive glands. (**A**).

to its exit into the oral cavity for the delivery of salivary secretions from the submandibular gland. Wharton's duct empties at the *sublingual caruncula,* an enlarged (Fig. 4.11) papilla adjacent to the lingual frenulum near its base. The *incisive glands,* a small group of minor accessory salivary glands, may also be found on the floor of the oral cavity on either side of the lingual frenulum just posterior to the mandibular incisors.

A more thorough discussion of the development, structure, vascularization, innervation, and function of the tongue is presented in Chapter 15.

Palate

The *palate,* representing the roof of the oral cavity is divided into the *hard palate,* comprising the anterior two-thirds, and *soft palate,* composing the remaining posterior third (Fig. 4.12). Mucoperiosteum covers part of the bony skeleton of the hard palate, while mucous membrane covers the muscular soft palate. Anterolaterally, the palatal mucosa blends into the alveolar and gingival mucosae surrounding the maxillary teeth on the lingual surface. Posteriorly, the palate blends into the anterior and posterior pillars of the fauces laterally. The free posterior border of the palate terminates in the inferiorly directed *uvula* located in the midline. The *palatine velum* is that area of the soft palate represented by the superiorly placed posterior free margin and the laterally placed pillars of the fauces.

The mucoperiosteum displays some specializations in its surface, especially anteriorly. A median *palatine raphe,* the developmental fusion of the palatine shelves, may be observed on the hard palate. Immediately behind the central incisors, in the midline, lies a small oval-shaped surface prominence termed the *incisive papilla* (Fig. 4.13). This structure covers the oral opening of the incisive canal through which the nasopalatine nerves are transmitted to the anterior palate. It is an important landmark for anesthesia of the anterior palate. Posterior to this region is a series of transverse folds which appear to radiate out from the incisive papilla. These are the *palatine rugae,* which are vestigial in man but may serve accessory masticating functions in some lower animals. Lateral to this area of the palate and beneath the covering mucosa is the *fatty region.* Moving posteriorly, the fatty region is replaced by a *glandular region,* wherein are located the palatine glands extending into the soft palate. Near the midline and just posterior to the hard palate is the *palatine fovea,* a small depression or pit which receives secretion from some of the *palatine glands* extending into the soft palate (Fig. 4.13).

The palate is formed by the fusion of the median nasal process, the palatine processes of the maxillae, and the horizontal plates of the palatine bones. This fusion is initiated early in development and serves to separate the common oronasal cavity into separate nasal and oral cavities which communicate through the pharynx only. A more thorough account of development and congenital anomalies associated with the palate is presented in Chapter 5.

Teeth

The teeth are arranged in a row on both the *maxillary dental arch* and the *mandibular dental arch* and form a boundary between the vestibule and the oral cavity proper. As discussed previously, the gingiva of the vestibule and the oral cavity proper becomes continuous in the interdental spaces.

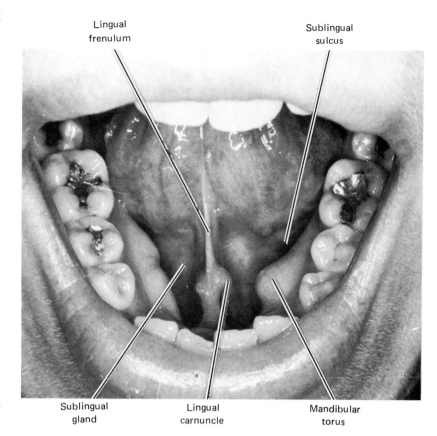

Lingual
frenulum

Sublingual
sulcus

Sublingual
gland

Lingual
carnuncle

Mandibular
torus

Figure 4.11.
Floor of mouth.
Observe large sub-
lingual caruncula
indicating opening
of the submandibu-
lar duct at the base
of the lingual
frenulum. Of spe-
cial interest are the
mandibular tori.

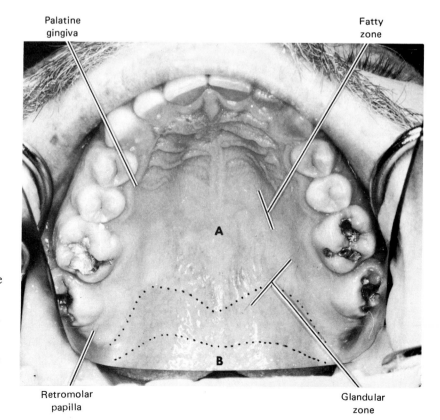

Palatine
gingiva

Fatty
zone

A

B

Retromolar
papilla

Glandular
zone

Figure 4.12.
Palate. Most of
area shown is hard
palate (**A**). Only the
most posterior as-
pect behind the
palatine bone (indi-
cated by dotted
line) is soft palate.
(**B**). Anterior aspect
is fatty, giving way
to a glandular re-
gion posteriorly.

Palatine   Incisive   Palatine
gingiva   papilla   rugae

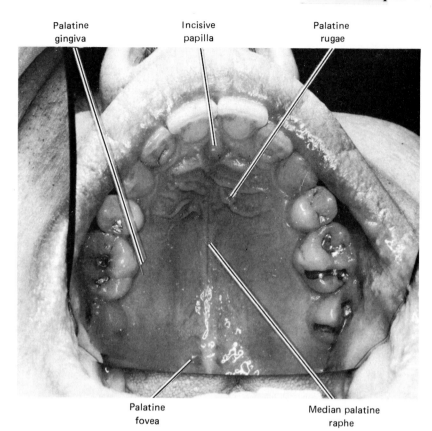

Palatine   Median palatine
fovea   raphe

Figure 4.13.
Palate illustrating incisive papilla, rugae, median palatine raphe, and fovea for receiving secretions of palatine glands.

The *permanent teeth,* beginning in the midline, are named similarly on each side and in the two arches. There are two *incisors,* one *canine* (cuspid), two *premolars* (bicuspid), and three *molars,* thus eight teeth in each quadrant of the jaw, for a total of thirty-two teeth. This is the normal complement of teeth found in a mature adult. The third molar, *wisdom tooth,* is often slow to erupt and may not present itself in the oral cavity. Occasionally it is congenitally absent, thereby reducing the total complement of teeth (Figs. 4.14, 4.15, 4.16).

Deciduous teeth, as the name implies, are those teeth eventually shed or replaced. Thus they represent the complement of teeth possessed in childhood. In each quadrant, there are two incisors, one canine, and two molars which lie in the same position as the premolars in the permanent teeth, or five in each quadrant for a total of twenty teeth (Fig. 4.17).

The two dentitions, deciduous and permanent, may be expressed in a dental formula as in the following diagrams.

		Deciduous								**Permanent**						
	M	C	I	I	C	M		M	P	C	I	I	C	P	M	
Maxilla	2	1	2	2	1	2	} = 20	3	2	1	2	2	1	2	3	} = 32
Mandible	2	1	2	2	1	2		3	2	1	2	2	1	2	3	

The teeth develop from substances elaborated by certain layers of the primitive oral ectoderm and certain specialized cells of the ectomesenchyme.

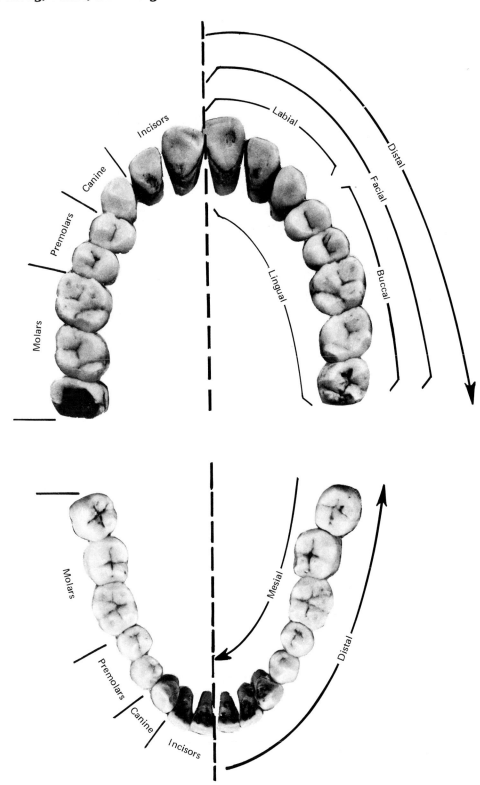

Figure 4.14. Dental arches. Terminology and relationships in dental anatomy.

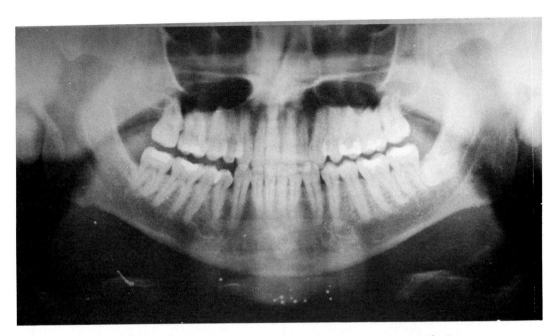

Figure 4.15. Panographic radiograph of the jaws. (Courtesy of Dr. Jon Park, Department of Oral Diagnosis, Dental School, University of Maryland, Baltimore.)

As the hard tissues of the tooth develop, the *alveolar processes* of either the maxilla or mandible form the bony socket surrounding it. The tooth is anchored in the *alveolus* by a calcified tissue, the *cementum,* and a soft tissue, the *periodontal ligament.* The clinical crown of the tooth is that part exposed in the oral cavity, whereas the root lies in the bony alveolus out of view. *Enamel* overlays *dentin* in the crown where it terminates just below the gingival line at the *neck.* The dentin in the root is overlaid by the cementum which anchors the tooth to the bone via the periodontal ligaments. The central core of the tooth is composed of pulp containing vessels, nerves, and lymphatics that reach the area through the apical formen at the tip of the root (Figs. 4.16, 4.18).

The tooth has an *occlusal surface* which contacts the same surface of its counterpart on the opposing dental arch upon closure of the mouth. *Buccal surface* and *lingual surface* refer to the vestibular surface and the oral cavity proper surface, respectively. The *incisal edge* is the cutting edge of the anterior teeth. The premolars and molars possess *cusps,* raised knobs on the occlusal surface. Also, since embryologically the teeth form from the midline laterally, that which most closely approximates the midline is considered to be the *mesial* aspect and that which is in the opposite direction, the *distal* aspect (Fig. 4.14).

Figure 4.18 depicts the major developmental stages in *odontogenesis* (tooth development) including eruption. Detailed information regarding developmental processes, as well as information on the complex anatomy and function of the individual teeth, is available in texts of oral histology and dental anatomy.

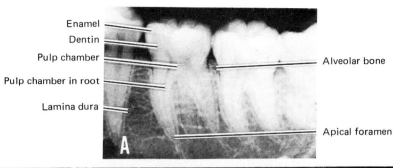

Enamel
Dentin
Pulp chamber
Pulp chamber in root
Lamina dura
Alveolar bone
Apical foramen

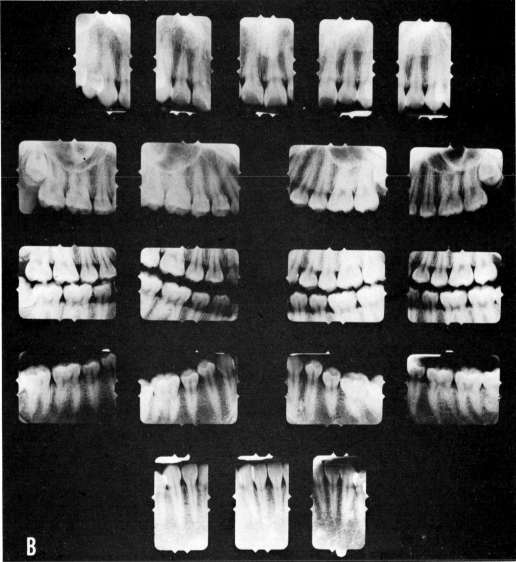

Figure 4.16. Radiographs of teeth. **A.** Enlargement of a molar tooth illustrating anatomy of the tooth and the alveolus. **B.** Full series of intra-oral radiographs of permanent teeth (Courtesy of Dr. Jon Park, Department of Oral Diagnosis, Dental School, University of Maryland, Baltimore.)

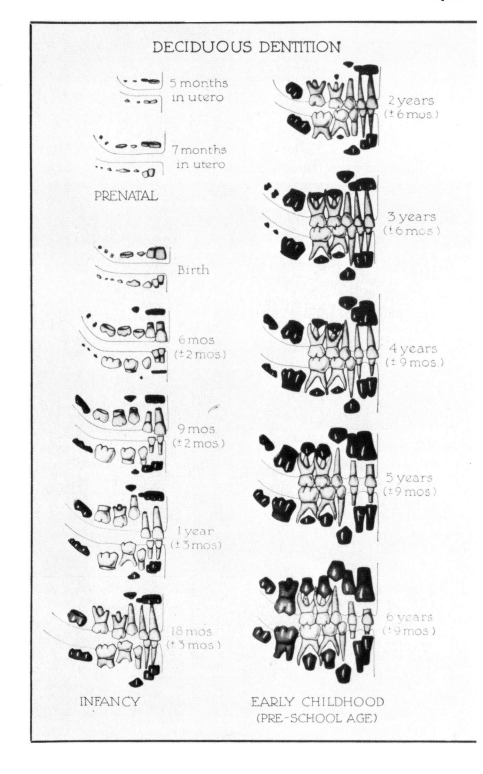

DECIDUOUS DENTITION

5 months in utero

7 months in utero

PRENATAL

Birth

6 mos. (±2 mos.)

9 mos. (±2 mos.)

1 year (±3 mos.)

18 mos. (±3 mos.)

INFANCY

2 years (±6 mos.)

3 years (±6 mos.)

4 years (±9 mos.)

5 years (±9 mos.)

6 years (±9 mos.)

EARLY CHILDHOOD
(PRE-SCHOOL AGE)

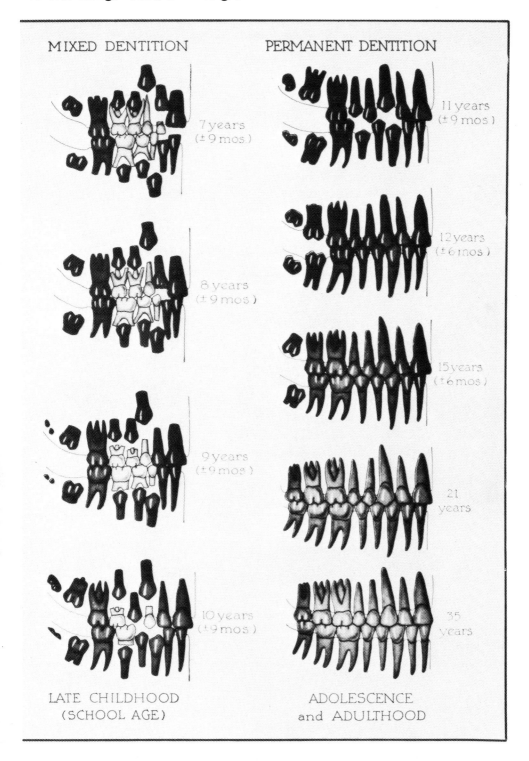

Figure 4.17. Development of the human dentition to maturity. Deciduous or primary teeth are darker in the illustration. (Copyright by the American Dental Association. Reprinted by permission.)

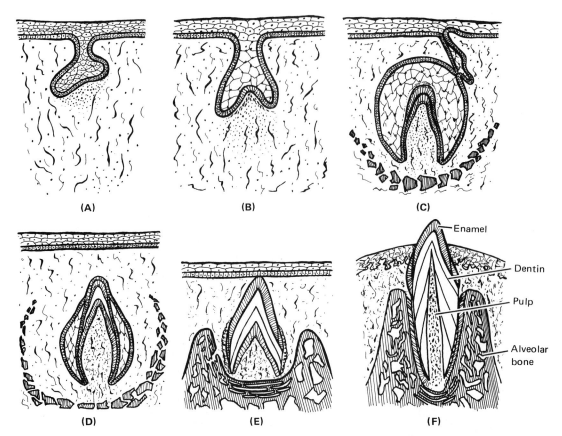

Figure 4.18. Tooth development in the human. **A.** Bud stage. **B.** Cap stage. **C.** Bell stage. **D.** Appositional stage. **E.** Beginning of eruption. **F.** Eruption into the oral cavity.

PHARYNX

The *pharynx* is a muscular tube lined with mucous membrane. It extends in an inferior direction from the base of the cranium to the level of the sixth cervical vertebra where it becomes continuous with the esophagus. Along its length it possesses several attachments so that its mobility is somewhat restricted. The pharynx lies behind the nasal cavity, oral cavity, and larynx. Though its posterior wall presents a continuous surface, superiorly its anterior wall is interrupted by the choanae of the nasal cavity and the isthmus of the oral cavity. Thus it serves to conduct air to the larynx from the nasal and oral cavities as well as food to the esophagus from the mouth.

The muscular wall of the tube is composed of three overlapping muscles, originating from several anatomical structures in their vicinity and all inserting into a longitudinal line, the *posterior median raphe,* in the dorsal wall of the pharynx. The muscles are the *superior pharyngeal constrictor, middle pharyngeal constrictor,* and *inferior pharyngeal constrictor,* each named for its relative location. Each muscle possesses fibers which ascend and descend from their origin to be inserted into the raphe. This fanned out arrangement provides for a strong but flexible multilayered wall whose muscle fibers course obliquely to each other (Fig. 4.19).

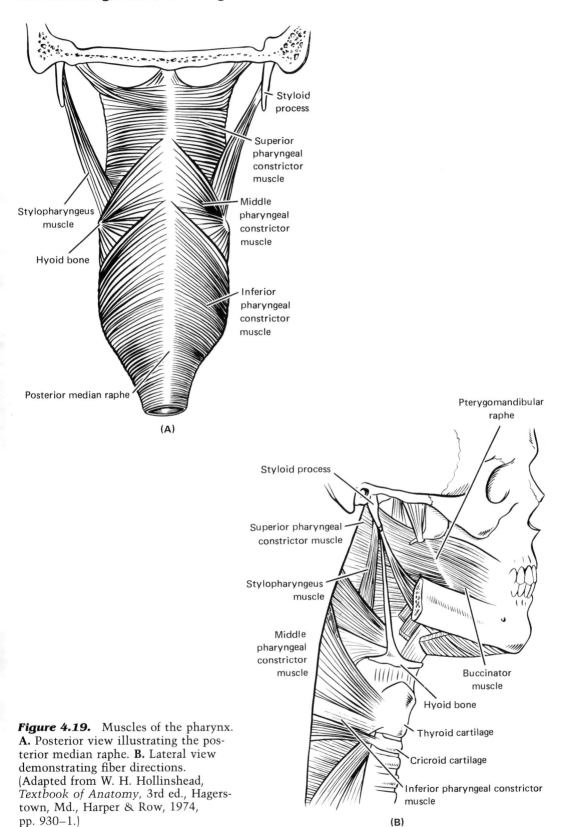

Figure 4.19. Muscles of the pharynx. **A.** Posterior view illustrating the posterior median raphe. **B.** Lateral view demonstrating fiber directions. (Adapted from W. H. Hollinshead, *Textbook of Anatomy*, 3rd ed., Hagerstown, Md., Harper & Row, 1974, pp. 930–1.)

The pharynx is divided into three anatomical regions for purposes of description. These are the *nasopharynx, oropharynx,* and the *laryngeal pharynx* (Fig. 4.20). The most superior portion, the nasopharynx, begins at the superior attachment to the sphenoid and occipital bones and ends at the soft palate. This is the widest part of the pharynx and is in communication with the nasal cavity via the choanae and with the middle ear cavity via the *auditory tube (Eustachian tube).* In the area of the auditory tube is a fold of mucous membrane covering the *salpingopharyngeus muscle* which blends into the pharyngeal wall. In the *pharyngeal recess,* behind the lip of the auditory tube, is the *nasopharyngeal tonsil* (Fig. 4.20).

During swallowing, the nasopharynx is sealed off from the oral cavity by the elevation of the soft palate superiorly and posteriorly against the posterior and lateral walls of the pharynx. This may be observed during an oral examination by having the patient open the mouth, protrude the tongue, and say "ah." This causes the palate to be elevated and permits observation of the oropharynx extending from the palate to the larynx.

The lateral wall is formed by the *palatopharyngeal fold* covering the palatopharyngeus muscle. This fold arising from the soft palate is also called the *posterior pillar of the fauces* (Fig. 4.21).

Anteriorly, the base of the dorsum of the tongue lies in the pharynx. Inferiorly, the epiglottis projects into the oral pharynx behind the tongue, separated by two small pouches *(valleculae)* located on either side of the epiglottis (Fig. 4.8).

A more thorough discussion of the pharynx will be undertaken in the regional descriptions that follow.

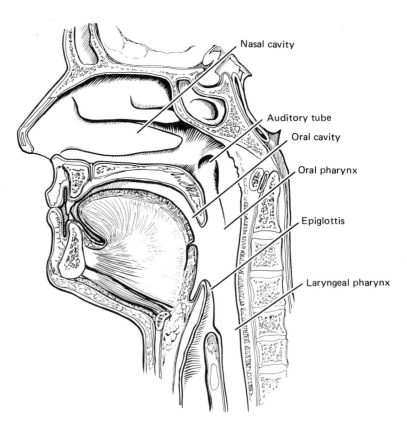

Nasal cavity

Auditory tube

Oral cavity

Oral pharynx

Epiglottis

Laryngeal pharynx

Figure 4.20. Regional divisions of the pharynx.

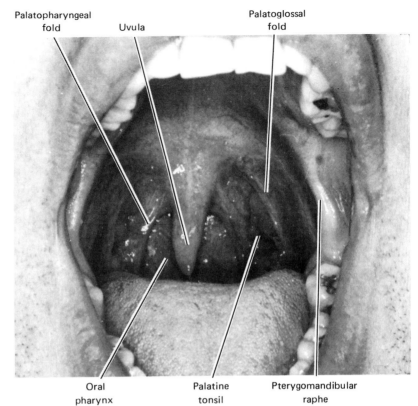

Palatopharyngeal fold   Uvula   Palatoglossal fold

Oral pharynx   Palatine tonsil   Pterygomandibular raphe

Figure 4.21. Oral pharynx and its lateral boundary formed by the palatopharyngeal fold overlying the muscle. Observe the pterygomandibular raphe delineating the tendinous inscription of the superior pharyngeal constrictor and buccinator muscles.

CLINICAL CONSIDERATIONS

Lips

Cleft lip, often associated with cleft alveolar and primary palate, is the result of a developmental defect and occurs in approximately 1 in 800 births. The terminology and severity of this and associated defects in the palate will be discussed in detail in Chapter 5.

Congenital commissural lip pits may be observed infrequently at the angle of the mouth in the commissure. These are remnants of development and are not clinically significant (Fig. 4.2).

The mouth from corner to corner normally spans between the first premolar teeth. As the mouth is opened the oral fissure becomes an oval to circular aperture.

Vestibule

A fold of mucosa in the posteriormost boundary of the vestibule connecting the maxillary and mandibular alveolar regions covers the *pterygomandibular raphe.* The raphe is a tendinous inscription between the buccinator and superior constrictor muscles which is attached to the pterygoid hamulus and the area of the *retromolar triangle* of the mandible (Figs. 4.21, 4.22).

The superior labial frenulum frequently possesses a tag of tissue located on its anterior surface approximately midway between its attachments at the lip and gingiva. This tissue, lending an irregular surface to the frenulum, was found to be present in 29 of 127 students in a recent class of the Dental School of the University of Maryland. This small mass is nonpathologic and may be regarded as a hyperplastic anomaly (Fig. 4.23).

The region of the buccal mucosa adjacent to the mandibular retromolar papilla contains an aggregation of accessory buccal glands which results in a prominence in the mucosa. This, along with the retromolar papilla, is often referred to incorrectly as the *retromolar pad* (Fig. 4.22).

Occasionally a white line, the *linea alba,* may be observed on the buccal mucosa representing that area of the mucosa in close proximity to the occlusal surfaces when the jaws are in the closed position (Fig. 4.22).

The space of the vestibule is somewhat reduced when the mouth is opened, by the forward movement of the coronoid process of the mandible as its condyle moves forward and downward. This may interfere with dental radiographic procedures in the maxillary molar area and in preparing study models and making maxillary dentures. The masseter muscle also impinges upon the vestibular space as the mouth is closed and teeth are clenched. The anterior edge of this muscle may be palpated in the clenched position by inserting a finger in the buccal vestibule. The presence of this muscle must be taken into account when fitting a mandibular prosthesis.

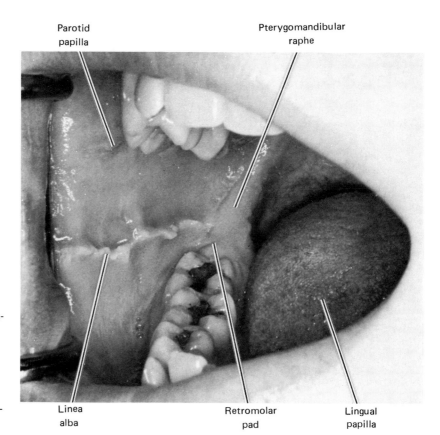

Parotid papilla

Pterygomandibular raphe

Linea alba

Retromolar pad

Lingual papilla

Figure 4.22. Buccal vestibule. Observe the linea alba, a nonpathologic condition resulting from the buccal mucosa fitting into the occlusal plane.

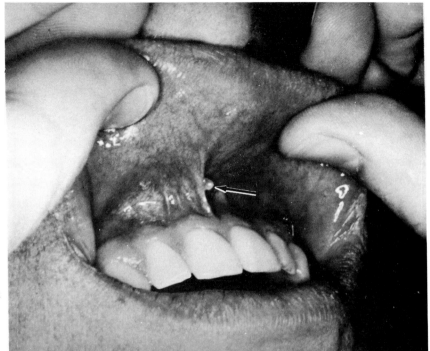

Figure 4.23. Superior labial frenulum. Observe the nonpathologic tissue tag on the free surface (arrow). (Courtesy of Dr. Mark Kutcher, Department of Ora Diagnosis, Dental School, University of Maryland, Baltimore.)

Tongue

Normally, the tongue varies considerably in size and surface presentation, this variation is often the result of developmental abnormalities. Some of the more common inconsequential anomalies are *microglossia* (small tongue), *macroglossia* (large tongue), *fissured tongue* (excessive fissures in dorsum) (Fig. 4.24), *median rhomboid glossitis* (an area devoid of papilla) (Fig. 4.25), and *crenated tongue* (indentations along the margins pressing on the teeth in occlusion) (Fig. 4.24). Other anomalies exist, particularly in the lingual papilla, and as such manifest themselves in many ways each of which has been supplied with a descriptive term. Space does not permit their descriptions here. Texts in oral diagnosis would contain this information.

If the lingual frenulum is attached to the tip of the tongue too far anteriorly, a condition known as *ankyloglossia* (tongue-tied) exists. This condition limits speech, due to the immobility of the tongue. Ankyloglossia may be surgically corrected by clipping the frenulum (frenectomy) to shorten its extent.

The thyroglossal duct normally atrophies during fetal life. Incomplete atrophy leads to formation of a midline cyst or accessory thyroid in the vicinity of the foramen cecum. Depending on the size of this *lingual thyroid*, other structures in the vicinity may be obliterated and/or hidden from view.

Floor of Mouth

The floor of the oral cavity proper frequently possesses bony swellings along the lingual surface of the mandible. These are known as *mandibular tori* (Fig.

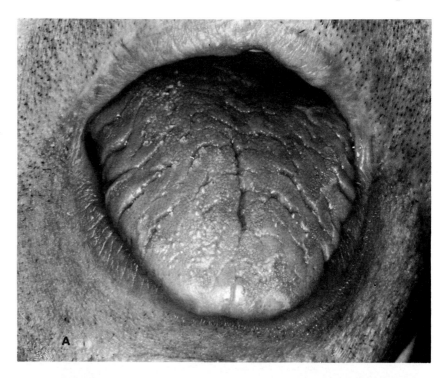

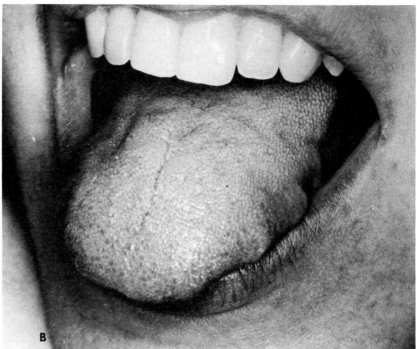

Figure 4.24. Tongue forms. **A.** Fissured tongue. Note the deep furrows on the surface. This represents a congenital anomaly rather than a pathology. **B.** Crenated tongue. Observe the scalloped regions along the lateral border apparently indicating the lingual aspect of the occlusal arch.

Fungiform papilla

Filiform papilla

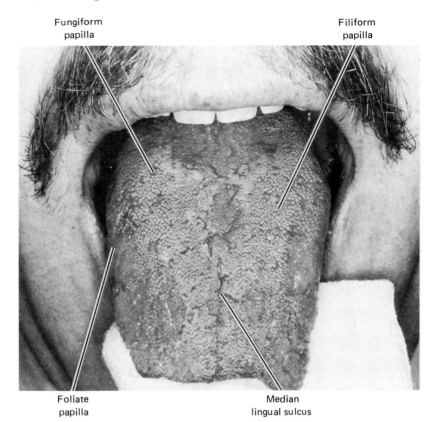

Figure 4.25. Median rhomboid glossitis. The area that appears to be inflamed is without lingual papilla. It is a congenital anomaly and has no clinical significance.

Foliate papilla

Median lingual sulcus

4.11). Additional *bony exostoses* may be present on the buccal surface of the mandible in the vicinity of the alveolar processes. The tori present radiographic opacity, while the buccal exostoses seldom demonstrate radiographic change. Neither of the two conditions presents problems, except in denture construction when they must be removed surgically. Difficulty may be encountered in placing films for dental radiographs and in preparing study models.

A *retrocuspid papilla*, a small papule, may often be observed located on the lingual gingiva adjacent to the mandibular cuspid. Such a papilla is not clinically significant.

Palate

The developmental defect of greatest concern to the dental profession is the cleft palate. Its incidence is in the vicinity of 1 in 900 births in the United States. Development, congenital anomalies, and terminology related to palate formation and clefting is discussed in detail in Chapter 5.

The normal shape of the palate is classically described as vault-like, but this varies between individuals from narrow to wide, flat or high, and so on.

Frequently, one may observe a midline bulge in the palate resulting from excess bone growth. This is termed *palatine torus* and presents no problem except during denture construction, at which time it must be removed surgically (Fig. 4.26).

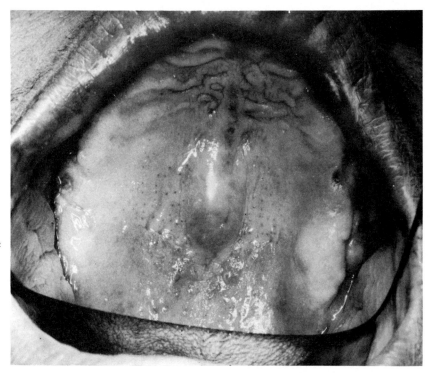

Figure 4.26.
Palatine torus. The bulges on the surface of the palate are bony exostoses and do not represent pathology. It may be necessary to remove them in preparing a denture.

Whenever anesthetic injections are to be administered in the palate, they should be given, if possible, in an area away from the mucoperiosteum. If an injection must be given in the area covered by mucoperiosteum (hard palate), care must be exercised and the injection must be given slowly to prevent tearing of the collagenous bundles away from the bone.

Oropharynx

Small clumps of lymphoid tissue surround the entry into the deep portions of the digestive tract at the oropharynx. This *lymphatic ring of Waldeyer* is well developed in the child and regresses with advancing age.

It is possible to view the posterior nasal choanae, the auditory tubes, and the larynx during an oral examination by illuminating the oropharynx and utilizing a dental mirror.

Upon examination of the oropharynx, a ridge of tissue located on the posterior pharyngeal wall may be observed on a plane with the soft palate. This ridge, known as *Passavant's bar*, represents the contact zone between the pharynx and the palate when it is elevated for sealing off the nasopharynx from the oropharynx.

Embryology of the Head and Neck

The head and neck comprise the most complicated portion of the human anatomy. The complex bony skull houses the brain, which is the control and coordination center for all body functions. Connected to the brain are the special sense organs of taste, hearing, smell, and sight. These organs perceive stimuli from the environment and transmit these sensations to the brain via the cranial nerves. Located in the head is the stomatognathic system for ingesting and masticating food. This system also articulates sounds produced by the larynx into speech for communication. In addition, the face possesses a special system of muscles whose coordinated contractions convey our emotions. And finally, the nose serves as the point of entry to the respiratory system, and incidentally as an entranceway for disease.

Indeed, no other region of the body is so complex or performs so many complicated functions as the head and neck. Because of its intricate nature, the compactness of the region, the ramifications of anomalies and congenital defects, and the disease manifestations arising in the head and neck, perhaps no other region of the body is served by so many areas of medicine and surgery.

Some understanding of the developmental processes which form the head and neck helps students assimilate and remember the vast amount of information necessary to master the study of head and neck anatomy. For example, understanding nerve-muscle relationships in development and subsequent muscle migrations away from their embryonic origin is of particular importance in the head and neck in relation to adult morphology and congenital defects. Understanding these elements of development helps one arrive at sound reasoning for diagnosis and treatment of disease manifestations.

Language utilized in describing the developmental anatomy of the head and neck may be particularly confusing for students who have not yet encountered the study of embryology. Early development within vertebrate animals is very similar; indeed to the untrained eye it would be difficult to distinguish an early human embryo from many of those of lower animals. For this reason, much of the terminology used in embryology is generally applied to all vertebrates, creating some confusion in the specific study of human development.

The term *branchia*, for example, literally means "gill" and is the term employed to describe the embryological development of gills in fish. This term is often employed in describing head and neck formation in human beings. Obviously, humans do not possess gills; however, the term is not utilized without reason. Many of the head and neck structures in humans are homologs

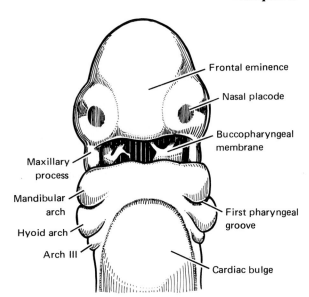

Figure 5.1. Frontal view of an embryo at 4–5 weeks of age. Observe the branchial arch formation and the ruptured buccopharyngeal membrane.

of gill structures in the primitive vertebrates. The equivalent term employed in descriptions of head and neck development in man is *pharyngeal*. This term, though not completely accurate, will be employed in this text. The terms *groove* and *cleft* may also be used interchangeably, but this should not create misunderstanding.

PHARYNGEAL ARCH, GROOVE, AND POUCH DEVELOPMENT

In a human embryo, the *stomodeum* or primitive mouth cavity, a shallow depression lined with ectoderm, is separated from the cephalic end of the pharyngeal gut by the *buccopharyngeal membrane*. This membrane ruptures during the fourth week of gestation (Fig. 5.1). Just anterior to the buccopharyngeal membrane, a midline diverticulum known as *Rathke's pouch* develops in the roof of the oral ectoderm. This evaginating pouch comes in contact with a pouch developing from the floor of the diencephalon. Further development of these two opposed structures gives rise to the pituitary gland. During the fourth and fifth weeks, outpouchings of the pharyngeal gut develop just posterior to the ruptured buccopharyngeal membrane, forming five *pharyngeal pouches* which invade the mesenchyme laterally. Concurrent with the formation of the pouches in the pharyngeal wall, four grooves develop around the stomodeal-neck area on the lateral surface of the embryo. These *pharyngeal clefts*, or *branchial grooves*, invade the underlying mesenchyme approximating the pharyngeal pouches, though contact never occurs. Invasion by the pouches and the clefts produces a condensation of mesodermal tissue interposed between successive pairs of pouches and clefts. These five bars of mesoderm are the *pharyngeal (branchial) arches*.

Continued development and growth of the arches medially, eventually to meet in the mideline anteriorly, provides each with its own cartilage, vascular, muscular, and nerve component. The arches form sequentially from rostral to caudal with the first arch being most highly developed and the last arch being

TABLE 5.1
Pharyngeal Arch Derivatives and their Innervation

Arch	Skeletal	Ligaments	Muscle	Nerve
I Mandibular	Meckel's cartilage Maxillae Mandible Malleus Incus	Sphenomandibular Anterior ligament of malleus	(Muscles of mastication) Temporalis Masseter Medial and Lateral Pterygoids Tensor veli palatini Tensor tympani Digastric (anterior belly) Mylohyoid	Cranial nerve V Trigeminal
II Hyoid	Reichert's cartilage Hyoid (part) Lesser cornu Body Styloid process Stapes	Stylohyoid	(Muscles of facial expression) Platysma Buccinator Frontalis Occipitalis Auricular Orbicularis Oris Oculi Stapedius Digastric (posterior belly) Stylohyoid	Cranial nerve VII Facial
III	Hyoid (part) Greater cornu Body		Stylopharyngeus Pharyngeal ⎫ ? ⎬ * Pharyngeal ⎭	Cranial nerve IX Glossopharyngeal Pharyngeal plexus**
IV ⎫ VI ⎭	Thyroid cartilage Laryngeal cartilages Cricoid Arytenoid Corniculate Cuneiform		Pharyngeal constrictors Laryngeal muscles	Cranial nerve X Pharyngeal plexus Recurrent laryngeal of the Vagus

*The origin of some of the muscles of the pharynx is yet unclear. The constrictors may in fact receive innervation from more than one source.
**Several of the pharyngeal and associated muscles including the levator palatini and palatopharyngeus muscles are innervated via a plexus derived from contributions of cranial nerves IX, X, XI.

poorly developed. The first two arches are named "mandibular" and "hyoid" arches respectively, while the remaining three are not named. The discussion of pharyngeal arch derivatives which follows is summarized in Table 5.1.

Derivatives of the Pharyngeal Arches

Mandibular Arch (Figs. 5.2, 5.3)
The first pharyngeal arch, the mandibular arch, is located between the stomodeum and the first pharyngeal groove. This arch divides early into two portions, the dorsally positioned *maxillary process* lying close to the eye and the

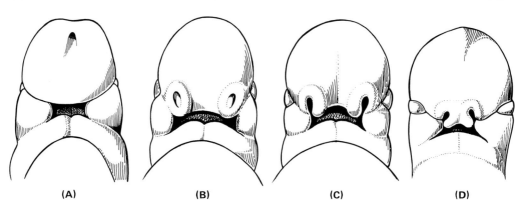

Figure 5.2. Developing face. **A.** Fourth week. **B.** Fourth–fifth week. **C.** Fifth–sixth week. **D.** Sixth–seventh week. Note how the nose develops and the eyes appear more anteriorly placed, illustrating the nasolacrimal groove.

ventrally placed *mandibular process. Meckel's cartilage* develops in this structure, forming a primitive support. Later Meckel's cartilage regresses and forms the incus and malleus of the middle ear dorsally, while ventrally the cartilage becomes incorporated into the mandibular symphysis. It should be noted, however, that most of the mandible is developed by intramembranous bone formation rather than by endochondral formation upon Meckel's cartilage.

Remnants of Meckel's cartilage become fibrous adjacent to the malleus, forming the anterior ligament of the malleus and the sphenomandibular ligament. The maxillary process grows forward to form the cheek and lateral part of the upper lip.

The musculature which develops within this arch are the muscles of mastication (masseter, temporalis, medial, and lateral pterygoids) and some muscles accessory to mastication, including the anterior belly of the digastric,

Figure 5.3. Early development of the pharyngeal grooves and pouches. **A.** Early development. **B.** Later development. Observe the second arch overgrowing the grooves of 2, 3, and 4 leaving a cyst in drawing **B**. Note the diverticula of pouches 3 and 4 as each develops dorsal and ventral prolongations.

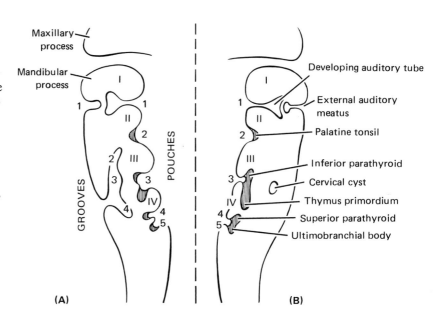

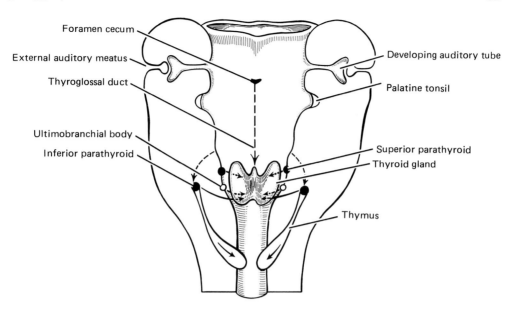

Foramen cecum

External auditory meatus

Thyroglossal duct

Developing auditory tube

Palatine tonsil

Ultimobranchial body

Inferior parathyroid

Superior parathyroid

Thyroid gland

Thymus

Figure 5.4. Late development of pharyngeal grooves and pouches illustrating migration of thymus primordia and parathyroids on the ventral side of the pharynx.

mylohyoid, as well as the tensor tympani and tensor veli palatini muscles. The cranial nerve providing innervation to the structures originating from this arch is the trigeminal nerve (cranial nerve V).

Hyoid Arch (Figs. 5.1, 5.3, 5.4)

The second or hyoid arch develops immediately behind the mandibular arch and is separated from it by the first pharyngeal groove. This arch assists in forming the anterior neck. The cartilage of the arch, *Reichert's cartilage*, gives rise to the styloid process of the temporal bone, the stylohyoid ligament, the lesser cornu, and part of the body of the hyoid bone and the stapes of the middle ear.

The muscle mass developed within this arch migrates over the superficial face and neck, forming the muscles of facial expression. Other muscles derived from the arch include the stapedius, attached to the stapes, the stylohyoid, attached to the styloid process, and the posterior belly of the digastric, attached to the hyoid bone anteriorly. Innervation to the structures derived from this arch is supplied by the facial nerve (cranial nerve VII).

Third Pharyngeal Arch (Figs. 5.1, 5.3, 5.4)

The unnamed third pharyngeal arch develops posterior to the hyoid arch just behind the second pharyngeal groove. From this arch develops the remainder of the hyoid bone. Only one muscle, the stylopharyngeus, originates from this arch. Controversy exists concerning the arch of origin of some of the other pharyngeal muscles. The developmental origin of the muscles of the pharynx has been difficult to elucidate since there is overlap of innervation via a complex of cranial nerves IX, X, and XI. This complex of nerves serving the muscles and mucous membranes of the third pharyngeal arch is termed the *pharyngeal plexus.* It is generally agreed that the stylopharyngeus muscle is the only muscle of this arch, its nerve supply being the glossopharyngeal nerve (cranial nerve IX).

Fourth and Sixth Pharyngeal Arches (Figs. 5.3, 5.4)
The fourth pharyngeal arch develops posterior to the third arch, separated from it by the third pharyngeal groove. The structures developing from the fourth arch include the thyroid cartilage, the pharyngeal constrictor muscles, and the cricothyroid muscle. These structures are innervated by the nerve of this arch, the superior laryngeal branch of the vagus nerve (cranial nerve X).

Technically, from the standpoint of comparative embryology, the fifth arch does not develop in humans, but a rudimentary sixth arch does. The sixth arch gives rise to the cricoid, arytenoid, and corniculate cartilages of the larynx. The intrinsic muscles of the larynx are developed from this arch as well. The nerve providing innervation is the recurrent laryngeal branch of the vagus.

Again, it must be remembered that the pharyngeal musculature presents an embryologic enigma in that the whole mass, with the exception of the stylopharyngeus muscle, is innervated by the pharyngeal plexus (cranial nerves IX, X, XI). A detailed discussion on each cranial nerve's contribution to the plexus appears in Chapter 18.

Continued differential growth of the second arch causes it to overgrow the three arches posterior to it, leaving a *cervical sinus* in the neck which is eventually obliterated.

Although the second, third, and fourth pharyngeal grooves become buried deep to the overgrowing second arch derivatives in the neck, the first pharyngeal groove continues to develop.

First Pharyngeal Groove (Figs. 5.1, 5.2, 5.3, 5.4)
The first pharyngeal groove, separating the mandibular and hyoid arches, continues to invade the mesenchyme opposite the evaginating first pharyngeal pouch. The groove gives rise to the external auditory meatus and the external ectoderm lining of the eardrum. Mesenchymal proliferations from the dorsal aspects of the first and second arches provide the tissues which later fuse and develop into the auricle.

Derivatives of the Pharyngeal Pouches

First Pharyngeal Pouch (Figs. 5.3, 5.4)
The first pharyngeal pouch, an endodermal lined, outpocketed pharyngeal wall located between the first and second arch mesoderm, evaginates into an elongated tubotympanic recess giving rise to the tympanic cavity and the mastoid antrum which remains connected to the pharynx as the auditory tube. The endodermal lining participates in the formation of the eardrum.

Second Pharyngeal Pouch (Figs. 5.3, 5.4)
The second pharyngeal pouch remains as the tonsillar fossa between the pillars of the fauces. Later the crypts of the fossa are invaded by lymphoid tissue which becomes organized into the palatine tonsils.

Third Pharyngeal Pouch (Figs. 5.3, 5.4)

The third pharyngeal pouch forms two diverticula, a dorsal one whose endoderm differentiates into the definitive inferior parathyroid tissue and a ventral one which develops into thymus primordium that then fuses with its counterpart of the opposite side forming the thymus gland. These primordia become detached from the wall and begin to migrate caudally. The thymus comes to lie in the superior thoracic cavity, while the parathyroid primordia migrating with it will occupy the inferior pole of the posterior surface of the thyroid gland—hence its name, *inferior parathyroid*.

Fourth Pharyngeal Pouch (Figs. 5.3, 5.4)

The fourth pharyngeal pouch, in a manner similar to the third, develops a dorsal and a ventral diverticulum. Developing from the dorsal diverticulum is the superior parathyroid, which eventually rests on the superior pole of the dorsal surface of the thyroid gland. The ventral portion soon disappears without contributing to a definitive structure, though some controversy exists on this point.

Fifth Pharyngeal Pouch (Figs. 5.3, 5.4)

This pouch is reported to give rise to the ultimobranchial body, which becomes incorporated into the substance of the thyroid gland. Several suggestions have been postulated regarding its function; however, whether these cells function at all is yet unclear.

FLOOR OF THE PHARYNX

The mouth is developed from the stomodeum and from the floor of the pharynx (foregut). The lips, gingiva, and teeth develop from the ectodermally lined stomodeum. The salivary glands also arise from the mouth cavity as ectodermal buds from the lining of the first arch. The parotid gland, the first to develop, appears between the maxillary and mandibular processes. It is followed by the submandibular gland and finally the sublingual gland in the floor of the mouth.

Tongue

The tongue forms in the floor of the pharynx first as a median swelling, the *tuberculum impar*, bounded by two *lateral lingual swellings* (Fig. 5.5). These structures develop in the dorsal aspects of the ventral ends of the mandibular arch. Shortly thereafter, another median swelling, the *copula*, develops just posterior to the tuberculum impar. It appears that this structure develops as a result of contributions from the second, third, and fourth arches. Posterior to the copula, yet another median swelling, which will become the epiglottis, develops from the fourth arch.

Continued growth in the lateral lingual swellings results in overgrowth of the tuberculum impar. Forward growth of the copula and the subsequent fusing with the lateral lingual swelling forms a V on the tongue surface separating, in the adult, the anterior two-thirds of the tongue (body) from the posterior

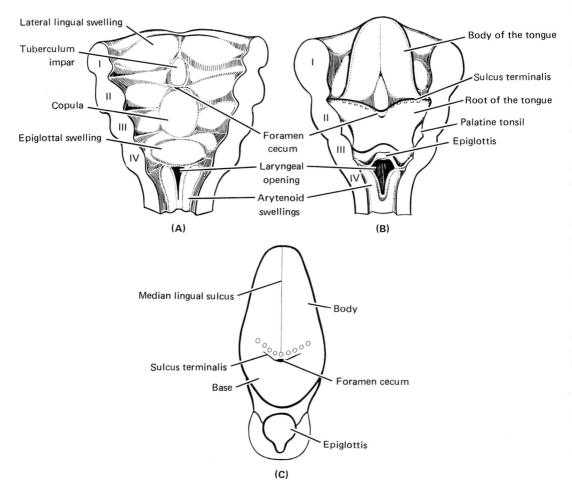

Figure 5.5. Tongue development. **A.** Early development (five weeks). **B.** Development at five months. **C.** Definitive tongue.

one-third (base) of the tongue. The V-shaped groove separating the two regions is the *terminal sulcus.* Located at the apex of the V is a small pit, the *foramen cecum,* demarcating the place where the primordium of the thyroid gland separated from the pharyngeal wall to migrate into the neck to be located ventral and inferior to the thyroid cartilage.

The tongue musculature does not arise from the pharyngeal arches. The muscle mass probably migrates from occipital somites, taking with it the hypoglossal nerve (cranial nerve XII).

The multiple origin of the tongue provides the reason for its multi-innervations. The anterior two-thirds, developing from the first arch ectoderm receives sensory innervation via the trigeminal nerve and special sensation (taste) from the facial nerve. The posterior one-third, developing from endoderm of arches two, three, and four, is served by the glossopharyngeal nerve for general and special sensation, while the very base of the tongue is supplied by branches of the vagus nerve. The motor components to the muscles are, however, supplied by the hypoglossal nerve. (See Table 5.2 for a summary of the discussion on the pharynx and its derivatives.)

TABLE 5.2
Derivatives of the Pharynx and the Pharyngeal Pouches

Region	Pouch I level	Pouch II level	Pouch III level	Pouch IV level	Pouch V level
Roof		Pharyngeal tonsils			
Lateral walls	Tympanic cavity lining of tympanum Mastoid air cells Auditory tube	Palatine tonsils and fossa	*Dorsal* Inferior parathyroid ——————— *Ventral* Thymus	*Dorsal* Superior parathyroid ——————— *Ventral* Thymus?	Ultimobranchial body— incorporated into lateral thyroid. Secretion of thyrocalcitonin?
Floor (Pharyngeal endoderm related to pharyngeal arch)	Body of tongue (anterior ⅔) Foramen cecum (Scar of rostral end of thyroglossal duct of thyroid)	Root of tongue (posterior ⅓) Lingual tonsil	Base of tongue (in part)	Base of tongue (in part) Epiglottis	

FACE, NOSE, AND PALATE DEVELOPMENT ════════════════════

During the fourth week of gestation, as the maxillary and mandibular processes of the first pharyngeal arch are developing and growing anteriorly, a median bulge covering the brain enlarges and grows forward. This *frontonasal prominence,* with its two lateral thickened areas, the *nasal placodes,* develops just above the stomodeum. Later, the medial and lateral rims of the nasal placodes grow around the placode leaving a depression, the *nasal pit.* Continued anterior growth of these rims through the fifth week causes a thinning of the epithelium covering the floor of the nasal pit. At this point the bucconasal membrane ruptures, thereby establishing a communication with the roof of the developing oral cavity. The *lateral nasal swelling* will become the ala of the nose. The two *median nasal swellings* will fuse and become the bulbus of the nose. Continued growth of this portion—now termed the *globular process*—anterior and inferior to the nose will give rise to the philtrum of the lip as well as the labial tubercle and the primary palate (premaxilla). The anterior teeth and gingiva will also develop in this structure (Fig. 5.6).

During this approximately two-week period, the maxillary swellings have moved anteriorly, meeting the median nasal swellings and fusing with them to seal the *nasolacrimal groove,* a deep furrow running between the eye and the primitive oral cavity on the face. The epithelium lining this groove separates from the surface ectoderm, finally forming the *nasolacrimal duct* (tear duct) opening in the nasal cavity (Fig. 5.7).

During this period, the mandibular processes have fused anteriorly, reducing the size of the primitive mouth. Mesoderm of the second arch has invaded the area, forming the muscles of facial expression over the entire face and frontal bulge of the forehead (Fig. 5.8).

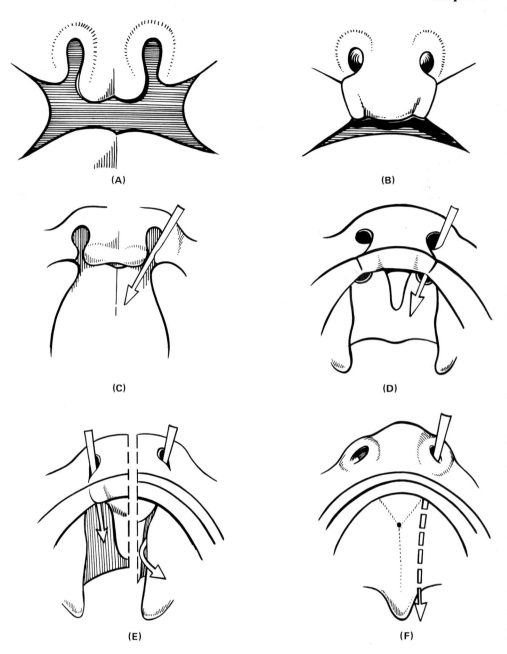

Figure 5.6. Development of nose, mouth, and palate. **A–B.** Formation of nose and upper lip. **C–F.** Formation of the philtrum, nose, and upper lip and the stages of palate formation and closure. Observe the steps of developing separate oral and nasal cavities from the early common oronasal cavity.

As the maxillary swellings grow medially, two shelf-like projections develop obliquely on either side of the tongue. These *palatine processes* ascend to a horizontal position above the tongue during the seventh week of development and fuse with each other in the midline forming the secondary palate.

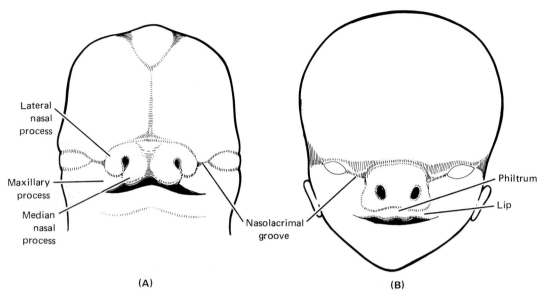

Figure 5.7. Face formation. **A.** The nasolacrimal groove is yet unsealed as are the maxillary/median nasal process seams. **B.** The nasolacrimal groove is sealing and the upper lip and philtrum have formed.

Fusion with the primary palate at the incisive foramen separates the oronasal pharynx into the nasal cavity and the oral cavity. The nasal septum develops as a downgrowth within the oronasal cavity, and as it fuses with the palatine shelves, it divides the nasal cavity into bilateral halves.

As the nasal wall continues to develop, diverticula form and invade the

Figure 5.8. Development of the face illustrating derivatives of embryological development. **A.** Approximately 8 weeks of development. **B.** Adult. Median nasal process (1). Lateral nasal process (2). Maxillary process (3). Mandibular process (4).

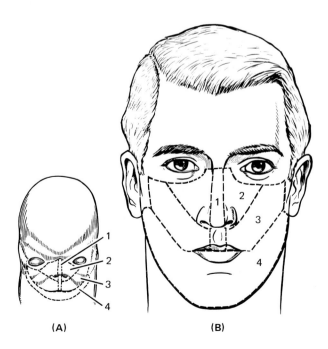

TABLE 5.3
Derivatives of Facial Components

Embryonic part	Facial derivatives	Skeletal derivatives
Frontal process	Forehead	Frontal bone
Fronto-nasal process	Bridge of nose	Nasal bones
Median nasal process	Globus of nose	Ethmoid-perpendicular plate
Globular process (Fused median nasal process)	Columella of nose	Vomer Primary palate (premaxilla)
	Philtrum Superior labial frenulum	
Lateral nasal process	Sides and ala of nose	
Maxillary process	Major portion of upper lip Upper cheek	Maxilla, zygoma Secondary palate
Mandibular process	Lower lip, lower cheek	Mandible

maxilla, frontal, ethmoid, and sphenoid bones, giving rise to the paranasal sinuses. (For a summary of the derivatives of facial components, see Table 5.3.)

CLINICAL CONSIDERATIONS

Abnormalities in the embryological development of the head and neck lead to a great variety of malformations with varying degrees of severity. The head and neck develop under the control of autosomal and sex-linked inheritance, modulated by the great influence of environmental factors.

The interdependence of events and the sequencing of development during this rather short embryonic period, perhaps before a woman is even aware of her pregnancy, contributes to the possibility of malformation.

Cysts and Fistulas

As the second arch overgrows the third and fourth arches to cover the neck, the grooves are normally buried and become obliterated. *Cervical cysts* develop if obliteration does not occur, thus connecting the surface of the neck with the pharynx via the *branchial fistula.* These cysts are usually found in the neck on a line just anterior to the sternocleidomastoid muscle. Often these are not found during childhood but may become apparent later as they enlarge. Surgery is necessary to repair the defect.

Preauricular pits may be observed in the external ear. These are usually inconsequential and result from incomplete covering of the sulci between the nodes of the first and second arch as these develop into the pinna of the ear.

Arch Defects

Defects of the first arch are the most common and of greatest significance since many structures develop from it. Because of the many possible defects, the term *first arch syndrome* is generally applied to anomalies from this arch.

Pouch Defects

Sometimes the thymus does not fuse together or descend into the chest cavity leaving thymic tissue behind in cords along its path. This may cause ectopic placement of the parathyroid tissue from its normal location on the dorsal aspect of the thyroid. Occasionally, supernumerary parathyroid glands develop or, infrequently, parathyroid development does not occur.

Thyroid

The epithelium destined to become the definitive thyroid tissue, which leaves a scar on the tongue (the foramen cecum), sometimes leaves a remnant along its migration path called the *thyroglossal duct* along which cysts and sinuses may develop. Should these ever become infected, they may enlarge and open onto the midline of the neck requiring corrective surgery. Rarely, the thyroid primordium fails to descend, thus forming a *lingual thyroid* at the base of the tongue. *Aberrant* or *accessory thyroid,* which may or may not be functional, may be found anywhere along the usual descent route.

Tongue

Since the tongue develops from several origins, several different malformations are possible.

Ankyloglossia (tongue-tie), perhaps the most common defect, results from a shortening of the lingual frenulum, thus restricting the tip of the tongue. It occurs in 1 in 300 infants. Simply clipping the frenulum relieves this condition. An excessively large or an unusually small tongue is relatively rare. *Macroglossia* is apparently the result of generalized hypertrophy of the tongue, while *microglossia* is usually associated with an underdeveloped mandibular process called *micrognathia.* Rarely, the tongue primordia fail to fuse, resulting in a *bifid tongue.*

Cleft Lip and Cleft Palate

These two malformations are the most common defects observed on the face. Cleft lip occurs in about 1 of every 900 births in the United States, being more prevalent in male children than in female children. The incidence also appears to be related to increasing maternal age. The incidence of cleft palate is about 1 in 2500 births. Unlike the differences noted with cleft lip, the cases observed in occurrence of cleft palate show females to be more prone to develop the defect than males. Some evidence points to the fact that the slower development in the female, with palatal fusion being delayed one week, may contribute to this condition.

Genetic and environmental factors play a large role in malformations of the lip and palate; however, space does not permit discussion of these factors here.

Cleft Lip (Fig. 5.9)

Cleft lip may be observed only as a small notching of the lip to a *unilateral cleft lip* revealing the unfused maxillary process with the median nasal process

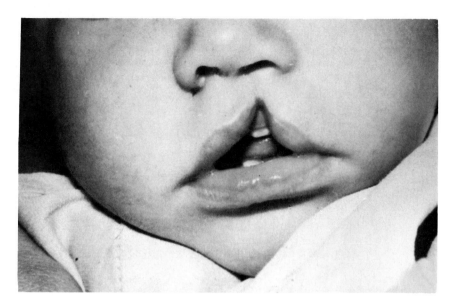

Figure 5.9. Cleft lip. The median nasal process and the maxillary process on the one side failed to fuse. (Courtesy of Hans Wilhelmsen, D.D.S., M.D., Baltimore.)

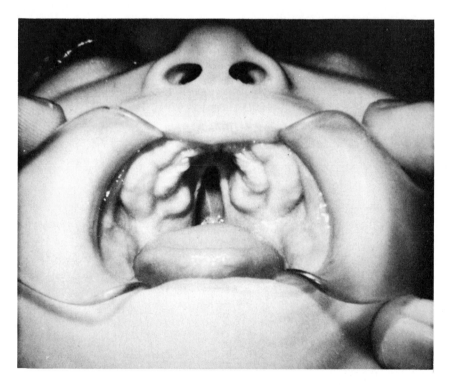

Figure 5.10. Cleft palate. Note the communication between the oral and nasal cavities. (Courtesy of Dr. Stefan Levin, The Johns Hopkins University School of Medicine, Baltimore.)

of one side. Malformation of more severe consequences results in *bilateral cleft lip* where neither of the maxillary swellings have fused with the globular process. Extremely severe cases of bilateral cleft lip display the philtrum and the entire undifferentiated globular process which would have developed into the primary palate. Many cases of cleft lip present malformation of the primary palate and the anterior teeth. Rarely, the median nasal processes fail to fuse and proliferate, resulting in *median cleft lip.*

Depending upon the severity of the cleft lip and the structures associated with it, surgical repair is very successful, though it may require several procedures.

Cleft Palate (Fig. 5.10)

Posterior (secondary) cleft palate results from failure of the lateral palatine processes to fuse in the midline with the median nasal process, thereby permitting a direct communication between the oral cavity and nasal cavity. *Unilateral cleft palate* results when one palatal shelf does not fuse. When both shelves fail to fuse with each other and the median septum, *bilateral cleft palate* results.

Anterior (primary) cleft palate is a consequence of fusion failure between the primary and secondary palatal processes. Clefts of both anterior and posterior palates result from failure of fusion between the primary palate, palatal shelves of the secondary palate, and the median nasal septum.

It should be noted that varying degrees of clefting exist, the last described being most severe, while the least severe is observed simply as a bifid uvula. It is also interesting to note that factors producing cleft lip, with or without cleft palate, are distinctly different from the factors producing cleft palate alone.

A team approach, involving specialists in medicine, dentistry, and speech therapy, are often employed to correct and rehabilitate the more serious cases of cleft palate and/or cleft lip. Though it may take several surgical and dental procedures over a number of years, along with therapy, the results are usually good.

CHAPTER **6**

Osteology

SKULL AND CERVICAL VERTEBRAE

The *skull* and *cervical vertebrae*, as well as the *hyoid bone*, comprise the bony skeletal system of the head and neck. Additionally, the viscera of the neck—specifically the larynx—contains a cartilaginous skeleton which will be discussed later. This chapter examines the skull, the cervical vertebrae, and the hyoid bone.

THE SKULL

The skull, excluding the six ossicles of the ear, is composed of twenty-two bones, some of which are paired, while others are single. Twenty-one of these bones are firmly attached to each other via sutures and are immovable. The only movable bone is the tooth-bearing mandible, which articulates with the paired *temporal bones* by a combined hinge and gliding (ginglymoarthrodial) joint, the temporomandibular joint (TMJ). Articulation at this joint permits the teeth of the mandible to interact with the teeth on the opposing tooth-bearing arch, the paired maxillae, and thus function in biting, mastication, and other actions.

It is convenient to divide the skull arbitrarily into two portions, namely the bones assisting in the formation of the face and those forming the cranium. Fourteen bones comprise the face: the paired *nasal, maxilla, palatine, lacrimal, zygoma,* and *inferior nasal concha,* along with the singular *vomer* and *mandible.* Those bones which compose the cranium, the portion housing the brain, are eight in number: the paired *temporal* and *parietal bones* and the singular *frontal, sphenoid, ethmoid,* and *occipital bones* (Table 6.1).

The examination of the skull is normally performed first externally, then internally. Externally, it is viewed from several perspectives—namely anterior, lateral, posterior, superior, and inferior views—while internally the base of the skull and the calvaria are studied.

External Aspect of the Skull

Anterior View (Figs. 6.1, 6.10)

From the anterior perspective, the skull is viewed face-on, making evident all of the bones which comprise the face as well as some of the bones which form the calvaria. At first glance, the most obvious landmarks are the paired orbits separated medially and inferiorly by the singular anterior nasal aperture. The

TABLE 6.1
Bones of the Skull

Cranial		Facial		Ossicles of the ears	
Ethmoid	1	Inferior concha	2	6	
Frontal	1	Lacrimal	2		
Occipital	1	Mandible	1		
Parietal	2	Maxilla	2		
Sphenoid	1	Nasal	2		
Temporal	2	Palatine	2		
		Vomer	1		
		Zygoma	2		
Total	8		14	6	28

bony prominence of the forehead is superior to the orbits, while the zygomatic arch is visible lateral and inferior to them. An additional obvious feature is the presence of the teeth located in the upper and lower jaws.

Bearing these landmarks in mind, one can now begin a thorough discussion of the anterior aspect of the skull. The forehead is formed by the squamous part of the *frontal bone* whose posterior aspect extends to the *coronal suture.* Here the frontal bone articulates with the right and left parietal bones, which are separated from each other by the midline *sagittal suture.* The paired *frontal eminences* are more or less prominent elevations on either side of the middle of the forehead just above the *superciliary arches.* These eminences may be palpated in the living individual as elevations superior to the eyebrows. Between the superciliary arches is a rather smooth depressed area, the *glabella.* Superior to the glabella, there is occasionally another suture, the *metopic frontal suture,* a remnant of the postembryonic fusion between the right and left halves of the frontal bone. Inferior to the superciliary arch is the superior rim of the orbit.

Orbit (Figs. 6.1, 6.2, 6.10). The orbit is a complex cavity, formed by seven bones: the maxilla, frontal, ethmoid, palatine, zygomatic, sphenoid, and lacrimal bones. It houses the eyeball and its associated muscles, vessels, nerves, and connective tissues. The medial walls of the orbits are parallel to each other (and to the sagittal suture), while the lateral walls are positioned approximately 45° from the medial walls. Consequently, each orbit is widest anteriorly and narrowest posteriorly and may be envisioned in the shape of a truncated pyramid.

The anteriormost aspect of the orbit (or its base), known as the *rim,* is formed by three bones: the frontal, the zygoma, and the maxilla. The whole superior aspect of the rim is formed by the frontal bone, which is interrupted by the *supraorbital foramen* (or frequently "notch") located medially. This foramen transmits the supraorbital vessels and nerves. Most of the medial and about half of the the inferior rim are formed by the maxilla, specifically its frontal and part of its orbital processes. The remaining inferior portion and most of the lateral portion of the rim are formed by the zygoma. The rest of the orbit will be described in relation to its roof, floor, lateral and medial walls, and apex.

The *roof* of the orbit is formed by a shelf of the frontal bone known as the *orbital plate*. Two depressions are located anteriorly on the roof, the smaller medial one, known as the *trochlear fovea*, for housing a small cartilage associated with the superior oblique muscle of the eye and a larger depression, the laterally positioned *lacrimal fossa*, to accommodate the lacimal gland. The roof is completed posteriorly by a small portion of the lesser wing of the sphenoid bone. The *lateral wall* is constituted by the greater wing of the sphenoid bone posteriorly and the zygomatic bone anteriorly. The line of fusion between the roof and the lateral wall is incomplete posteriorly, creating the *superior orbital fissure*, which is bounded also by the lesser wing and body of the sphenoid and the orbital plate of the frontal bone. The superior orbital fissure is traversed by cranial nerves III, IV, VI, and the ophthalmic division of V, as well as small arterial branches and the superior ophthalmic vein. Similarly, there is a space between the lateral wall and the floor of the orbit, the *inferior orbital fissure*, formed by the greater wing of the sphenoid bone, the maxilla, the palatine, and the zygoma. The inferior orbital fissure transmits the maxillary division of cranial nerve V, the zygomatic nerve, infraorbital vessels, and the vein to the pterygoid plexus.

The *floor* of the orbit is composed of the maxilla, palatine bone, and zygoma. In the middle of the floor, located mostly on the orbital plate of the maxilla, is a depression, the *infraorbital groove* which communicates with the *infraorbital foramen* via the *infraorbital canal*. The infraorbital vessels and nerve leave the orbit through the infraorbital canal. The *medial wall* of the orbit is formed by four bones: the maxilla, lacrimal, ethmoid, and sphenoid. Bordering the rim of the orbit medially, the frontal process of the maxilla and the lacrimal bone both participate in the formation of a depression, the *fossa* for the *lacrimal sac*. This fossa is continuous inferiorly with the *nasolacrimal canal*. Two small foramina, evident on the medial wall of the orbit at the ethmoidal-frontal suture, are the *anterior* and *posterior ethmoidal foramina*. The anterior ethmoidal foramen transmits the anterior ethmoidal nerve and vessel, while the posterior ethmoidal nerve and vessel pass through the posterior ethmoidal foramen.

The *apex* of the orbit consists of a single, round opening, the *optic foramen*, through which cranial nerve II, the ophthalmic artery, a branch of the internal carotid artery, as well as autonomic nerve fibers enter the orbit from the cranial vault.

Nasal Cavity (Figs. 6.1, 6.2, 6.3, 6.4, 6.10). The nasal cavity is below and between the two orbits. Anterosuperiorly, it is covered by the paired *nasal bones*, which articulate with each other in the midline, with the perpendicular plate of the ethmoid internally, as well as with the frontal process of the maxilla and the frontal bone. The nasal bones along with cartilages form the bony and cartilaginous bridge of the nose. The cavity opens at its anterior extent via the *anterior nasal aperture* (piriform aperture), whose boundary is formed by the two nasal bones superiorly and the maxillae laterally and inferiorly. Inferiorly, at the midline of the anterior nasal aperture, the right and left maxillae fuse forming a small, bony nipple, the *anterior nasal spine*. Posteriorly, the nasal cavity extends to the *posterior nasal aperture*, or *choanae*, where similarly, the *horizontal plates* of the *palatine bones* fuse in the midline to form the *posterior nasal spines*.

The cavity is divided in the midline into right and left halves by the *nasal septum,* composed of the *perpendicular plate* of the *ethmoid* anteriorly and superiorly and the *vomer bone* inferiorly and posteriorly. The sphenoid, maxillae, and palatine bones also make minor contributions to the bony nasal septum. The floor of each nasal cavity is formed by the horizontal plate of the palatine bone posteriorly and by the palatine process of the maxilla anteriorly. The *incisive canals* are located at the junction of the vomer with the anteriormost portion of the palatine process of each maxilla. These canals transmit the descending septal arteries and the nasopalatine nerves, which course along on both sides of the nasal septum. The two incisive canals open on the oral palatal surface of the maxillae in the midline just posterior to the interproximal aspect of the central incisors, at the *incisive foramen.*

The lateral wall of the nasal cavity is rather complex, for it contains foramina communicating with the sinuses, *meatuses* (which form air passages in an anteroposterior direction), and their overlying turbinate bones, known as *conchae.* Several bones participate in the formation of the lateral wall, these in an anteroposterior direction: the maxilla, lacrimal, ethmoid, and palatine bones, the medial pterygoid plate of the sphenoid, and the *inferior nasal concha.* The ethmoid bone has turbinate bones, the *superior* and *middle conchae,* protruding into the nasal cavity. Lateral, deep, and inferior to these conchae are air passages, the meatuses. The *superior meatus* extends as far as the middle concha, and it communicates with the *posterior ethmoid air cells.* The space below and deep to the middle nasal concha and superior to the inferior nasal concha is the *middle meatus.* This meatus communicates indirectly with the anterior ethmoidal air cells, directly or indirectly with the frontal sinus, and, with the *maxillary sinus* via the opening (ostium) of the maxillary sinus. The space lateral and inferior to the inferior nasal concha is the *inferior meatus,* which extends as far inferiorly as the floor of the nasal cavity. The *nasolacrimal canal* opens into the anterior portion of the inferior meatus.

Face (Figs. 6.1, 6.2, 6.10). That portion of the face between the inferior rim of the orbit and the upper teeth is formed primarily by the maxillae. Just inferior to the rim is the *infraorbital foramen.* Lateral to this is the suture between the *zygomatic process of the maxilla* and the *maxillary process of the zygoma,* both contributing to the bony cheek prominence.

The inferiormost aspects of the two maxillae house the 16 maxillary teeth, forming the upper *dental arch.* Each maxilla contains a central and a lateral incisor, and a canine, whose single root forms a prominent tuberosity on the maxilla, known as the *canine eminence.* Medial to the canine eminence is a fossa superior to the two incisors, the *incisive fossa,* and a similar fossa located lateral to the canine eminence, known as the *canine fossa.* There are also two premolars and three molars in the maxillary dental arch. Teeth of this arch articulate with those of the mandible, the only bone of the skull which possesses the capacity to move. The right and left halves of the mandible each contain a central and lateral incisor and a canine, whose single root is demarcated on the mandible as the canine eminence. Similarly to the maxillae, medial to this eminence, is the *incisive fossa.* Two premolars and three molars complete the mandibular dental arch. At the level of the second premolar is the *mental foramen,* through which the mental nerve and vessels exit the *mandibular canal.*

Occasionally, a line indicating the *mental symphysis* may be observed in the midline inferior to the interdental septum between the two central incisors, extending through the *mental protuberance* or point of the chin. This represents the line of fusion of the right and left halves of the mandible during embryogenesis. The *oblique line,* the *angle,* and the anterior border of the mandible are also evident from this view.

Lateral View (Figs. 6.2, 6.5).

From the lateral aspect, the skull is viewed in profile. The large cranial vault is very evident, as are the bones of the face. Various suture lines may be observed, namely the *coronal suture,* between the frontal and parietal bones, which ends in the *sphenoparietal suture* at the greater wing of the sphenoid. Another suture, separating the squama of the temporal bone from the parietal bone, is the *squamosal suture,* which arches posteriorly, ending in the *lambdoidal suture* separating the occipital and parietal bones. Continuous with the lambdoidal suture inferiorly is the *occiptomastoid suture,* separating the mastoid portion of the temporal bone from the occipital bone. The anterior border of the temporal squama participates in the formation of the *sphenosquamosal suture,* delineating its fusion with the greater wing of the sphenoid. Two lines, the *superior* and *inferior temporal lines* arch across the frontal and parietal bones, indicating sites of attachment of the temporal fascia and muscle, respectively. This region of the skull lies deep to the zygomatic arch and constitutes the medial wall of a large region known as the *temporal fossa.*

Temporal Fossa (Figs. 6.5, 6.6). Muscles, vessels, and nerves occupy the temporal fossa, which is bounded by the zygoma and the zygomatic process of the frontal bone anteriorly and the superior temporal lines superiorly and posteriorly. Inferiorly, its boundary is delineated by the supramastoid crest, the posterior root of the zygomatic arch, a line connecting the posterior and anterior roots of the zygomatic arch, the infratemporal crest of the greater wing of the sphenoid, and its posterior continuation on the temporal bone to the anterior root of the zygomatic arch. The zygomatic arch marks the boundary of the lateral aspect of this fossa, while the bony structures of the skull form its medial wall or floor. The anteromedial aspect of the temporal fossa presents the inferior orbital fissure. The temporal fossa is superior to and continuous with another deep space, the *infratemporal fossa.*

Infratemporal Fossa (Fig. 6.6). This space is located inferior and deep to the zygomatic arch. Its contents include the muscles of mastication, their vascular and nerve supply, as well as other structures of the deep face. The anterior boundary of the infratemporal fossa is the infratemporal surface of the maxilla and the deep surface of the zygomatic bone. Medially, it is bounded by the lateral surface of the lateral pterygoid plate of the sphenoid, the maxillary alveolar border, and a space, the pterygomaxillary fissure. Superiorly, its boundary is the infratemporal crest of the sphenoid (the boundary between the temporal and infratemporal fossae), the inferior aspect of the temporal squama and the infratemporal surface of the greater wing of the sphenoid, housing the *foramen ovale* and the *foramen spinosum.* Posteriorly the infratemporal fossa is poorly defined by the anterior limits of the mandibular fossa while inferiorly it is completely open.

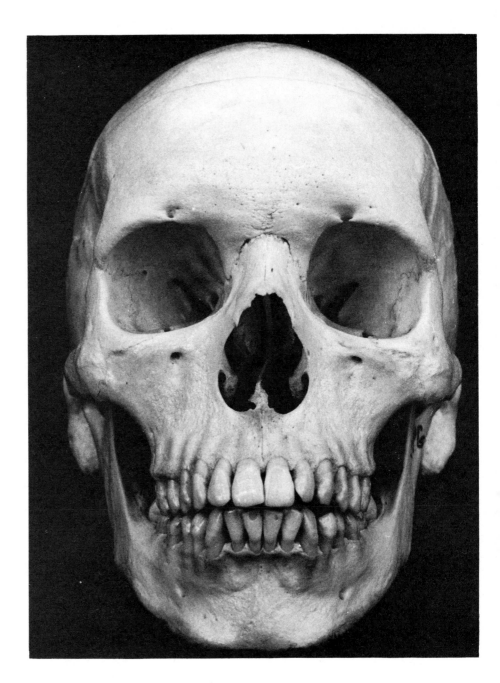

Figure 6.1. Frontal view of the skull.

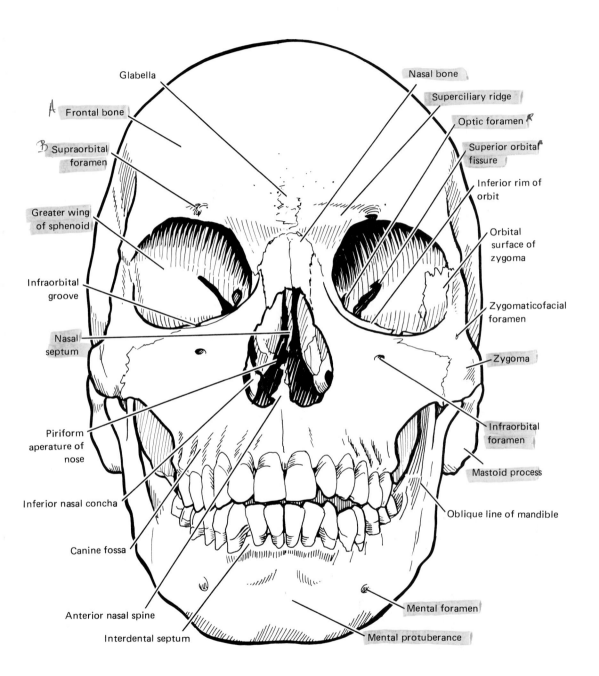

Glabella

Nasal bone

Superciliary ridge

A Frontal bone

Optic foramen

B Supraorbital foramen

Superior orbital fissure

Greater wing of sphenoid

Inferior rim of orbit

Orbital surface of zygoma

Infraorbital groove

Zygomaticofacial foramen

Nasal septum

Zygoma

Piriform aperature of nose

Infraorbital foramen

Mastoid process

Inferior nasal concha

Oblique line of mandible

Canine fossa

Anterior nasal spine

Mental foramen

Interdental septum

Mental protuberance

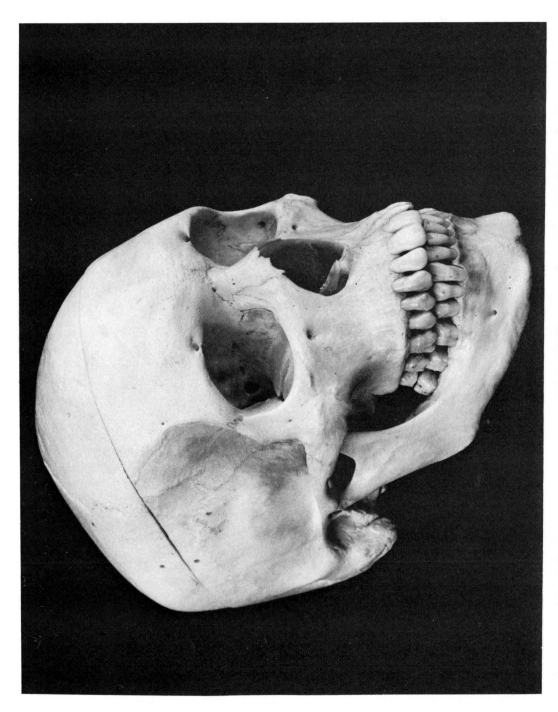

Figure 6.2. Anterior oblique view of the skull.

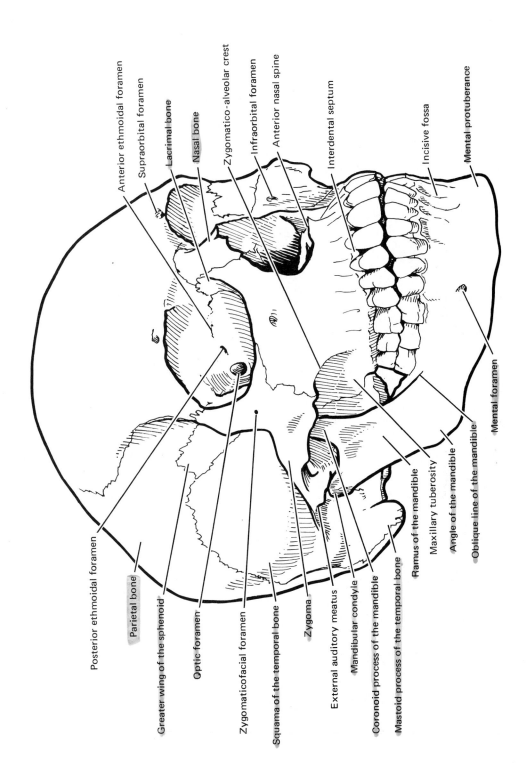

Posterior ethmoidal foramen

Anterior ethmoidal foramen

Supraorbital foramen

Lacrimal bone

Nasal bone

Zygomatico-alveolar crest

Infraorbital foramen

Anterior nasal spine

Interdental septum

Incisive fossa

Mental protuberance

Parietal bone

Greater wing of the sphenoid

Optic foramen

Zygomaticofacial foramen

Squama of the temporal bone

Zygoma

External auditory meatus

Mandibular condyle

Coronoid process of the mandible

Mastoid process of the temporal bone

Ramus of the mandible

Maxillary tuberosity

Angle of the mandible

Oblique line of the mandible

Mental foramen

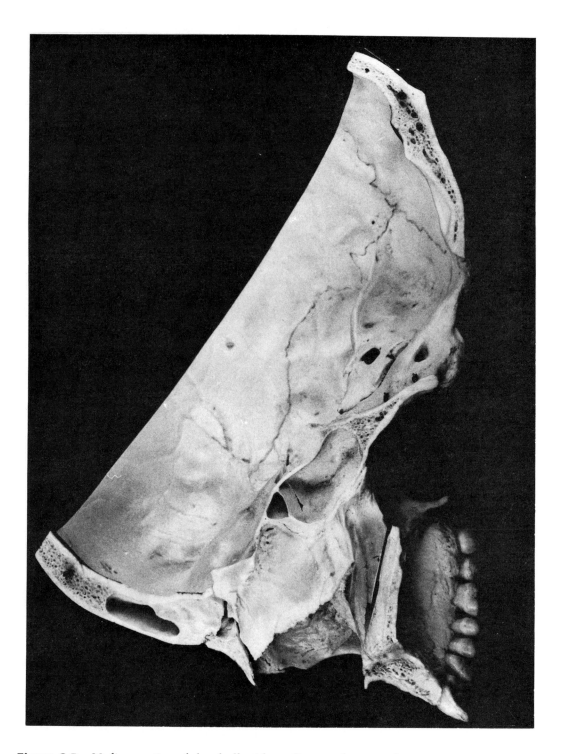

Figure 6.3. Median section of the skull with median nasal septum intact.

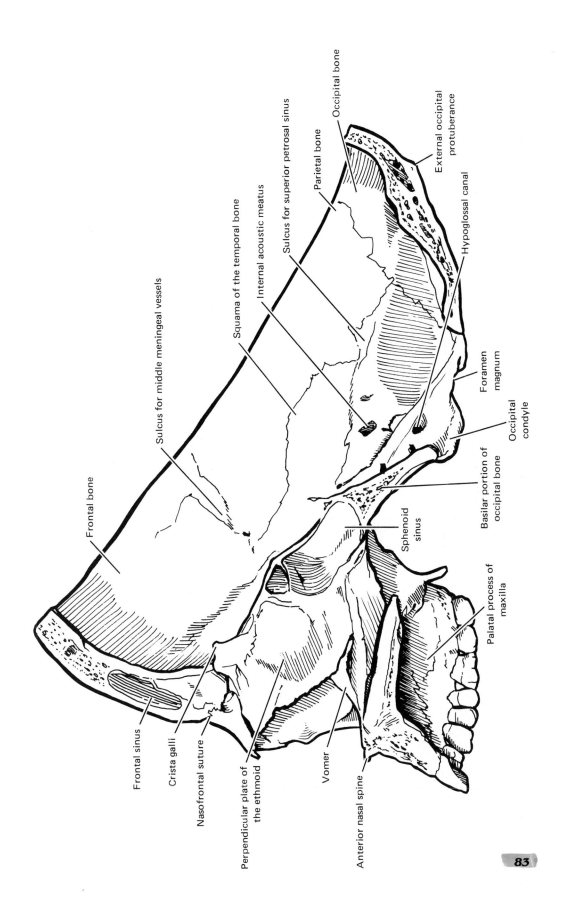

Frontal bone

Sulcus for middle meningeal vessels

Squama of the temporal bone

Internal acoustic meatus

Sulcus for superior petrosal sinus

Parietal bone

Occipital bone

External occipital protuberance

Hypoglossal canal

Foramen magnum

Occipital condyle

Basilar portion of occipital bone

Palatal process of maxilla

Sphenoid sinus

Vomer

Anterior nasal spine

Perpendicular plate of the ethmoid

Nasofrontal suture

Crista galli

Frontal sinus

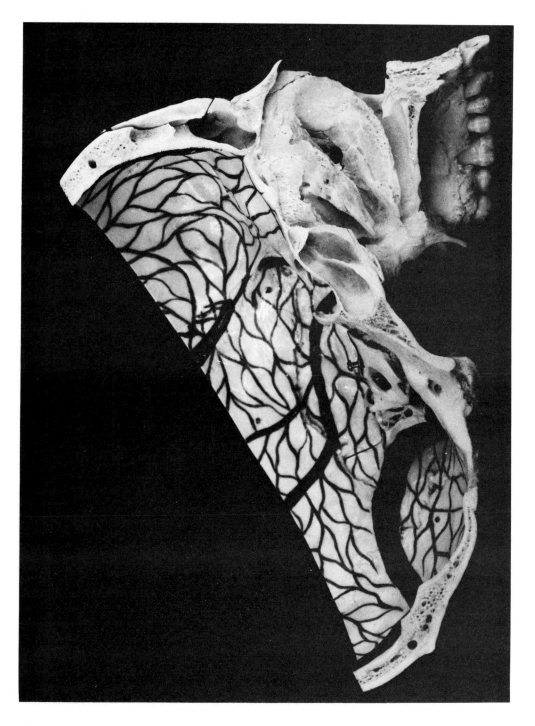

Figure 6.4. Median section of the skull with the median nasal septum removed.

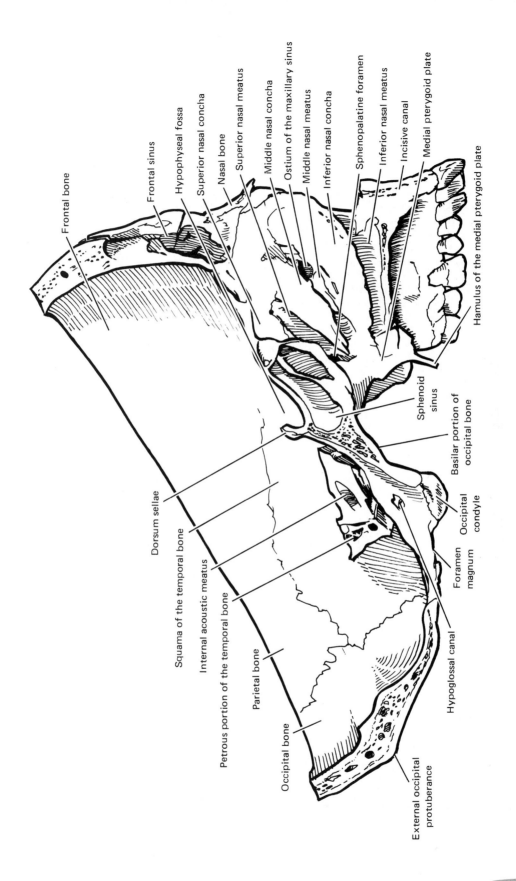

Frontal bone

Frontal sinus

Hypophyseal fossa

Superior nasal concha

Nasal bone

Superior nasal meatus

Middle nasal concha

Ostium of the maxillary sinus

Middle nasal meatus

Inferior nasal concha

Sphenopalatine foramen

Inferior nasal meatus

Incisive canal

Medial pterygoid plate

Hamulus of the medial pterygoid plate

Sphenoid sinus

Basilar portion of occipital bone

Occipital condyle

Foramen magnum

Hypoglossal canal

External occipital protuberance

Occipital bone

Parietal bone

Petrous portion of the temporal bone

Internal acoustic meatus

Squama of the temporal bone

Dorsum sellae

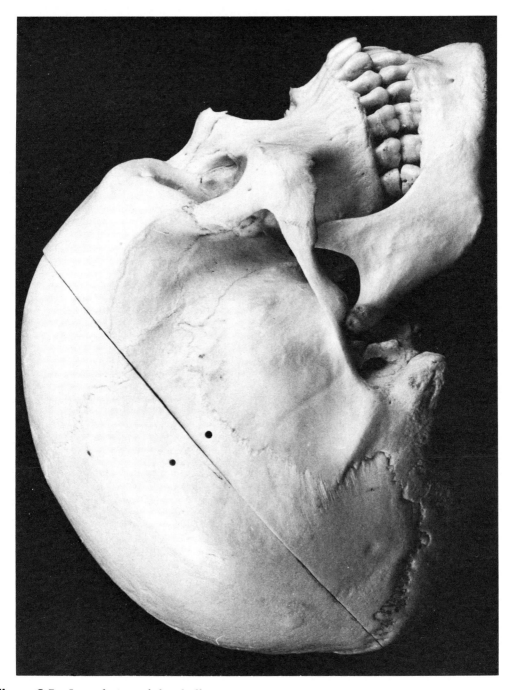

Figure 6.5. Lateral view of the skull.

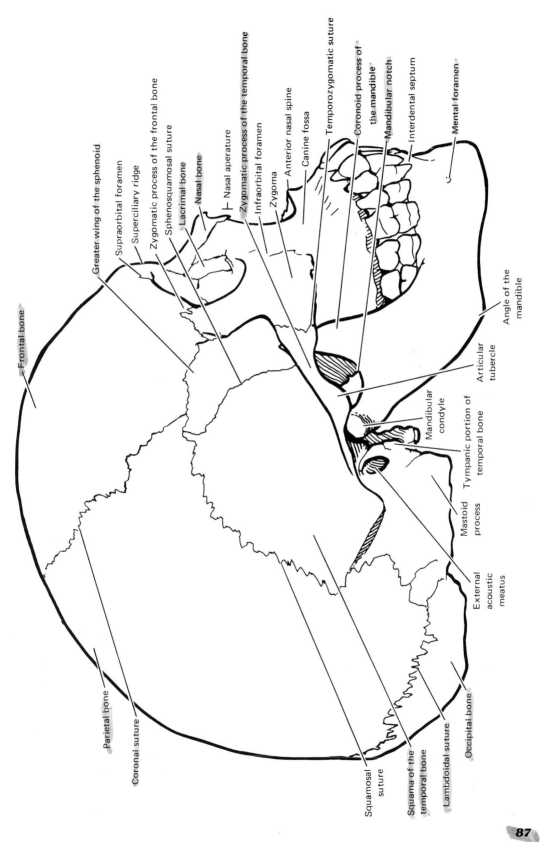

Frontal bone

Greater wing of the sphenoid

Supraorbital foramen

Superciliary ridge

Zygomatic process of the frontal bone

Sphenosquamosal suture

Lacrimal bone

Nasal bone

Nasal aperature

Zygomatic process of the temporal bone

Infraorbital foramen

Zygoma

Anterior nasal spine

Canine fossa

Temporozygomatic suture

Coronoid process of the mandible

Mandibular notch

Interdental septum

Mental foramen

Angle of the mandible

Articular tubercle

Mandibular condyle

Tympanic portion of temporal bone

Mastoid process

External acoustic meatus

Parietal bone

Coronal suture

Squamosal suture

Squama of the temporal bone

Lambdoidal suture

Occipital bone

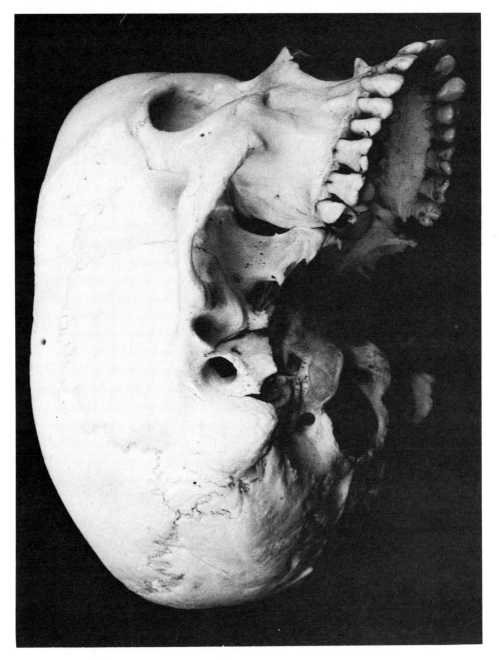

Figure 6.6. Lateroinferior view of the skull.

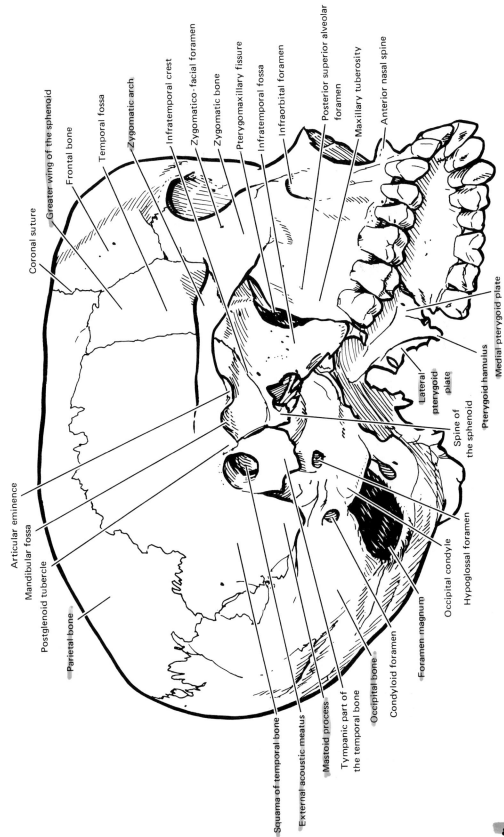

Coronal suture

Greater wing of the sphenoid

Frontal bone

Temporal fossa

Zygomatic arch

Infratemporal crest

Zygomatico-facial foramen

Zygomatic bone

Pterygomaxillary fissure

Infratemporal fossa

Infraorbital foramen

Posterior superior alveolar foramen

Maxillary tuberosity

Anterior nasal spine

Lateral pterygoid plate

Pterygoid hamulus

Medial pterygoid plate

Spine of the sphenoid

Occipital condyle

Hypoglossal foramen

Foramen magnum

Condyloid foramen

Occipital bone

Tympanic part of the temporal bone

Mastoid process

External acoustic meatus

Squama of temporal bone

Parietal bone

Postglenoid tubercle

Mandibular fossa

Articular eminence

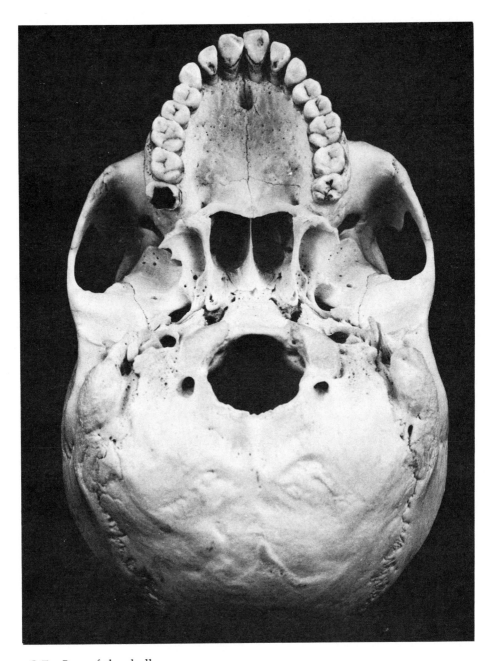

Figure 6.7. Base of the skull.

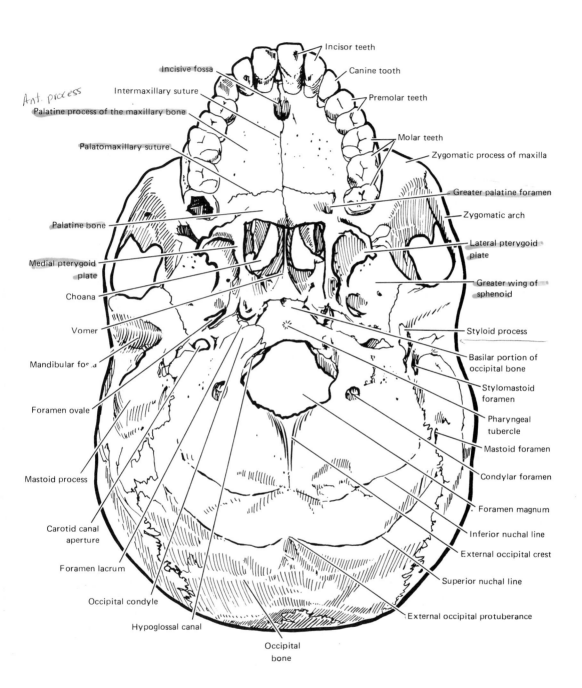

Ant. process

Incisor teeth

Incisive fossa

Canine tooth

Intermaxillary suture

Premolar teeth

Palatine process of the maxillary bone

Palatomaxillary suture

Molar teeth

Zygomatic process of maxilla

Greater palatine foramen

Palatine bone

Zygomatic arch

Lateral pterygoid plate

Medial pterygoid plate

Greater wing of sphenoid

Choana

Vomer

Styloid process

Mandibular fossa

Basilar portion of occipital bone

Foramen ovale

Stylomastoid foramen

Pharyngeal tubercle

Mastoid foramen

Condylar foramen

Mastoid process

Foramen magnum

Carotid canal aperture

Inferior nuchal line

Foramen lacrum

External occipital crest

Occipital condyle

Superior nuchal line

Hypoglossal canal

External occipital protuberance

Occipital bone

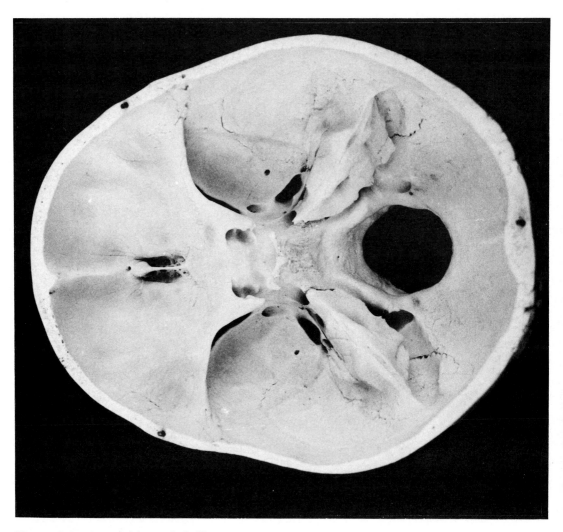

Figure 6.8. Internal base of skull.

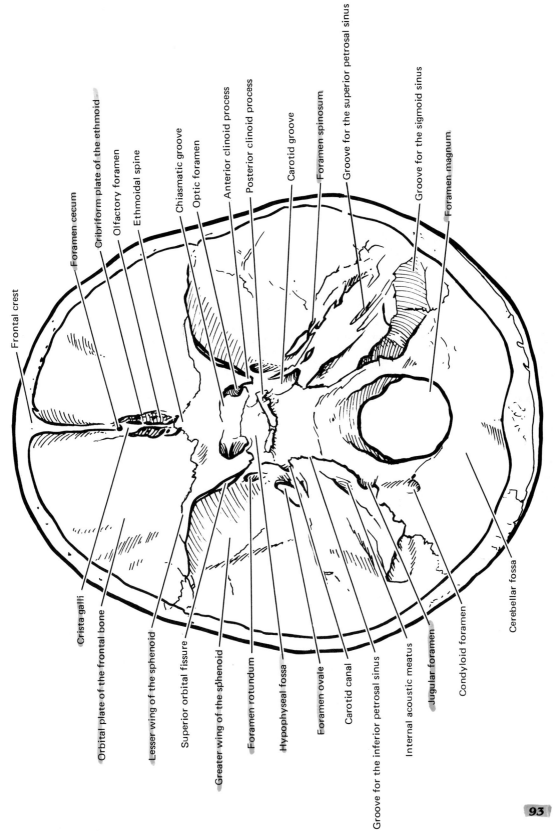

Frontal crest

Foramen cecum

Cribriform plate of the ethmoid

Olfactory foramen

Ethmoidal spine

Chiasmatic groove

Optic foramen

Anterior clinoid process

Posterior clinoid process

Carotid groove

Foramen spinosum

Groove for the superior petrosal sinus

Groove for the sigmoid sinus

Foramen magnum

Crista galli

Orbital plate of the frontal bone

Lesser wing of the sphenoid

Superior orbital fissure

Greater wing of the sphenoid

Foramen rotundum

Hypophyseal fossa

Foramen ovale

Carotid canal

Groove for the inferior petrosal sinus

Internal acoustic meatus

Jugular foramen

Condyloid foramen

Cerebellar fossa

93

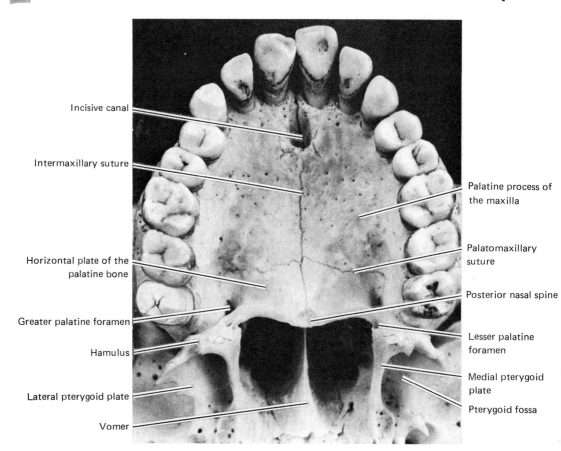

Incisive canal

Intermaxillary suture

Palatine process of the maxilla

Horizontal plate of the palatine bone

Palatomaxillary suture

Greater palatine foramen

Posterior nasal spine

Hamulus

Lesser palatine foramen

Lateral pterygoid plate

Medial pterygoid plate

Vomer

Pterygoid fossa

Figure 6.9. Palate and associated area.

Pterygopalatine Fossa (Fig. 6.6). Entrance into the pterygopalatine fossa is gained via the *pterygomaxillary fissure,* which transmits the maxillary vessels. This fissure is located on the medial wall of the infratemporal fossa and is formed by the interval between the pterygoid process of the sphenoid and the convex posterior aspect of the maxilla. The fossa is pyramidal in shape and is enclosed by three bones, the maxilla and palatine bones, and the pterygoid process of the sphenoid. It communicates with the interior of the skull through the *foramen rotundum,* transmitting the maxillary branch of the trigeminal nerve, with the orbit via the inferior orbital fissure, and with the nasal cavity by the *sphenopalatine foramen.* Extending posteriorly from this fossa is the *pterygoid canal* which transmits the nerve of the pterygoid canal. Inferiorly, the fossa becomes constricted and ends in the *pterygopalatine canal* (greater palatine canal) conducting the greater palatine vessels and nerves. The fossa contains an autonomic ganglion and its associations and blood vessels.

Zygomatic Arch (Figs. 6.5, 6.6). The zygomatic arch assists in the formation of the bony prominence of the cheek and provides attachments for the temporalis fascia and the masseter muscle. The arch is formed by the *temporal process of the zygomatic bone* and the *zygomatic process of the temporal bone,* which are joined to each other by a suture positioned more or less 45° to the vertical. Just medial to this suture, in the temporal fossa, the temporalis muscle passes to insert on the mandible. The zygomatic process of the temporal bone arises from two or (according to some) three roots. The anterior root ends in front of the *mandibular (glenoid) fossa* in a round prominence, the articular eminence, which is the point of articulation of the mandibular condyle with the temporal bone. The posterior root continues further posteriorly, passing above the exter-

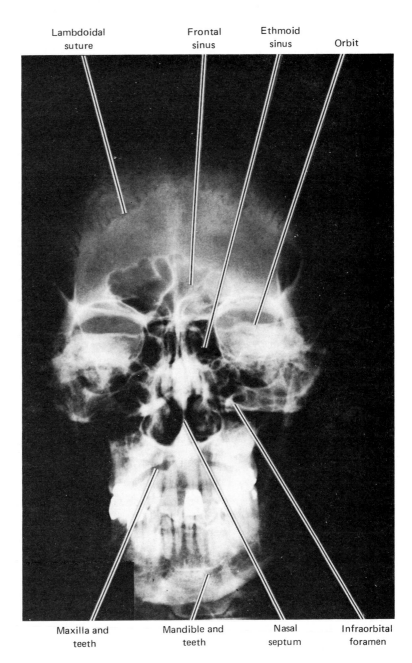

| Lambdoidal suture | Frontal sinus | Ethmoid sinus | Orbit |

| Maxilla and teeth | Mandible and teeth | Nasal septum | Infraorbital foramen |

Figure 6.10.
Posterior-anterior radiograph of the head. (Courtesy of Mary Jane Thommen, RT, Department of Radiology, University of Maryland Hospital, Baltimore.)

nal auditory meatus and lateral to the mandibular fossa. The *post-glenoid tubercle*, a bony structure posterior to the mandibular fossa which assists in preventing backward excursion of the condyle out of the fossa, is considered by some to be the third root of the zygomatic process of the temporal bone.

The zygomatic arch is continuous medially with the *zygoma*, a quadrilateral-shaped bone constituting a part of the inferior and lateral border of the orbit. The superior border is formed by the frontal process of the zygoma and the inferior border by its maxillary process. The *zygomaticofacial foramen* (frequently two foramina) pierces the body of the zygoma and transmits the zygomaticofacial nerve and vessels. On its orbital aspect, the zygomatic bone presents the two *zygomaticoorbital foramina*, which transmit nerves and vessels to the zygomaticofacial and *zygomaticotemporal* foramina. The last foramen opens on the medial (temporal) surface of the zygomatic bone, and through it the zygomaticotemporal nerve and vessels enter the temporal fossa. The zygomatic bone articulates with the zygomatic process of the maxilla. The zygomatic process of the maxilla describes an arched line, the *zygomaticoalveolar crest* as it curves inferiorly to meet the alveolar portion of the maxilla.

Mastoid and Styloid Processes (Fig. 6.6). The *external acoustic meatus* and the surrounding lateral aspect of the tympanic portion of the temporal bone are wedged between the mastoid process and the posterior root of the zygomatic process of the temporal bone just posterior to the mandibular fossa. This oval opening transmits the cartilaginous external ear canal leading to the tympanic membrane. Behind and inferior to the external acoustic meatus is the *mastoid process*, which serves as a point of attachment of several muscles. On its posterior aspect, a foramen, the *mastoid foramen* is frequently present transmitting *emissary veins*. Between the mastoid and *styloid process* is a constant foramen, the *stylomastoid foramen*, transmitting the facial nerve. The *styloid process* is a long, sharp, pointed structure directed inferiorly and anteriorly. It gives attachment to several muscles and ligaments, which serve to assist in the regulation of the excursion and movements of the mandible, hyoid bone, tongue, and pharynx.

Posterior View (Fig. 6.7)

Observing the skull from a posterior view, the *foramen magnum* is completely out of view. The most obvious features present are the posterior aspects of the *sagittal suture* and the *lambdoidal suture,* the former separating the paired parietal bones from each other and the latter acting as the dividing line between the occipital and parietal bones. Occasionally, one or more small islands of bone, known as sutural bones (Wormian), are present in the apex of the lambdoidal suture where it is met by the inferior extent of the sagittal suture. Enclosed by the diverging lines of the lambdoidal suture is the flat, shell-shaped portion of the occipital bone, the squama. A thick ridge, known as the *superior nuchal line* extends to bisect the occipital squama into superior and inferior halves. At the midpoint, the right and left superior nuchal lines meet in a bony point, the *external occipital protuberance.* A thin ridge of bone on the occipital squama runs directly inferiorly to terminate at the posteromedial ridge of the foramen magnum. It is known as the *external occipital crest* or *median nuchal line.* At the midpoint of the external occipital crest, the *inferior nuchal line* extends laterally, representing the superior border of attachment for three muscles of the back of the neck. Occasionally, the *highest nuchal lines,* positioned just above the superior nuchal lines, are evident. These serve as lines of attachment for the galea aponeurotica.

Superior View

The skull, observed from a superior view, has more or less the outline shape of an egg. It is narrower anteriorly and broader posteriorly where the broadest region is the *parietal eminence.* This view reveals the portions of those bones which form the skullcap, consisting of the frontal squama, two parietal bones, and a small portion of the occipital squama. The frontal eminences and, if present, the metopic frontal sutures are evident. The coronal suture, indicating the border between the frontal and paired parietal bones, is met at its midline by the anterior extent of the sagittal suture at the bregma. This suture separates the right and left parietal bones from each other, terminating posteriorly at the lambda, the apex of the lambdoidal suture. Anterior to the lambda, just lateral to the sagittal suture, are the paired *parietal foramina,* through which *emissary veins* pass. The bones comprising the calvaria (skullcap) are somewhat unusual in that they present two tables of compact bone, the outer and inner plates, which sandwich between them a layer of spongy (cancellous) bone, known as the *diploë.*

Inferior View (Figs. 6.7, 6.9)

The inferior aspect of the skull is usually observed with the mandible detached to permit an unobstructed view of the various structures. The anteriormost border includes the central incisors, while the posterior border is said to be the superior nuchal line. The lateral extent includes the two zygomatic arches and the two mastoid processes.

The base of the skull will be examined in three sections, the anterior portion, which extends as far back as the hard palate, the middle portion, which stops at a tangent drawn along the anteriormost point of the foramen magnum, and the posterior portion, which entails the rest of the base of the skull.

Anterior Portion. The anterior portion is a flat-topped, dome-shaped region which houses the 16 maxillary teeth arranged peripherally in a horseshoe-shaped configuration. It is the inferiormost portion of the skull, with the exception of the mandible. The teeth are embedded in the *alveolar arch* and between any two teeth, known as the interproximal region, is a bony extension, the *interdental septum.* Posterior to the third molars, the buccal and lingual alveolar arches fuse, and the area of fusion is known as the *alveolar tubercle.* Superior to the alveolar tubercle, the broad, posterior extent of the maxilla is the *maxillary tuberosity.* In the anterior portion (and at this point it should be appreciated that, while this view observes the skull upside down, the descriptive terms refer to the normal anatomical position) the roof is arched and is separated into four segments by two intersecting sutures, the *cruciform suture.* The longer suture is the combination of the intermaxillary/interpalatine sutures which separate the *hard palate* into right and left halves. The shorter suture is made up of the palatomaxillary sutures which separate the horizontal plates of the palatine bones from the palatine processes of the maxillae. The anteriormost part of the intermaxillary suture lies in a depression, the *incisive fossa* (not to be confused with the same-named depression on the external aspect of the maxilla), into which the *incisive foramen* opens. The incisive foramen receives the right and left *incisive canals*, each of which transmits the nasopalatine branch of the sphenopalatine artery and the nasopalatine nerve. Posteriorly, on the lateral aspect of the hard palate, normally within the palatomaxillary suture, is the *greater palatine foramen*, through which the greater palatine vessels and nerves pass. Usually two, sometimes three smaller foramina, the *lesser palatine foramina*, are present. They permit the passage of the lesser palatine vessels and nerves. These foramina are contained in the *pyramidal process* of the palatine bone, which juts out posteriorly and laterally and is interposed between the *lateral* and *medial pterygoid plates* of the sphenoid bone. The posterior aspect of the hard palate ends in a midline, bony projection known as the *posterior nasal spine*, the origin of the muscle of the uvula.

Middle Portion. This is the most complex portion of the base of the skull. It is composed of parts of the sphenoid, palatine, temporal, vomer, and occipital bones, housing several foramina which present passageways from and to the exterior of the skull. The pyramidal portion of the palatine bone has already been discussed. It covers a portion of the maxillary tuberosity and is interposed between the alveolar tubercle and the medial and lateral pterygoid plates of the sphenoid.

The medial pterygoid plate presents a short, wedge-shaped structure at its inferior free edge, the *pterygoid hamulus*, around which the tendon of the tensor veli palatini muscle passes. This muscle originates in the *scaphoid fossa*, a small depression at the base of the pterygoid processes. Above this fossa, at the root of the medial pterygoid plate, is the opening of the *pterygoid canal (vidian canal)*, through which the like-named nerve passes. Below this fossa is a larger depression, between the lateral and medial pterygoid plates, known as the *pterygoid fossa*. It contains the medial pterygoid and tensor veli palatini muscles.

Between the right and left medial pterygoid plates is the choana, the posterior entrance into the nasal cavity which is separated into right and left compartments by the nasal septum. The posterior aspect of this midline septum is the vomer, whose superior, broadened portion, evident in the inferior view, is met by a horizontal projection from the base of the medial pterygoid plate known as the *vaginal process*. This process forms the floor of the *pharyngeal canal* which transmits the like-named nerve. Posterior to the vomer is a thick bridge-like bone, the *basilar portion of the occipital bone*, which flares out laterally as it extends back to the foramen magnum and the *occipital condyles*. A bony protuberance in the middle of the basilar portion of the occipital bone is known as the *pharyngeal tubercle*. It acts as a point of suspension for the entire pharynx, via the pharyngeal raphe. Shallow depressions and slight ridges on either side of the pharyngeal tubercle represent attachments for some of the muscles of the posterior neck. The occipital bone approximates the jagged *petrous portion* of the temporal bone, which houses the *carotid canal* through which the *internal carotid artery* gains entrance into the cranial cavity. This canal terminates anteromedially at the apex of the temporal petrous, at the *foramen lacerum*. This foramen, enclosed in the live individual by a cartilaginous plate, is formed by the junction of the temporal, occipital, and sphenoid bones. Small arterial branches to the meninges and emissary veins from the cavernous sinus are said to pass through it.

The petrous portion of the temporal bone articulates anteriorly with the sphenoid, forming a groove which passes backwards and laterally, finally disappearing as a canal in the petrous bone. This groove and canal house the cartilaginous portion of the Eustachian tube. A ridge of bone, the *spine of the sphenoid,* forms the lateral border of this groove and also contains the *foramen spinosum,* through which the middle meningeal artery and recurrent meningeal branch of the mandibular branch of cranial nerve V gains entrance into the cranial cavity. The *foramen ovale,* located just anterior and medial to the foramen spinosum, pierces the greater wing of the sphenoid and permits the passage of the accessory meningeal artery and the mandibular division of the trigeminal nerve.

Lateral to the foramen ovale is the flat portion of the greater wing of the sphenoid and part of the root of the zygomatic arch of the temporal bone. These form part of the roof of the infratemporal fossa. The lateral border of this table turns upwards at nearly a right angle, and this ridge, the *infratemporal crest,* marks the boundary of the infratemporal and temporal fossae. The sphenotemporal suture passes diagonally across this ridge. Posterior to this table is a deep depression, housed in the tympanic and squamous portions of the temporal bone, the *mandibular fossa (glenoid fossa).* This depression accepts the articular disc and, indirectly, the condyle of the mandible, thus participating in the formation of the temporomandibular joint. The *squamotympanic fissure* passes diagonally across the mandibular fossa. Approximately halfway through its course, a thin wedge of bone, the inferior-most tip of the *tegmen tympani,* protrudes through this fissure, thus creating two new fissures, an anterior *(petrosquamous)* and a posterior *(petrotympanic)* fissure. The petrotympanic fissure transmits the chorda tympani branch of the cranial nerve VII and the anterior tympanic branch of the maxillary artery. The anterior border of the mandibular fossa is represented by the articular eminence of the zygomatic process and the posterior extent by the postglenoid tubercle, which is, according to some, the posterior root of the zygomatic arch. Curving inferiorly and posteriorly from the postglenoid tubercle is the free edge of the tympanic portion of the temporal bone.

Posterior Portion. This portion contains the *foramen magnum,* the *occipital condyles,* styloid and mastoid processes, as well as the region of the occipital squama as far superiorly as the superior nuchal line. On either side of the anterior portion of the foramen magnum are located the occipital condyles which articulate with the atlas. Directly in front of and superior to the condyle is a canal which traverses the bone in a posteromedial direction. This is the *hypoglossal canal,* which transmits cranial nerve XII and a meningeal artery. Just posterior to the condyle is a depression, the *condylar fossa* which may or may not be perforated by the *condylar foramen,* through which emissary veins pass. Lateral to the hypoglossal canal is a large foramen, the *jugular foramen,* formed by the *jugular notch of the occipital* and *jugular notch of the temporal bones.* Several important structures pass through this foramen, namely cranial nerves IX, X, and XI, the inferior petrosal and transverse sinuses (draining into the jugular bulb, the expanded terminus of the internal jugular vein), as well as some meningeal arteries. Just lateral to the large jugular foramen is a small foramen, wedged between the needle-shaped styloid process and the thick cone-shaped mastoid process. This is the *stylomastoid foramen* through which cranial nerve VII leaves the skull. The mastoid process also gives rise to several muscles, one of which originates from a deep cleft, the *mastoid notch,* on the medial aspect of the process. Medial to this cleft is the *groove* for the *occipital artery.* This groove is bordered medially by the *temporo-occipital suture* and laterally by the ridge of bone separating the groove from the mastoid notch. Frequently, above and behind the mastoid process is the *mastoid foramen* transmitting emissary veins.

The most obvious structure in this part of the base of the skull is the foramen magnum, which transmits the medulla oblongata and associated meninges, the spinal roots of cranial nerve XI, the vertebral arteries, anterior and posterior spinal arteries, as well as autonomic fibers traveling on the vertebral arteries. The remaining outstanding features of the occipital bone were described in the posterior view.

Internal Aspect of the Skull

The internal aspect of the skull may be divided into two major regions, namely the superior aspect—that is the internal surface of the calvaria—and the internal base of the skull.

Internal Surface of the Calvaria
The calvaria, or skullcap, is a dome-shaped structure which protects the superior aspect of the brain. It is composed of the frontal and two parietal bones as well as a small portion of the occipital bone. The anteriormost aspect may or may not contain the superiormost extent of the two *frontal sinuses* housed between the external and internal plates of the frontal bone. A thin, wedge-shaped ridge of bone, the *frontal crest,* juts out, its sharp edge pointing posteriorly to which the *falx cerebri* attaches while its superior aspect flares out before blending into the surrounding frontal squama. As it flares out, it is grooved, indicating the location of the superior sagittal sinus. This groove, the *sagittal sulcus,* becomes deeper as it continues posteriorly in the midline. The coronal, saggital, and lambdoidal sutures are also evident. Lateral to the sagittal sulcus, a few shallow, irregular excavations, the *foveolae granularis,* are present, indicating the location of the lacunae lateralis, structures associated with arachnoid granulations. The lateral aspects of the cranial vault are grooved by branches of the meningeal vessels.

Internal Base (Fig. 6.8)
The internal base of the skull is arranged as three depressions positioned in an anterior-posterior direction, each lower than the one preceding it. These are named the *anterior, middle,* and *posterior cranial fossae.* In the living individual, the internal base (as well as the calvaria) is lined by a periosteo-dural membrane, which is reflected onto itself to form venous sinuses (discussed in Chapter 17). These sinuses leave their marks on the bones as grooves, one of which, the sagittal sulcus, was mentioned in the previous section. Additional

marks on these bones are due to the presence of blood vessels, cranial dura, sulci and gyri of the brain, and foramina permitting the passage of structures into and out of the cranial cavity.

Certain foramina, viewable in the internal base of the skull were described in the previous section, and their contents were noted there. The relative locations of these will be indicated in the present section, but further description will not be repeated. Table 6.2, as well as the previous section, provides that information.

Anterior Cranial Fossa. The anterior cranial fossa is composed of portions of the frontal, ethmoid, and sphenoid bones. The frontal lobes of the cerebrum lie on this floor. The anterior and lateral extents are formed by the frontal bones, while the posterior boundary is formed by the lesser wings and body of the sphenoid. The frontal bone has a wedge-shaped midline structure, the frontal crest, which ends in a point inferiorly demarcating part of the contribution of the frontal bone to the *foramen cecum*. This foramen, if patent, transmits emissary veins, and it is here that the superior sagittal sinus originates. The posterior part of the foramen cecum is formed by the ethmoid bone. Just behind this foramen is a triangular wedge of bone, the *crista galli* (cock's comb) of the ethmoid, which provides attachment for the falx cerebri. The base of the crista galli sits in a depression between the two orbital plates of the frontal bone. The floor of this midline depression is known as the *cribriform plate* of the *ethmoid*. As its name implies, this plate is perforated by numerous *olfactory foramina* which transmit the *olfactory nerves* to the *olfactory bulbs* that occupy this depression.

A small, triangular-shaped plate of bone extends from the body of the sphenoid anteriorly. The apex of this bony triangle, the *ethmoidal spine* of the sphenoid bone, contacts the posteriormost part of the crista galli. Thus it is interposed between the orbital plates of the frontal bone and the cribriform plate of the ethmoid. The ethmoidal spine blends laterally into the lesser wings of the sphenoid. Posteriorly, the lesser wings terminate in a curved knife-edge, the inferior aspect of which contains the *sphenoparietal sinus*. The lesser wing of the sphenoid becomes broader medially, ending in a blunt, rounded process, the *anterior clinoid process*, forming a ledge above the middle cranial fossa. This process forms the most anterior attachment of the *tentorium cerebelli*.

Middle Cranial Fossa. The floor of the middle cranial fossa, which supports the temporal lobes of the brain, is at a lower level than and extends anteriorly underneath the anterior cranial fossa. Anteriorly, it is limited by the lesser wings of the sphenoid, the anterior border of the *groove* for the *optic chiasma*, and the anterior clinoid processes. Laterally, it extends to the greater wing of the sphenoid, squamous portion of the temporal, and inferior part of the parietal bones. Posteriorly, it is limited by the dorsum sellae of the sphenoid and the superior aspect of the petrous portion of the temporal bone. Most of the center of this fossa is occupied by the *sella turcica* of the sphenoid, spreading antero- and posterolaterally to its wall. The body of the sphenoid is sculpted in the midline to form the sella turcica whose deepest portion is known as the *hypophyseal fossa*. The anterior wall of the sella turcica, the *tuberculum* *sellae,* is almost vertical and bears a lateral projection on each side, the *middle clinoid process.* The posterior wall of the sella turcica, the *dorsum sellae,* juts up and bears two small knoblike projections known as the *posterior clinoid processes.* These processes provide attachment for the tentorium cerebelli.

The chiasmatic groove leads laterally into the optic foramen, through which the optic nerve, central artery of the retina, and the ophthalmic branch of the internal carotid artery, with its associated sympathetic plexus, enter the orbit. Immediately lateral to the optic foramen, the diagonal slit between the lesser and greater wings of the sphenoid is known as the *superior orbital fissure* which transmits cranial nerves III, IV, VI, and the ophthalmic division of V, along with the ophthalmic veins. Posterior to the superior orbital fissure is the *foramen rotundum,* through which the maxillary division for the trigeminal nerve exits the cranial fossa. Two additional foramina, the *foramen ovale* and *foramen spinosum,* lie posterolateral to the foramen rotundum in the sphenoid bone. Medial to the foramen ovale is the *foramen lacerum,* which is, at times, formed into an incomplete canal by a piece of bone, the *lingula,* jutting out posteriorly from the body of the sphenoid. The lingula, at its origin, participates in the formation of a ridge forming the lateral border of a shallow groove for the internal carotid artery. Posteriorly, the lingula approximates the medialmost region of the petrous portion of the temporal bone, the anterior surface of which bears a slight depression known as the *trigeminal impression* (for the trigeminal ganglion). Lateral to this impression is a small groove on the anterior, deep surface of the petrous portion of the temporal bone. The groove opens posteriorly into the canal, the *hiatus* of the *facial canal.* Above and lateral to the hiatus is a bony prominence, the *arcuate eminence,* overlying the superior semicircular canal. The thin bony roof of the tympanic cavity partly surrounds (laterally and anteriorly) the arcuate eminence and is known as the *tegmen tympani.* The superiormost portion of the petrous portion of the temporal is a thin ridge, which constitutes part of the posterior border of the middle cranial fossa. This ridge contains the *groove* for the *superior petrosal sinus.*

Posterior Cranial Fossa. The remainder of the internal base of the skull is referred to as the *posterior cranial fossa.* It is composed of the occipital, temporal, and parietal bones, along with a small contribution from the sphenoid. It is both deeper and larger than the other two fossae and houses the brain stem, cerebellum, and occipital lobe of the cerebrum. The most obvious structure is the *foramen magnum,* which occupies the deepest part of the posterior cranial fossa. Immediately anterior to the foramen magnum, the somewhat concave *clivus* extends upward to articulate with the sphenoid. Along the lateral aspect of this basilar portion, as it approximates the petrous portion of the temporal bone, is the groove for the *inferior petrosal sinus.* An oval foramen, the *internal auditory (acoustic) meatus,* pierces the posterior face of the petrous temporal bone, leading to the internal ear. Cranial nerves VII and VIII, as well as the internal auditory arteries and veins, pass through it. Directly inferior to the internal auditory meatus is the large *jugular foramen* conducting various nerves and vessels. Medial to the jugular foramen is a bony elevation, the jugular tubercle, whose superior surface is grooved for the passage of cranial nerves IX, X, and XI to the jugular foramen. The *hypoglossal foramen,* leading to the *hypoglossal canal,* pierces the occipital bone just inferior to the jugular tubercle. This canal transmits cranial nerve XII and the meningeal branch of the ascending pharyngeal artery. Occasionally, the condylar canal also pierces the occipital bone, ending at the mouth of the jugular foramen where it is met by the *groove for the sigmoid sinus.* This groove describes a sigmoid-shaped curve on the occipital and neighboring temporal and parietal bones, where it continues as the *groove for the transverse sinus.* Usually the groove on the left is somewhat shallower than the one on the right. Near the midline of the posterior wall of the posterior cranial fossa, the groove for the transverse sinus makes a 90° arc, turns superiorly to end in the *groove for the superior sagittal sinus.* At the region where the transverse sinus turns superiorly is a large protuberance, the *internal occipital protuberance,* which marks the intersection of two linear bony elevations forming a cross, the *cruciate eminence.* The cruciate eminence divides the region into four concavities. The lower concavities serve as the housing of the two cerebellar hemispheres and are known as the *cerebellar fossae,* while the two superior depressions indicate the location of the occipital lobes of the cerebrum. The lower leg of the cruciate eminence, extending from the internal occipital protuberance to the posterior lip of the foramen magnum, is the *internal occipital crest,* to which the falx cerebelli attaches.

MANDIBLE

The mandible, forming the skeleton of the chin, is one of the largest bones of the skull and the only moveable one. The mandible houses the 16 lower teeth and, via its articulation with the temporal bone, brings the lower dentition into intimate contact with the upper dental arch. The mandible consists of a horseshoe-shaped, horizontally placed *body* and two *rami* projecting upward and backward. The two rami are suspended from the skull by a series of bilateral ligaments and muscles. These limit the excursion of the bone and simultaneously provide great versatility of motion by permitting a plethora of movements, including opening, closing, protrusion, retraction, lateral excursion, and a limited degree of rotation.

The mandible presents an external and internal surface (Fig. 6.11). The *external surface* will be described first. The horseshoe-shaped body presents a fusion line in the anterior midline, between the two central incisors, known as the *symphysis menti* (mandibular symphysis), the inferior extent of which is triangular and is referred to as the *mental protuberance,* or the point of the chin. The base of the mental protuberance forms the anteriormost portion of the inferior border of the mandible and is somewhat concave in the midline but presents two small bony projections laterally, the *mental tubercles.* Above the mental tubercles, on either side of the symphysis menti, the body of the mandible presents two slight concavities, the *incisive fossae.* On the lateral surface, the *mental foramen* is evident, located inferior to the interproximal region between the first and second premolars. It opens in a posterior direction and transmits the mental nerve and vessels.

A line, the *oblique line,* connects the mental tubercle with the anterior border of the ramus. This oblique line is very faint until it reaches the first molar, where it becomes prominent and, at the level of the second molar,

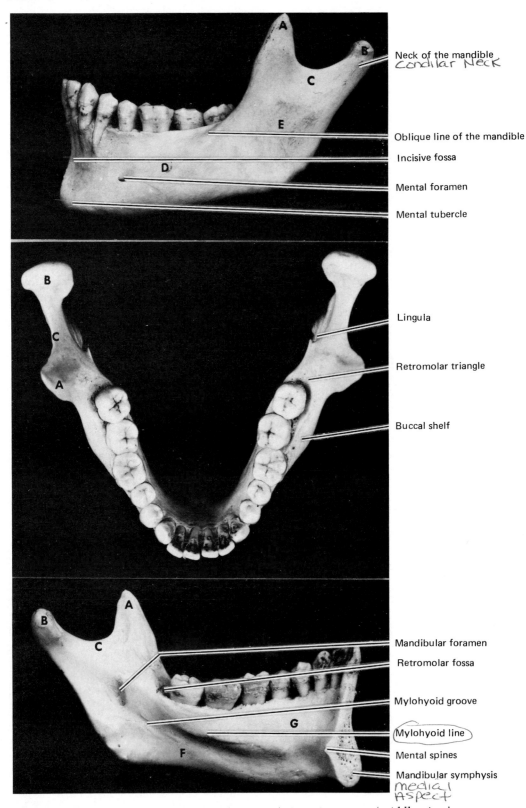

Neck of the mandible
Condilar Neck

Oblique line of the mandible

Incisive fossa

Mental foramen

Mental tubercle

Lingula

Retromolar triangle

Buccal shelf

Mandibular foramen

Retromolar fossa

Mylohyoid groove

Mylohyoid line

Mental spines

Mandibular symphysis
medial
Aspect

Figure 6.11. Mandible. Lateral aspect (top view). Superior aspect (middle view). Medial aspect (bottom view). **A.** Coronoid process. **B.** Mandibular condyle. **C.** Mandibular notch. **D.** Body of the mandible. **E.** Ramus of the mandible. **F.** Submandibular fossa. **G.** Sublingual fossa.

begins to arch upward to become continuous with the sharp, anterior edge of the ramus.

Medial to the oblique line, just lateral and distal to the third molar, is a shallow depression, the *retromolar fossa*. Medial to the retromolar fossa is another shallow depression, triangular in shape, the *retromolar triangle*. The lateral border of the retromolar triangle becomes continuous with the *lateral (buccal) alveolar crest*, while the medial border is continuous with the *medial alveolar crest* of the third molar. These crests then continue forward to form the buccal and lingual alveolar plates of the mandible. In the interproximal regions, these plates are connected to each other by bony connections, the *interdental septa*.

The *internal surface* in the midline bears two, or sometimes four, bony tubercles. The two superior are constant and are the mental spines (also referred to as *superior mandibular spines* or *genial tubercles*) from which the genioglossus muscles originate. The two lower tubercles, the *inferior mandibular spines*, serve as the origins of the geniohyoid muscles. The medial aspect of the body of the mandible bears a bony ridge, the *mylohyoid line*, extending from the symphysis menti to the region of the third molar. The mylohyoid line delineates the origin of the mylohyoid muscle. Superior to the mylohyoid line anteriorly is a shallow fossa, the *sublingual fossa*, while the *submandibular fossa* projects posteriorly below this line. Each fossa is named after the major salivary gland that occupies it.

Posterior to the body of the mandible is the ramus. The region where the posterior border of the ramus is continuous with the posterior extent of the base of the mandible is the *angle* of the *mandible*. The buccal (external) aspect of the ramus is marked with tuberosities and depressions, indicating the site of attachment of the masseter muscle. Just anterior to the attachment of the masseter is a slight groove on the body of the mandible, the *groove for the facial artery*, indicating the route that artery takes as it curves upward to enter the face. The upward extension of the ramus ends in the *coronoid* and the *condylar processes*. The flattened, triangular coronoid process serves as the insertion for the temporalis muscle. The insertion of this muscle also occupies the anterior border of the ramus on its medial aspect. The condylar process flares out and ends in an articular surface, the *condyle of the mandible*, which articulates with the temporal bone. The region just below the condyle is the *neck of the mandible*, on whose medial aspect the *lateral pterygoid muscle* inserts onto a slight depression, the pterygoid fovea. The arciform region between the two processes is known as the *mandibular notch*, through which the masseteric nerve and vessels pass into the masseter muscle.

Near the middle of the medial surface of the ramus is the *mandibular foramen* which opens into the *mandibular canal* housing the inferior alveolar vessels and nerve. The opening is guarded anteriorly by a sharp ridge of bone, the *lingula*, whose free apex points posteriorly toward the condyle. The lingula serves as the region of attachment of the sphenomandibular ligament. Inferior to the lingula is the *mylohyoid groove*, extending from the mandibular foramen in an anteroinferior direction and indicating the course of the mylohyoid nerve. The angle of the mandible and the region posterior to the mylohyoid groove presents a roughened, craggy appearance, indicating the insertion of the medial pterygoid muscle.

TABLE 6.2
Foramina of the Skull and Their Contents

Foramen	Location on skull	Bone(s)	Location on bone	Contents
Anterior ethmoidal	Medial wall of orbit	Ethmoidal and frontal	Fronto-ethmoidal suture	Anterior ethmoidal nerve and vessels
Carotid canal	Middle cranial fossa	Temporal	Petrous portion of temporal	Internal carotid artery and associated sympathetic plexus
Cecum	Anterior cranial fossa	Frontal and ethmoidal	Between the base of the frontal crest and crista galli	Emissary veins
Condyloid	Posterior cranial fossa	Occipital	In condylar fossa just behind the condyle	Emissary veins
Greater palatine	Anterior base of the skull	Palatine and maxilla	Between the palatomaxillary suture; lingual to the third molar	Greater palatine vessels and nerve
Hiatus of the facial canal	Middle cranial fossa	Temporal	Petrous portion of temporal, lateral to trigeminal impression	Greater petrosal nerve
Hypoglossal canal	Posterior cranial fossa	Occipital	Directly above the anterior aspect of the occipital condyle	Cranial nerve XII; meningeal branch of the ascending pharyngeal artery
Incisive	Palatal midline	Maxillae	Opens into the incisive fossa just behind the interdental septum between the two central incisors	Nasopalatine nerves and nasopalatine branch of the sphenopalatine artery
Incisive canal	Palatal midline	Maxilla	Opens into the incisive foramen	Descending septal artery and nasopalatine nerve
Inferior orbital fissure	Orbit	Sphenoid, Maxilla, palatine, and zygoma	Between lateral wall and floor of orbit	Maxillary division of cranial nerve V2; zygomatic nerve; infraorbital vessels and veins to the pterygoid plexus; ophthalmic vein
Infraorbital	Inferior to rim of orbit	Maxilla	Inferior to rim of orbit, lateral to nasal aperture, above canine fossa	Infraorbital vessels and nerve
Internal auditory meatus	Posterior cranial fossa	Temporal	Posterior aspect of the petrous portion of temporal	Cranial nerves VII and VIII, nervus intermedius and internal auditory vessels

(handwritten annotations: "nerve going" next to Hypoglossal canal; "V2" next to Inferior orbital fissure)

TABLE 6.2 (CONTINUED)

Foramen	Location on skull	Bone(s)	Location on bone	Contents
Jugular	Posterior cranial fossa	Occipital and temporal	Lateral to the foramen magnum, medial to the styloid process	Cranial nerves IX, X, and XI; inferior petrosal and transverse sinuses; meningeal arteries; jugular bulb of internal jugular vein
Lacerum	Middle cranial fossa	Temporal, occipital, and sphenoid	Medial to the apex of the petrous part of the temporal; lateral to basilar part of occipital	Covered by cartilaginous plate which is pierced by meningeal arteries and emissary veins
Lesser palatine	Palate (posterior part)	Palatine	Pyramidal process of palatine	Lesser palatine vessels and nerves
Magnum	Posterior cranial fossa	Occipital	Posterior to the clivus	Medulla oblongata and associated meninges; spinal roots of cranial nerve XI; vertebral arteries; anterior and posterior spinal arteries; postganglionic sympathetic fibers
Mandibular	Medial surface of the mandible	Mandible	Medial surface of ramus, inferior to lingula	Inferior alveolar vessels and nerve
Mastoid	Posterior external surface	Temporal	Above and behind the mastoid process, near temporooccipital suture	Emissary veins; mastoid branch of the occipital artery
Mental	Anterior surface of mandible	Mandible	Inferior to interproximal region between first and second premolar	Mental nerve and vessels
Nasolacrimal canal	Anteromedial aspect of orbit	Maxilla and lacrimal	Region of articulation between the frontal process of the maxilla and the lacrimal bone	Nasolacrimal duct
Olfactory	Anterior cranial fossa	Ethmoid	Cribriform plate of ethmoid surrounding the crista galli	Olfactory nerves
Optic	Middle cranial fossa	Sphenoid	Apex of the orbit; between the two roots of the lesser wing of the sphenoid	Optic nerve; ophthalmic artery and associated postganglionic sympathetic fibers; central artery of retina

TABLE 6.2 (CONTINUED)

Foramen	Location on skull	Bone(s)	Location on bone	Contents
Ovale	Middle cranial fossa	Sphenoid	Greater wing of sphenoid; anteromedial to the foramen spinosum	Mandibular division of cranial nerve V; accessory meningeal artery; sometimes the lesser petrosal nerve
Parietal	Anterior to lambda on either side of the sagittal suture	Parietal	On superior aspect near the sagittal suture	Emissary vein to superior sagittal sinus; sometimes a branch of the occipital artery
Pharyngeal canal	External base of skull; medial to medial pterygoid plate	Sphenoid and palatine	Between the vaginal process of the sphenoid and the sphenoidal process of the palatine	Pharyngeal nerve; pharyngeal artery
Posterior ethmoidal	Medial wall of orbit	Frontal and ethmoidal	Fronto-ethmoidal suture, posterior to the anterior ethmoidal foramen	Posterior ethmoidal nerve and vessels (when present)
Posterior superior alveolar	Anterior to the pterygomaxillary fissure	Maxilla	Infratemporal surface and maxillary tuberosity	Posterior superior alveolar nerves and vessels
Pterygoid canal (Vidian canal)	Extends from foramen lacerum to pterygopalatine fossa	Sphenoid	Body of sphenoid just above the pterygoid processes	Nerve and vessels of the pterygoid canal (vidian nerve and vessel)
Rotundum	Middle cranial fossa	Sphenoid	Greater wing	Maxillary branch of the trigeminal
Sphenopalatine	Medial wall of pterygopalatine fossa	Sphenoid and palatine	Between sphenoidal and orbital processes	Sphenopalatine artery and posterior superior nasal branches (nasopalatine) nerves
Spinosum	Middle cranial fossa	Sphenoid	Spine of the sphenoid	Middle meningeal vessels and recurrent meningeal branch of mandibular division of cranial nerve V
Stylomastoid	Between styloid and mastoid processes	Temporal	Posterior to the base of the styloid process	Facial nerve; stylomastoid vessels
Superior orbital fissure	Posterior superior aspect of orbit	Sphenoid and frontal	Between roof and lateral wall, lateral to apex	Cranial nerves III, IV, VI, ophthalmic division of V; sympathetic fibers; branches of middle meningeal artery; recurrent branch of lacrimal artery; superior ophthalmic vein
Supraorbital	Superior rim of orbit	Frontal	Below superciliary arch	Supraorbital nerve and vessels

TABLE 6.2 (CONTINUED)

Foramen	Location on skull	Bone(s)	Location on bone	Contents
Zygomaticofacial	Lateral to the inferolateral angle of the orbital rim	Zygoma	Malar surface, above the origin of zygomaticus major muscle	Zygomaticofacial nerve and vessels
Zygomaticoorbital	Anterior floor of orbit	Zygoma	Orbital surface	Zygomaticofacial and zygomaticotemporal nerves and vessels
Zygomaticotemporal	Temporal fossa	Zygoma	Temporal surface	Zygomaticotemporal nerve and vessels

HYOID BONE

The hyoid is a small, U-shaped bone which, at first appearance, is of insignificant size. However, each bilateral half gives attachment to three ligaments and as many as ten and sometimes eleven muscles. This bone is suspended by ligaments and muscles between the temporal bones and the sternum. It consists of five parts, the quadrilateral, median *body (corpus)* and four *cornua (horns),* the two *greater* and two *lesser cornua.* The two greater horns, directed posteriorly, end in a tubercle and are attached by a cartilaginous connection earlier in life. The cartilage ossifies in middle-aged individuals. The lesser cornua, small nipple-like structures pointing cranially and posteriorly, are attached to the articulation of the greater cornua with the body (Fig. 6.12).

Frequently, an anterior midline vertical ridge divides the body into right and left halves. The inferior border of the body is flat, except for a small, cranially directed midline concavity. The following muscles attach to the body: genioglossus (via a few tendinous slips), geniohyoid, hyoglossus, levator of the thyroid gland (when present), mylohyoid, omohyoid, sternohyoid, and thyrohyoid. Two ligaments, the hyoepiglottic and thyrohyoid (in part) are also attached to the body of the hyoid.

The following muscles are attached to the greater cornu: digastric (via a tendinous loop), hyoglossus, middle pharyngeal constrictor, stylohyoid, and thyrohyoid. The thyrohyoid membrane is attached, in part, to the tubercle of the greater cornu.

The lesser cornu gives attachment to the chondroglossus portion of the hyoglossus muscle, as well as to the stylohyoid membrane.

CERVICAL VERTEBRAE

There are seven cervical vertebrae, and they constitute the most superior extension of the vertebral column. The superior two, the atlas and axis, are greatly modified to support the head and permit its rotation at the atlanto-axis joint. The seventh cervical vertebra (C7) is also modified, but will not be treated separately here. Interposed between any two vertebrae is an intervertebral disc, as well as other cartilaginous structures involved in regions of facets

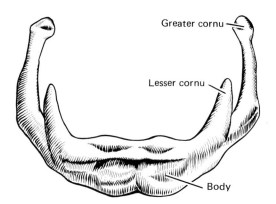

Figure 6.12. Hyoid bone.

to facilitate smooth, frictionless movement and provide cushioning and support for the whole vertebral column.

Typical Cervical Vertebra (Fig. 6.13)

The typical cervical vertebra, as any other typical vertebra, has a large, anteriorly directed *body* from which the *posterior vertebral arch* is directed dorsally. This arch encloses the *vertebral foramen.* All the vertebral foramina together constitute the *vertebral canal,* which houses the spinal cord, meninges, and associated vessels. The posterior vertebral arch consists of two short, anterior *pedicles* and two broader, posterior *laminae.* Jutting out from the two laminae are two *superior articular processes,* two *inferior articular processes,* two *transverse processes,* and a single posteriorly and inferiorly directed *spinous process.*

The superior and inferior aspects of the pedicles bear *vertebral notches* known as the *superior* and *inferior vertebral notches.* As two vertebrae articulate with each other, the superior notch of the lower vertebra and the inferior notch of the upper vertebra form the *invertebral foramen,* through which the spinal nerves leave the vertebral canal.

The transverse processes of all cervical vertebrae (except the seventh) are pierced by a large foramen, the *foramen transversarium,* housing the vertebral vessels and associated sympathetic plexus. The seventh cervical vertebra has a small or doubled foramen transversarium. The superior articular processes project cranially, bearing the posteriorly directed *articular facets.* The inferior articular processes project caudally with their articular facets directed anteriorly.

The superior surface of the body is somewhat concave and presents an upward-curving lip on either side. The inferior surface of the body is slightly concave in an anteroposterior direction, while being convex in the transverse plane. The bifid spinous process (longest in C7) projects posteriorly and inferiorly.

Atlas (Fig. 6.14)

The atlas, or first cervical vertebra, is greatly modified. The body is replaced by an *anterior arch,* whose ventral surface possesses an anterior tubercle, while the dorsal surface presents the *facet* for the *dens* of the axis. The anterior arch

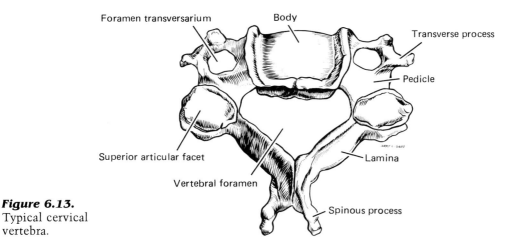

Figure 6.13.
Typical cervical
vertebra.

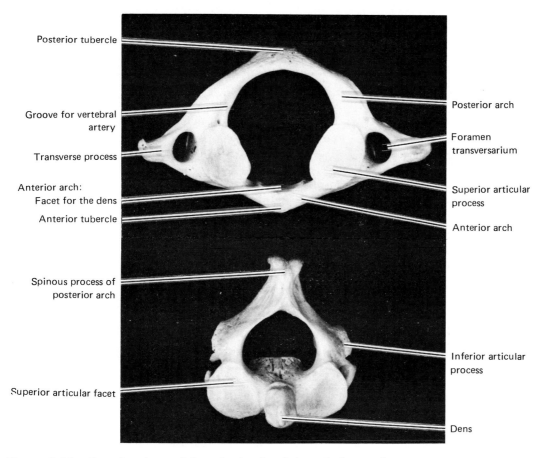

Figure 6.14. Superior views of the atlas (top) and the axis (bottom).

is connected to the *posterior arch* via the right and left *lateral masses,* which bear the *superior* and *inferior articular facets.* The superior facets articulate with the occipital condyles, while the inferior facets articulate with the superior articular facets of the axis. The dens is retained in the atlas by the transverse ligament of the atlas, a fibrous sling which is attached to a tubercle on the medial surface of each lateral mass.

The transverse processes of the atlas are very long and bear the foramina transversarium for the passage of the vertebral artery and associated structures. The superior surface of the posterior arch possesses a groove for the passage of the vertebral artery to enter the foramen magnum. The posterior arch ends in the small *posterior tubercle,* representing the spinous process.

Axis (Fig. 6.14)

The axis, or second cervical vertebra, is also modified to participate in the formation of the atlanto-axis joint. The body of the axis is modified superiorly to present a cranial tooth-like projection, the *dens,* which is notched posteriorly to accept the transverse ligament of the atlas. Anteriorly, the dens possesses an articular facet which meets the articular facet of the atlas' anterior arch.

The pedicles are modified superiorly, since they are overlaid by the superior articular facets, and the vertebral notches of this surface are very shallow. The inferior vertebral notches, however, are very deep. The transverse processes of the axis are short and possess only a single tubercle, but they otherwise are unremarkable. The spinous process is large and bifid and it serves for the attachment of many muscles responsible for various movements of the head.

Neck

This is the first of several chapters utilizing the regional approach for the examination of the head and neck. The chapter moves from superficial to deeper layers, almost as if the structures were being dissected for the reader. Hence, if a structure passes through the region being discussed, its detailed description will be confined only to that portion which resides in the area being treated. The remainder of that structure will be detailed in the appropriate chapters.

SURFACE ANATOMY (Fig. 7.1)

The neck is a more or less cylindrical structure connecting the head to the trunk. Anteriorly, it extends from the inferior border of the mandible to the superior surfaces of the manubrium and laterally along the clavicles to the point of the shoulders, or acromion. Posteriorly, it is bounded inferiorly by a somewhat irregular surface, described by an imaginary line between the two acromions passing through the intervertebral disc between the seventh cervical (C7) and first thoracic vertebrae (T1), and superiorly by the superior nuchal line of the occipital bone. The posterior aspect of the neck is composed mostly of muscle masses on either side of the spinous processes of the cervical vertebrae. These muscle masses are more properly considered the deep muscles of the back, since they function in the extension of the atlanto-occipital and other vertebral joints, in addition to supporting the head. These masses are covered by the *trapezius muscle,* which helps in shaping the posterior aspect of the neck.

The anterior midline of the neck presents a bulge whose size reflects sexual dimorphism, in that it is considerably larger in the male than in the female. This prominence is the *larynx* (Adam's apple), specifically the *thyroid cartilage,* whose superior aspect is marked by an easily palpable notch, the *thyroid notch,* above which lies the less palpable body and greater cornu of the *hyoid bone.* Inferior to the thyroid notch is the *laryngeal prominence,* which is formed by the fusion of the right and left plates of the thyroid cartilage. Immediately inferior to the thyroid cartilage is the *cricoid cartilage,* below which the superior two or three cartilaginous rings of the trachea may be palpated. The inferiormost point in the midline of the anterior neck is the *jugular notch* of the manubrium. Tensing the neck reveals the bellies and the tendons of origin of the *sternocleidomastoid muscle* just lateral to this notch. This muscle may be palpated along its entire length as it passes posteriorly and obliquely to insert on the mastoid process of the temporal and superior nuchal line of the occipital bones.

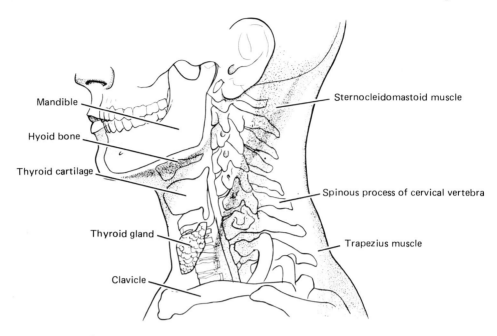

Figure 7.1. Anatomic landmarks of the neck.

SUPERFICIAL STRUCTURES OF THE NECK (Fig. 7.2)

The skin covering the neck is arranged in such a fashion that *Langer's lines* run horizontally to encircle it. Deep to the dermis is a very thin fascial layer, consisting of an areolar type of connective tissue known as the hypodermis or *superficial fascia.* This superficial fascia envelopes the neck, just as the overlying skin, and contains within it a paper-thin sheet of skeletal muscle, the *platysma.* This muscle originates from the deltoid and pectoralis fasciae and passes cranially, overlying the anterior triangle as well as the inferior part of the posterior triangle. The muscle inserts onto the inferior border of the body of the mandible as well as into the skin and hypodermis of the face. The platysma intermingles with and assists muscles which depress the lower lip and corner of the mouth. The platysma, since it is derived from the second branchial arch, is innervated by the cervical branch of the facial nerve (cranial nerve VII).

Superficial Drainage

The superficial venous drainage consists of the *external jugular vein* and its tributaries, which drain a very limited area of tissue—specifically, the region superficial and immediately deep to the investing layer of the deep cervical fascia. During this discussion of venous drainage, the great variability of venous size and distribution must be kept in mind. This section will concern itself only with the classical description.

The external jugular vein is formed by the union of the *posterior auricular* and *retromandibular veins* just posterior to the angle of the mandible, sometimes within the body of the parotid gland. It passes straight down the neck,

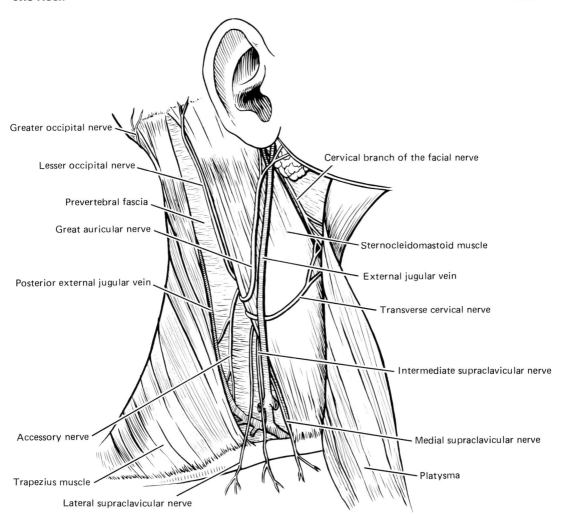

Greater occipital nerve

Lesser occipital nerve

Prevertebral fascia

Great auricular nerve

Posterior external jugular vein

Accessory nerve

Trapezius muscle

Lateral supraclavicular nerve

Cervical branch of the facial nerve

Sternocleidomastoid muscle

External jugular vein

Transverse cervical nerve

Intermediate supraclavicular nerve

Medial supraclavicular nerve

Platysma

Figure 7.2. Posterior triangle of the neck (superficial view). The platysma muscle has been reflected to expose veins and cutaneous nerves of the cervical plexus.

under the cover of the platysma muscle and associated superficial fascia, superficial to the fleshy belly of the sternocleidomastoid. In its path along this muscle, it crosses the muscle at an oblique angle (Figs. 7.1, 7.2). Once it reaches the subclavian triangle, the external jugular pierces the investing fascia, parallels the posterior border of the sternocleidomastoid, and dives deep to the clavicle to deliver its blood to the *subclavian vein,* which it joins. The external jugular vein has two pairs of incompetent valves just before it empties into the subclavian vein. Several tributaries join the external jugular vein along its path, namely the *posterior external jugular,* which drains the superficial aspect of the back of the neck, and two others, the *transverse cervical* and *suprascapular veins.* The last two veins drain the region of the shoulder. Another superficial vessel, the *anterior jugular vein,* occasionally empties into the external jugular vein, but usually it joins the subclavian vein directly. The anterior jugular is quite variable, but normally it begins at the level of the body of the hyoid bone and descends parallel to the anterior midline of the neck. Inferiorly, near the origin of the medial head of the sternocleidomastoid, the vein pierces the superficial lamina of the investing layer and turns laterally, pierces the posterior lamina, and joins the subclavian (or occasionally, the external jugular) vein. While it is between the two laminae of the investing fascia, the anterior jugular vein communicates with its corresponding vein on the other side via a venous connection, the *jugular arch*, which occupies the suprasternal space.

The external jugular, posterior external jugular, and anterior external jugular veins have numerous smaller named and unnamed tributaries, which drain the areas in their immediate vicinity.

Sensory Innervation of the Neck

Cutaneous innervation of the neck is mediated by branches of the dorsal and ventral primary rami of cervical spinal nerves. It is important to remember the following concepts concerning cutaneous innervation of the neck: the first cervical spinal nerve probably has no cutaneous branches; the side and front of the neck receive their sensory fibers from branches of the ventral primary rami of C2, C3, and C4; the ventral primary rami of C1, C2, C3, and most of C4 form the *cervical plexus;* the ventral primary rami of parts of C4, all of C5, C6, C7, and C8, and most of T1 participate in the formation of the *brachial plexus;* hence, the cutaneous supply of the side and front of the neck is derived from branches of the cervical plexus (C2, C3, and C4).

Sensation to the back of the neck is mediated by the medial branches of the dorsal primary rami of C2, C3, C4, and infrequently, C5. The medial branch of the dorsal primary ramus of the second cervical nerve is known as the *greater occipital nerve.* It passes between the semispinalis capitis and the obliquus capitis inferior and perforates the former muscle and the overlying trapezius to supply sensation to the superiormost portion of the neck and the back of the head. Medial to the greater occipital nerve is the major sensory branch of the medial branch of the primary dorsal ramus of the third cervical spinal nerve, also known as the *third occipital nerve.* This nerve also supplies sensory innervation to the superior portion of the back of the neck and the lower occipital region of the scalp. The rest of the back of the neck receives sensory innervation via the medial branch of the dorsal primary ramus of the fourth, and occasionally the fifth, cervical spinal nerves.

The front and side of the neck receive their sensory supply from branches of the cervical plexus containing fibers derived from the ventral primary rami of C2, C3, and C4. These branches of the cervical plexus are the lesser occipital, great auricular, transverse cervical, and supraclavicular nerves (Fig. 7.2). These nerves emerge in the posterior triangle, pierce the investing layer of the deep cervical fascia, and distribute to the regions they serve. They all appear very close to each other at the posterior border of the sternocleidomastoid muscle at midbelly. The *lesser occipital nerve* (C2) closely follows the posterior border of the sternocleidomastoid as it ascends towards the mastoid process. Near the insertion of this muscle, the lesser occipital nerve perforates the investing layer of the deep cervical fascia, crosses over the sternocleidomastoid muscle, and distributes to the back of the auricle of the ear and to the region of the scalp behind and superior to it.

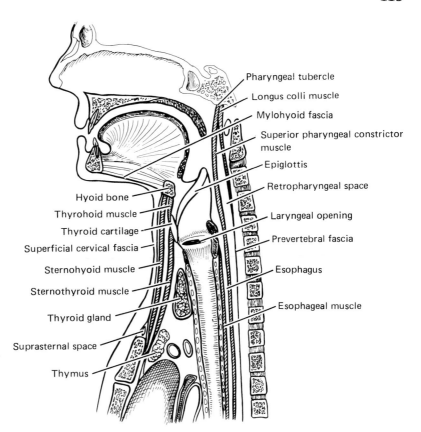

Pharyngeal tubercle

Longus colli muscle

Mylohyoid fascia

Superior pharyngeal constrictor muscle

Epiglottis

Retropharyngeal space

Laryngeal opening

Prevertebral fascia

Esophagus

Esophageal muscle

Hyoid bone

Thyrohoid muscle

Thyroid cartilage

Superficial cervical fascia

Sternohyoid muscle

Sternothyroid muscle

Thyroid gland

Suprasternal space

Thymus

Figure 7.4. Cervical fascia in midsagittal view. Note that the retropharyngeal space continues into the thorax.

cipital protuberance, the superior nuchal line, and the inferior extent of the mastoid process. Here it splits to enclose the parotid gland, where it continues superiorly as the *parotid fascia.* The superficial lamina of the parotid fascia is attached to the inferior border of the zygomatic arch. The deep lamina extends along the temporal bone to the carotid canal. A part of this deep lamina is thickened and extends from the styloid process to the mandible. It is aptly named the *stylomandibular ligament.* This ligament effectively separates the parotid and submandibular glands from each other.

Inferiorly, the investing layer is attached to the spinous process of the seventh cervical vertebra, spine of the scapula, acromion, the clavicle, and the manubrium. In places, it is attached to both the anterior and posterior aspects of the clavicle, and scapula, following the course of the attachment of the sternocleidomastoid and trapezius muscles. The fascia also splits into two laminae to envelop and fix the intermediate tendon of the omohyoid muscle. Immediately above the suprasternal notch, the two laminae of the investing layer remain separated, forming the small *suprasternal space.* This space contains adipose tissue as well as the *jugular arch,* a venous connection between the two anterior jugular veins.

Prevertebral Fascia (Figs. 7.3, 7.4)

The prevertebral fascia of the cervical fascia envelops the vertebrae and the deep cervical muscle masses surrounding the vertebral column, thus forming the floor of the posterior cervical triangle. Posteriorly, it is attached along the entire length of the ligamentum nuchae, where it merges with the origin of the investing layer. The prevertebral fascia is attached superiorly to the basilar portion of the occipital bone, jugular foramen, and carotid canal. It passes along the mastoid process of the temporal bone onto the superior nuchal line to the external occipital protuberance, where it meets its counterpart from the other side. This cylindrical layer of fascia forms attachments to the anterior surfaces of the transverse processes and bodies of the seven cervical vertebrae. Passing from the transverse process of one side to the other, it forms two laminae, with a loose connective tissue between them. This potential space constitutes the "danger space," a term explained in this chapter's section on clinical considerations. As the prevertebral fascia passes laterally, it covers the deep muscles of the neck, as well as all of the cutaneous nerves which eventually pierce it. This fascia attaches to the transverse processes of the cervical vertebrae and continues deep to the trapezius muscle as a thin film of fascia. The accessory nerve is the only cranial nerve lying superficial to this fascia. Inferiorly, this fascia continues into the thorax with the muscles of the neck as they insert onto the bones surrounding the superior thoracic aperture.

Pretracheal Fascia (Figs. 7.3, 7.4)

The pretracheal fascia forms a small, thin cylindrical fascial layer surrounding the viscera of the neck. Its posterior lamina is referred to as the *buccopharyngeal fascia.* The pretracheal fascia forms a complete investment for the thyroid gland, and the deep layer of this envelope encircles the larynx and trachea, as well as covers the lateral aspects of the esophagus. Posteriorly, the esophagus is separated from the prevertebral fascia by the buccopharyngeal portion of the pretracheal fascia. The superior attachment of the pretracheal fascia is the body and lesser and greater cornua of the hyoid bone, the stylohyoid ligament, medial pterygoid plate of the sphenoid bone, and the pharyngeal tubercle of the occipital bone, where it is met by its counterpart from the other side. Inferiorly, its boundaries include the oblique line of the thyroid cartilage, and it subsequently merges with the fasciae of the aorta and pericardium. Its fate dorsal to the esophagus is not clear, since it merges with the fascial layers of the posterior thoracic wall.

Carotid Sheath (Fig. 7.3)

The carotid sheath is a consolidation of connective tissue derived from the three fascial layers of the deep cervical fasciae and encloses the major neurovascular bundle of the neck. Compartments exist within this cylindrical connective tissue sheath which separate constituent parts of the neurovascular bundle. The contents of the carotid sheath are the common carotid artery, internal carotid artery, internal jugular vein, and the vagus nerve. The ansa cervicalis, a nerve complex, may be found on the surface of, embedded in, or just within the carotid sheath. Superiorly, the sheath is attached to the area of the jugular foramen and carotid canal, while inferiorly it is continuous with the fasciae of the great vessels and heart.

POSTERIOR ASPECTS OF THE NECK

The back of the neck consists of several bundles of muscles which, essentially, keep the head erect and partly control the atlanto-occipital and atlanto-axial articulations (Table 7.1).

Muscles

Trapezius (Figs. 7.2, 7.3)

The most superficial muscle of the back of the neck is the trapezius, a flat, triangular muscle extending from the superior nuchal line and external occipital protuberance, down the midline of the back of the neck, along the ligamentum nuchae to the spinous processes of vertebrae C7 through T12. Its fibers originating from the thoracic vertebral spines insert onto the scapula; fibers from the cervical and upper thoracic region insert onto the lateral one-third to one-half of the clavicle. This muscle is innervated by the spinal accessory nerve (XI) and also receives proprioceptive fibers from spinal nerves C3 and C4.

The muscle bundles deep to the trapezius are innervated by dorsal rami of cervical nerves. These muscles may be grouped in various manners, but due to the fusions of their embryonic segmented origins, no single classification suffices. This section will treat them in the simplest possible manner by dividing the muscles into groups according to their size and fiber direction. These are the splenius, erector spinae, transversospinal, and the suboccipital muscles.

Splenius (Figs. 7.3, 7.5)

There are two splenius muscles, the splenius capitis and splenius cervicis (the "bandage" of the head and neck, respectively). The splenius muscles are the most superficial of the muscles of the back of the deep neck proper. The *splenius capitis* originates on the lower region of the ligamentum nuchae and the spinous processes of vertebrae C7 through T4. The fibers pass craniad, deep to the trapezius and sternocleidomastoid, to insert on the mastoid process of the temporal bone and inferior to the attachment of the sternocleidomastoid muscle on the lateral third of the superior nuchal line. The *splenius cervicis* is a thin muscle whose fibers follow the inferior and lateral portion of the splenius capitis. It originates on the spines of vertebrae T3 through T6 and inserts on the transverse processes of vertebrae C1 through C3. Lateral branches of dorsal primary rami of the cervical nerves innervate both of these muscles. Their combined actions are antagonistic to the action of the sternocleidomastoid muscle in that they pull the head posteriorly. Individually, they incline the head, tilting it in the same direction as the side on which the muscle is positioned.

Erector Spinae (Figs. 7.3, 7.5)

The erector spinae muscles are not well represented in the neck, for they are composed of a few muscle fibers, some of which blend with neighboring muscles, forming longitudinally arranged columns. The *iliocostalis cervicis* arises from the angles of ribs three through six to insert on the transverse processes of vertebrae C4 through C6. Bilaterally, they act to extend the cervical spine, while unilaterally they tilt the cervical vertebrae back and to the side.

TABLE 7.1
Muscles of the Back of the Neck

Name	Location	Origin
Trapezius	Most superficial layer covering the back of the neck and upper back	External occipital protuberance, superior nuchal line, ligamentum nuchae, and spinous processes of C7–T12
Splenius capitis	Immediately deep to the trapezius	Ligamentum nuchae; spinous processes of vertebrae C7–T4
Splenius cervicis	Lateral and inferior to splenius capitis	Spines of the vertebrae T3–T6
Iliocostalis cervicis	Back of neck to the angle of upper few ribs	Angles of ribs 3, 4, 5, and 6
Longissimus cervicis	Medial to iliocostalis cervicis	Transverse processes of vertebrae T1–T5
Longissimus capitis	Medial to the longissimus cervicis	Transverse processes of T1–T5 and articular processes of vertebrae C4–C7
Spinalis cervicis	Inconstant	Inferior portion of ligamentum nuchae; spine of vertebrae C7, T1, and T2
Spinalis capitis	Usually fused with the medial part of the semispinalis capitis	Transverse processes of vertebrae T5 and T6
Semispinalis capitis	Deep to the splenius capitis	Transverse processes of vertebrae C7–T6 and articular processes of vertebrae C4–C6
Semispinalis cervicis	Deep to the semispinalis capitis	Transverse processes of T1–T6
Multifidus (cervical portion)	On either side of the spinous process of each cervical vertebra	Articular processes of vertebrae C4–C7
Rotatores longus and brevis spinae (cervical portion)	Dorsal aspect of vertebrae	Transverse processes of C3–C7
Interspinales (cervical portion)	Between the spines of cervical vertebrae	Spine of each cervical vertebra, except C2
Intertransversarii anterior (cervical portion)	Between transverse processes of cervical vertebrae, placed anteriorly	Anterior tubercle of transverse process of vertebrae C2–T1
Intertransversarii posterior (cervical portion)	Behind the intertransversarii anterior	Posterior tubercles of transverse processes of vertebra C2–T1

Insertion	Innervation	Action
Lateral ⅓ of the clavicle; acromion, spine, and tubercle of the spine of the scapula	Accessory nerve and ventral primary rami of C3, C4	Most of its action is on the shoulder in suspending, squaring, shrugging, and pulling it in. It is also a rotator of the scapula. Fixing the shoulder, it assists in pulling the head posteriorly and laterally.
Mastoid process of temporal bone and lateral ⅓ of superior nuchal line of occipital bone	Dorsal primary rami of middle cervical nerves	Pulls head back and rotates.
Transverse processes of vertebrae C1–C3	Dorsal primary rami of lower cervical nerves	Pulls head back and rotates.
Transverse processes of vertebrae C4–C6	Dorsal primary rami of lower cervical nerves	Extends and rotates cervical spine.
Transverse processes of vertebrae C2–C6	Dorsal primary rami of cervical nerves	Extends and inclines cervical spine laterally.
Posterior aspect of mastoid process of temporal bone	Dorsal primary rami of cervical nerves	Extends and inclines head laterally.
Spine of vertebrae C2–C4	Dorsal primary rami of cervical nerves	Extends cervical vertebral column.
Lateral to the external occipital crest, between superior and inferior nuchal lines	Dorsal primary rami of cervical nerves	Extends the head.
Occipital bone between superior and inferior nuchal lines	Branches of dorsal primary rami of cervical nerves	Extends head and, acting unilaterally, tilts it to one side.
Spinous processes of vertebrae C2–C5	Branches of dorsal primary rami of upper thoracic nerves	Extends cervical vertebrae and, acting unilaterally, tilts it to one side.
Spine of vertebrae C2–C7	Branches of dorsal primary rami of upper thoracic and cervical nerves	Extends cervical vertebral column, and, acting unilaterally, tilts it to one side.
Base of spinous processes of vertebrae above	Branches of dorsal primary rami of cervical nerves	Pull back spinal column & rotate neck to opposite side.
Spine of cervical vertebrae immediately above except C1	Branches of dorsal primary rami of cervical nerves except C1	Extends the cervical spinal column.
Anterior tubercles of the transverse processes of vertebrae C1–C7	Ventral primary ramus of nerves C2–T1	Tilts the cervical spinal column to one side. Acting in concert with the other side, they fix the cervical spinal column.
Posterior tubercles of transverse processes of vertebrae C1–C7	Ventral primary rami of nerves C2–T1	Tilts the cervical spinal column to one side. Acting in concert with the other side, they fix the cervical spinal column.

TABLE 7.1 (CONTINUED)

Name	Location	Origin
Obliquus capitis superior	Deep to semispinalis capitis	Transverse process of atlas
Obliquus capitis inferior	Deep to semispinalis capitis and inferior to obliquus capitis superior	Spinous process of axis
Rectus capitis posterior major	Medial to the obliquus capitis superior	Spine of the axis
Rectus capitis posterior minor	Medial to the rectus capitis posterior major	Tubercle of the posterior arch of the atlas

The *longissimus cervicis,* located just medial to the iliocostalis cervicis, originates on the transverse processes of vertebrae T1 through T5 and inserts onto the transverse processes of vertebrae C2 through C6. Bilaterally, they draw the cervical vertebrae back and, contracting unilaterally, to one side.

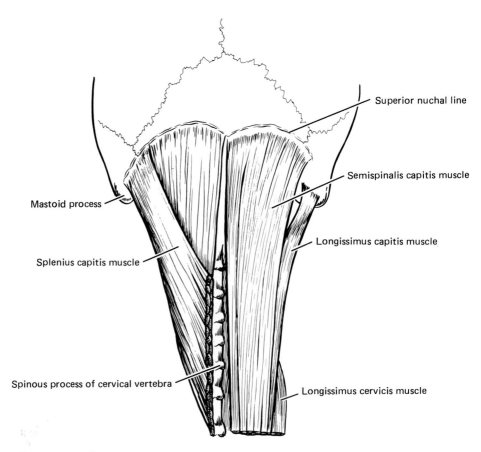

Figure 7.5. Posterior neck.

Insertion	Innervation	Action
Inferior to the superior nuchal line of the occipital bone	Dorsal primary ramus of suboccipital nerve (C1)	Pulls head back and, acting unilaterally, tilts it to one side.
Transverse process of the atlas	Dorsal primary ramus of suboccipital nerve (C1)	Rotates atlanto-axis joint to turn the face laterally.
Below and on the inferior nuchal line of the occipital bone	Dorsal primary ramus of suboccipital nerve (C1)	Draws the head back and turns the face laterally.
Above superior lip of foramen magnum to inferior nuchal line	Dorsal primary ramus of suboccipital nerve (C1)	Pulls head directly posteriorly.

The *longissimus capitis*, located medial to the longissimus cervicis, also originates on the transverse processes of vertebrae T1 through T5, as well as on the articular processes of vertebrae C4 through C7. The fibers of this muscle pass directly craniad to insert onto the posterior aspect of the mastoid process, just deep to the insertion of the sternocleidomastoid. The function of this muscle is to draw the head back, and when acting with its counterpart or unilaterally, to draw the head back and to one side.

Two insignificant muscles represent the medial column of the erector spinae in the neck, the *spinalis cervicis* and *spinalis capitis.* The first is usually not present and the second is fused with the semispinalis capitis. This entire group is innervated by dorsal primary rami of cervical spinal nerves.

Transversospinal Group (Figs. 7.3, 7.5)

The transversospinal group of muscles consists of several muscle groups, the semispinalis, multifidus spinae, rotatores spinae, interspinales, and the intertransversarii. These muscle groups extend along either side of the vertebral column, interconnecting contiguous and/or skipping one or more contiguous vertebrae. The most superficial of these is the semispinalis capitis, which is partly covered by the splenius capitis. The *semispinalis capitis* originates from the transverse processes of vertebrae C7 through T6 and the articular processes of vertebrae C4, C5, and C6, to insert onto the occipital bone between the superior and inferior nuchal lines, just below the attachment of the trapezius muscle. The medial aspect of the semispinalis capitis is usually fused with the spinalis capitis. This muscle serves to pull the head back and, if acting unilaterally, to one side. The *semispinalis cervicis* muscle lies deep to the semispinalis capitis. It originates from the transverse processes of vertebrae T1 through T6 and inserts onto the spinous processes of vertebrae C2 through C5. The muscle functions in extending the cervical vertebrae and, if acting unilaterally, tilts them to one side.

The *multifidus spinae* muscle runs the length of the spinal column, but only its cervical region will be described. It is lodged in the interval located on either side of the spinous process of each vertebra. The fasciculi of this muscle originate, in the cervical region, from the articular processes of vertebrae C4 through C7 and insert on the spines of vertebrae C2 through C7. The function of the multifidus is to extend the vertebral column and, if contracting unilaterally, to tilt it to one side.

The *rotatores spinae* occupy the deepest portion of the interval between the spinous and transverse processes of each vertebra. This muscle group is composed of a series of short and long muscles, the rotatores brevis, which arise from the transverse processes of each vertebra and insert on the spinous process of the vertebra directly craniad. The rotatores longus muscles also arise on the transverse processes of each vertebra and insert on the spinous process of the second vertebra craniad. The superficial fibers of the rotatores spinae quite often are fused to the multifidus. The rotatores spinae in the neck act to pull back the spinal column and rotate the neck to the opposite side.

The cervical portions of the *interspinales* are composed of short, fleshy fibers, extending between the spinous processes of all but the first cervical vertebra. They function in extending the cervical vertebral column.

The *intertransversarii* muscles of the neck region are also short, fleshy fibers located between the transverse processes of contiguous vertebrae from the atlas through T1. The fascicles may be grouped into intertransversarii anteriors and intertransversarii posteriors, depending upon whether they extend between the anterior or posterior tubercles of contiguous transverse processes. The interval between each intertransversarii anterior and posterior is used as a pathway by the ventral primary ramus of the corresponding cervical nerve. These muscles act to tilt the cervical vertebral column laterally.

When the multifidus spinae, rotatores spinae, interspinales, and intertransversarii act in concert, their probable primary role is the stabilization of the vertebral column. This entire group of deep cervical muscles receives its innervation via dorsal primary rami of cervical and upper thoracic spinal nerves.

Suboccipital Muscles (Fig. 7.6)

The suboccipital muscles lie immediately deep to and are completely covered by the splenius capitis muscle. Four muscles are found in this area and they play a very important role, for they bridge the atlanto-axial and atlanto-occipital joints. Three of the four muscles form the boundaries of the *suboccipital triangle*. The four muscles are the laterally positioned obliquus capitis superior and inferior, the medially located rectus capitis posterior major, and the rectus capitis posterior minor. All four muscles receive their nervous supply from branches of the dorsal primary ramus of the *suboccipital* (first cervical) *nerve.*

The *obliquus capitis superior* muscle arises from the transverse process of the atlas and is inserted just below the superior nuchal line of the occipital bone between the insertions of the semispinalis capitis and the rectus capitis posterior major. Its function is to pull the head back and, acting unilaterally, to tilt it laterally.

The *obliquus capitis inferior* muscle runs almost horizontally from its origin on the lamina and the spinous process of the axis to insert, in common with the origin of the obliquus capitis superior, on the transverse process of the atlas. This muscle rotates the atlanto-axial joint to turn the face laterally.

The *rectus capitis posterior major* muscle originates on the spinous process of the axis to insert below and on the inferior nuchal line between the regions of insertion of the obliquus capitis superior and rectus capitis posterior

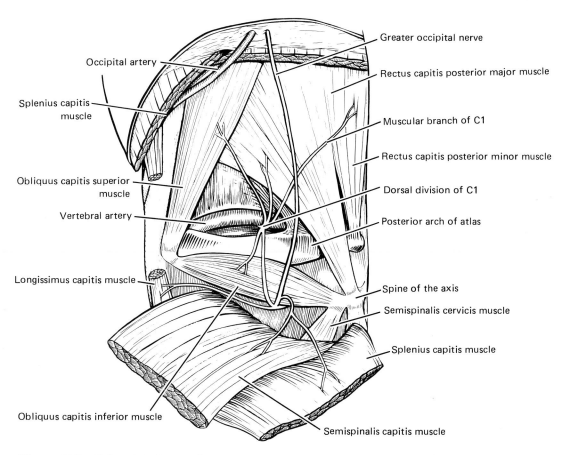

Occipital artery

Splenius capitis muscle

Obliquus capitis superior muscle

Vertebral artery

Longissimus capitis muscle

Obliquus capitis inferior muscle

Greater occipital nerve

Rectus capitis posterior major muscle

Muscular branch of C1

Rectus capitis posterior minor muscle

Dorsal division of C1

Posterior arch of atlas

Spine of the axis

Semispinalis cervicis muscle

Splenius capitis muscle

Semispinalis capitis muscle

Figure 7.6. Suboccipital triangle.

minor. The action of the rectus capitis posterior major is to draw the head back and turn the face laterally.

The *rectus capitis posterior minor* is a shorter muscle, since it takes its origin from the tubercle of the posterior arch of the atlas and inserts medially in the region of insertion of the rectus capitis posterior major just above the superior lip of the foramen magnum. Medially, its insertion is bounded by the external occipital crest, and its superior boundary is the medial one-quarter of the inferior nuchal line and the insertion of the semispinalis capitis. The rectus capitis posterior minor pulls the head directly backwards.

Suboccipital Triangle (Fig. 7.6; Table 7.2)

Three muscles circumscribe the triangular area called the *suboccipital triangle.* The borders of this triangle are, superomedially, the lateral border of the rectus capitis posterior major; superolaterally, the medial border of the obliquus capitis superior; and inferiorly, the superior border of the obliquus capitis inferior. The roof is composed of a dense collagenous but fatty connective tissue, which is covered by the semispinalis capitis muscle. The floor of the triangle is part of the atlanto-occipital membrane and the posterior margin

TABLE 7.2
Boundaries and Contents of the Suboccipital Triangle

Borders	
Inferior	Obliquus capitis inferior muscles
Medial	Rectus capitis posterior major muscle
Lateral	Obliquus capitis superior muscle
Roof	Dense collagenous and fatty connective tissue deep to the semispinalis capitis muscle
Floor	Atlanto-occipital membrane and the posterior arch of the atlas
Contents	Vertebral artery, suboccipital nerve and its branches, and the greater occipital nerve

of the arch of the atlas. The vertebral artery passes on its way to the foramen magnum and the first cervical (suboccipital) nerve enters the triangle at this point. The suboccipital nerve pierces the atlanto-occipital membrane between the posterior arch of the atlas and the vertebral artery to supply the suboccipital muscles.

The dorsal primary ramus of the second cervical nerve emerges between the atlas and the axis, just below the obliquus capitis inferior. It passes between the semispinalis capitis and obliquus capitis inferior muscles, crosses the medial aspect of the suboccipital triangle to pierce the semispinalis and trapezius muscles in order to supply sensation to the back of the scalp. Immediately lateral to the obliquus capitis superior muscle and passing between the splenius capitis and semispinalis capitis muscles, thus skirting the superior apex of the suboccipital triangle, is the occipital artery on its way to the occipital groove of the temporal bone.

TRIANGLES OF THE NECK (Fig. 7.7)

The quadrilateral area between the anterior midline of the neck and the anterior border of the trapezius muscle is subdivided into two triangular areas, the anterior and posterior triangles. This division is accomplished by a thick, strap-like muscle, the sternocleidomastoid, whose oblique path extends from the manubrium of the sternum to the region behind the ear. Inferiorly, the *sternocleidomastoid muscle* has two heads of origin, a lateral and a medial, which demarcate a triangular interval between them. Superior to this origin the fibers of the two heads intermingle, forming a thick, muscular belly. The lateral (clavicular) head springs from musculo-tendinous fibers attached to the medial one-third of the clavicle; it is a flattened, quadrilateral-shaped structure. The medial (sternal) head arises from a conical tendon attached to the anterosuperior border of the manubrium just lateral to the jugular notch. The lateral head passes deep to the medial head, and their fibers merge a few centimeters above their origins. The fleshy belly continues to its wide insertion, becoming tendinous just before reaching the mastoid process of the temporal bone and the lateral one-half of the superior nuchal line of the occipital bone. This insertion, in conjunction with the medialmost point of insertion of the trapezius muscle, forms the superior apex of the posterior triangle. The sterno-cleidomastoid muscle receives motor fibers from the spinal accessory nerve, which pierces the deep surface of its belly. Proprioceptive fibers derived from the second and third cervical spinal nerves also enter the muscle's deep surface.

The sternocleidomastoid acts on the head to approximate the ear of the same side to the shoulder, while acting in concert with its counterpart to assist the deep muscles of the back of the neck in pulling the head back, thus raising the chin.

Muscular and bony structures located in the triangles further subdivide the anterior and posterior triangles into smaller triangular compartments, as is detailed in Table 7.3. The boundaries of the posterior triangle are, posteriorly, the anterior border of the trapezius muscle; anteriorly, the posterior edge of the sternocleidomastoid muscle; and inferiorly, the middle third of the clavicle. A thin, fusiform muscle, the posterior belly of the omohyoid, enters the posterior triangle at its inferoposterior apex. It traverses the lower aspect of this triangle and disappears deep to the sternocleidomastoid, thus subdividing the posterior triangle into an inferior *subclavian* (supraclavicular, omoclavicular) *triangle* and a superior *occipital triangle.*

The limits of the anterior triangle are, anteriorly, an imaginary line along the anterior midline of the neck extending from the inferiormost portion of the symphysis menti of the mandible down to the center of the jugular notch of the manubrium; posteriorly, the anterior edge of the sternocleidomastoid; and superiorly, the inferior border of the mandible.

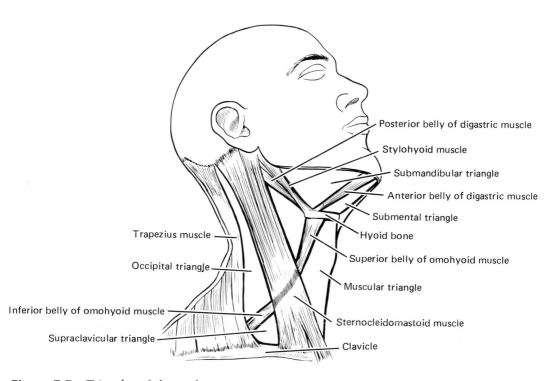

Figure 7.7. Triangles of the neck.

TABLE 7.3
Boundaries of the Cervical Triangles

Name of Triangle	Borders			
	Superior	*Inferior*	*Medial*	*Lateral*
Anterior	Inferior border of the mandible		Anterior midline of the neck from the symphysis menti to the center of jugular notch	Anterior border of the sternocleidomastoid
Submandibular (digastric)	Inferior border of the mandible		Superior border of anterior belly of digastric	Superior border of posterior belly of digastric
Carotid	Inferior border of the posterior belly of the digastric		Superior border of superior belly of omohyoid	Anterior border of sternocleidomastoid
Muscular	Inferior border of superior belly of omohyoid		Anterior midline of the neck from inferior border of body of hyoid to the jugular notch	Anterior border of sternocleidomastoid
Submental		Superior border of body of hyoid bone (between two slings for intermediate tendon of right and left digastrics)		Inferior borders of the anterior bellies of the digastrics
Posterior		Middle one-third of the clavicle	Posterior border of sternocleidomastoid	Anterior border of the trapezius
Subclavian (omoclavicular, supraclavicular)	Inferior border of inferior belly of the omohyoid	Middle one-third of the clavicle	Posterior border of the sternocleidomastoid	
Occipital		Superior border of the inferior belly of the omohyoid	Posterior border of the sternocleidomastoid	Anterior border of the trapezius

The superior belly of the omohyoid muscle enters the anterior triangle and inserts onto the body of the hyoid bone. The posterior belly of the digastric muscle also enters the anterior triangle, at the interval between the angle of the mandible and the mastoid process. It becomes tendinous as it reaches the greater cornu of the hyoid bone (near its junction with the body of the hyoid) and is attached to the hyoid bone by a fascial sling. The muscle, now known as the anterior belly of the digastric muscle, becomes fleshy again and continues to its insertion into the digastric fossa of the mandible. These muscles, in conjunction with the hyoid bone and the inferior border of the mandible, subdivide the anterior triangle into several smaller triangular components. The anterior and posterior bellies of the digastric muscle enclose a space, the *submandibular triangle* (digastric), just below the body of the mandible. The posterior belly of the digastric, superior belly of the omohyoid, and the anterior border of the sternocleidomastoid muscles enclose the *carotid triangle.* The superior belly of the omohyoid, the anterior midline of the neck (and body of the hyoid bone), as well as the anterior border of the sternocleidomastoid circumscribe the *muscular triangle.* Finally, the two anterior bellies of the digastric muscle (one on either side) and the intervening body of the hyoid bone delimit the *submental triangle.* This is the only triangle which encompasses both sides of the neck and is, therefore, unpaired.

Posterior Triangle of the Neck (Figs. 7.2, 7.7, 7.8; Table 7.3)

The boundaries of the posterior triangle are the anterior border of the trapezius, posterior border of the sternocleidomastoid, and the superior border of the middle one-third of the clavicle. The inferior belly of the omohyoid muscle crosses the floor of the posterior triangle, subdividing it into the inferiorly located, small *subclavian* and the superiorly positioned, larger *occipital triangles.* The posterior triangle is covered by skin, the underlying superficial

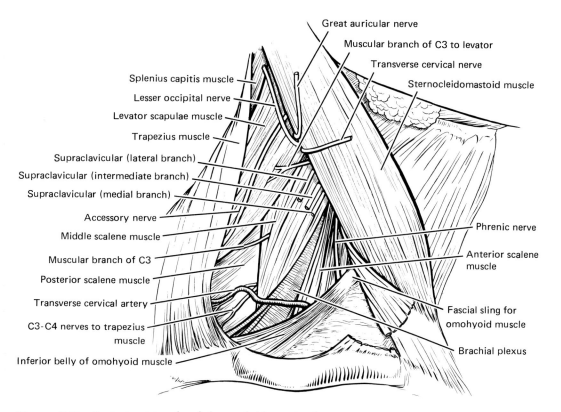

Figure 7.8. Posterior triangle of the neck (deep view).

TABLE 7.4
Muscles Associated With the Posterior Triangle

Name	Location	Origin
Sternocleidomastoid	Bisects the lateral aspect of the neck	Lateral head: medial one-third of clavicle; medial head: manubrium
Platysma	Anterior and posterior triangle of the neck	Epimysium of the deltoid and pectoralis major muscles
Omohyoid	Posterior and anterior triangles of the neck	Superior border of scapula, just medial to the scapular notch
Splenius capitis	Superior apex of posterior triangle	Ligamentum nuchae; spinous processes of vertebrae C7–T4
Levator scapulae	Below floor of posterior triangle	Transverse processes of vertebrae C1–C4
Anterior scalene	Just deep to the clavicular head of the sternocleidomastoid	Transverse processes of vertebrae C3–C6
Middle scalene	Lateral to the anterior scalene	Transverse processes of vertebrae C2–C7
Posterior scalene	Deep and lateral to the middle scalene	Transverse processes of vertebrae C4–C6

fascia, and the platysma muscle. It is roofed over by the investing layer of the deep cervical fascia, superficial to which is the external jugular vein and its tributaries, which were described earlier in this chapter.

The cutaneous nerves, derived from the cervical plexus, appear in the posterior triangle and were described previously along with the superficial veins (Fig. 7.2).

Spinal Accessory Nerve (Figs. 7.2, 7.8)

The spinal accessory nerve has two component fiber groups: the cranial root derived from the brainstem and the spinal root arising from the spinal cord. The two roots unite and later become separated. The cranial root joins the vagus nerve, while the spinal root becomes the distinct peripheral spinal accessory nerve. This nerve then pierces the deep surfaces of the sternocleidomastoid muscle, which it supplies, and emerges in the occipital triangle at the posterior border of that muscle just superior to the appearance of the cutaneous branches of the cervical plexus. The spinal accessory nerve then traverses diagonally across the posterior triangle, passing in the fatty connective tissue between the investing and prevertebral layers of the deep cervical fascia. The spinal accessory nerve has no branches in this triangle but dives deep to the trapezius muscle, where it forms the *subtrapezial plexus* in conjunction with spinal nerves C3 and C4 to innervate that muscle.

Insertion	Innervation	Action
Mastoid process of temporal bone and lateral half of superior nuchal line	Spinal accessory and C2, C3	Unilaterally: approximates ear of the same side to shoulder. In unison with its counterpart: tips head back, raising the chin.
Inferior border of body of mandible; skin and hypodermis of face	Cervical branch of the facial nerve	Assists in depressing mandible, corner of the mouth, and lower lip.
Inferior border of the body of the hyoid bone	Superior ramus of ansa cervicalis (C1, C2) and the ansa itself (C2, C3)	Depresses the hyoid bone.
Mastoid process of temporal; lateral ⅓ of superior nuchal line	Branches of dorsal primary rami of middle cervical spinal nerves	Pulls head back; acting unilaterally, it rotates the head.
Medial border of spine of scapula, from superior angle to spine	C3–C5	Elevates scapula; if the scapula is fixed, it tilts head backwards.
Ridge and the scalene tubercle of the first rib	Ventral primary rami of spinal nerves C4–C6	Function in respiration by lifting the thoracic cage. If thoracic cage is fixed, they flex cervical vertebral column to one side or bend it anteriorly when acting in concert.
First rib, between tubercle and groove for subclavian artery	Ventral primary rami of spinal nerves C3–C8	
Outer surface of second rib	Ventral primary rami of spinal nerves C5–C7	

Muscles Associated with the Posterior Triangle (Table 7.4)

The muscles directly associated with the posterior triangle are the trapezius, sternocleidomastoid, and inferior belly of the omohyoid. In addition, the fascial carpet forming the floor of the posterior triangle lies on a series of muscles which are associated with the triangle though not located in it. These prevertebral muscles are the splenius capitis, levator scapulae, and the posterior, middle, and anterior scalenes (Fig. 7.8). The trapezius, sternocleidomastoid, and splenius capitis muscles located in the posterior triangle were described earlier.

Omohyoid. The omohyoid muscle is thin and consists of two bellies, *inferior* and *superior*, connected to each other by an intermediate tendon. The inferior belly originates on the superior border of the scapula, just medial to the scapular notch, and passes ácross the inferior aspect of the posterior cervical triangle, where it is enveloped by the investing layer of the deep cervical fascia. This fascia forms a fascial sling which fixes the intermediate tendon to the clavicle and the first rib. The superior belly of the muscle passes obliquely, deep to the sternocleidomastoid, to emerge in the anterior triangle. It inserts onto the inferior border of the body of the hyoid bone. Branches of the ansa cervicalis (C1, C2, C3) supply the two bellies of this muscle. The omohyoid acts to depress the hyoid bone, thus countering the actions of the suprahyoid muscles.

Levator Scapulae. The levator scapulae is not properly considered a muscle of the neck. It serves as one of the muscles attaching the superior extremity to the trunk, but its location requires at least a cursory description. It arises from the transverse processes of the first four cervical vertebrae from where it proceeds as one or more fleshy fascicles along the side of the neck to insert into the medial border of the scapula. It receives its innervation from spinal nerves C3 and C4 directly and from C5 indirectly. The levator scapulae acts to elevate the scapula, and when the scapula is fixed, its contraction tilts the head backwards.

Scalenes. The *anterior scalene* is covered, to a great extent, by the clavicular head of the sternocleidomastoid muscle. The anterior scalene originates from the transverse processes of the third through sixth cervical vertebrae. The fibers pass inferolaterally to form a fleshy belly, which inserts as a flat, tendinous sheath on the scalene tubercle of the first rib and on its ridge, just anterior to the groove for the subclavian artery. The nerve supply comes via branches from ventral primary rami of spinal nerves C4, C5, and C6. The muscle functions in respiration by initially lifting the first rib. If the thoracic cage is fixed, the muscle then flexes the cervical vertebral column to one side. Acting in concert with its counterpart on the other side, the anterior scalene bends the cervical spinal column anteriorly, provided the thoracic cage is immobilized.

Several important anatomical landmarks are associated with the anterior scalene muscle. The subclavian artery is described conveniently in three segments as it curves around the deep aspect of this muscle on its path to the axilla. Likewise, the trunks of the brachial plexus traverse the interval between the anterior and middle scalene muscles in passing to the axilla. Additionally, the phrenic nerve lies directly on the anterior scalene muscle, deep to its blanket of prevertebral fascia.

The *middle scalene* is longer than the anterior and originates from the transverse processes of vertebrae C2 through C7. The fibers become tendinous as the muscle inserts on the first rib between the tubercle and the groove for the subclavian artery. The middle scalene receives its nerve supply from branches of ventral primary rami of the spinal nerves C3 through C8. Its action is the same as that of the anterior scalene (primarily related to respiration).

The *posterior scalene* is the smallest of the three scalene muscles, and it is usually intimately related to the deep and lateral aspect of the middle scalene. The fibers of the two muscles are frequently intermingled so that complete separation cannot be effected. The posterior scalene originates on the transverse processes of the fourth, fifth, and sixth cervical vertebrae and inserts via a slender, narrow tendon on the external aspect of the second rib. Ventral primary rami of spinal nerves C5 through C7 innervate the muscle, whose action is the same as those of the other two scalenes.

Brachial Plexus (Figs. 7.3, 7.8)

The ventral primary rami of some spinal nerves appear not to retain their metameric (segmental) identities. Instead, they unite shortly after their origins to form bundles of nerve fibers which become intermixed forming plexuses for redistribution. In this form, the resultant fibers can reach their intended fields whose original locations became altered. The *brachial plexus* is one such intermixing of ventral primary rami of spinal nerves C4 through T1 (and occasionally T2). Although the plexus is primarily responsible for innervation of the upper limb and associated structures, it also supplies some muscles of the neck. A thorough discussion of this important plexus is found in any general textbook of anatomy.

Cervical Plexus (Table 7.5; Fig. 7.9)
Ventral primary rami of the first four cervical spinal nerves participate in the formation of the cervical plexus. The ventral primary rami of all but the first cervical spinal nerve bifurcate into ascending and descending branches. These branches then join each other and become united, forming simple loops that lie deep to the prevertebral fascia. Branches arising from the cervical plexus are arranged in a superficial and deep division.

The superficial division is completely sensory and consists of ascending and descending branches. The lesser occipital (C2), great auricular (C2, C3), and transverse cervical (C2, C3) compose the ascending branch, while the supraclaviculars (C3, C4) comprise the descending branches.

The deep division of the cervical plexus is mostly motor, though it does contain sensory components. This division supplies the muscle masses deep to the floor of the posterior triangle, as well as proprioceptive fibers to the sternocleidomastoid and trapezius muscles. Further, the division supplies the anterior vertebral muscles. A summary of the specific innervations may be found in Table 7.5. Two additional important components of this division must be given special consideration. These are the ansa cervicalis and the phrenic nerve.

The *ansa cervicalis* (Figs. 7.9, 7.13) and its two roots are derived from C1, C2 (superior root), sometimes incorrectly referred to as the descending hypo-

TABLE 7.5
Branches of the Cervical Plexus

	Name	Origin	Function
Superficial branches			
Ascending	Lesser occipital	C2	Sensory
	Great auricular	C2,C3	Sensory
	Transverse cervical	C2,C3	Sensory
Descending	Supraclaviculars	C3,C4	Sensory
Deep branches			
Medial	Superior root of ansa cervicalis	C1,C2	Motor
	Branch to rectus capitis lateralis	C1	Motor
	Branch to rectus capitis anterior	C1,C2	Motor
	Branch to longus capitis	C1,C2,C3	Motor
	Branch to longus colli	C1,C2,C3,C4	Motor
	Inferior root of ansa cervicalis	C2,C3	Motor
	Phrenic	C3,C4,C5	Motor and some sensory
Lateral	Branch to trapezius	C3,C4	Proprioception (?)
	Branch to sternocleidomastoid	C2,C3	Proprioception (?)
	Branch to levator scapulae	C3,C4	Motor
	Branch to scalenus medius	C3,C4	Motor

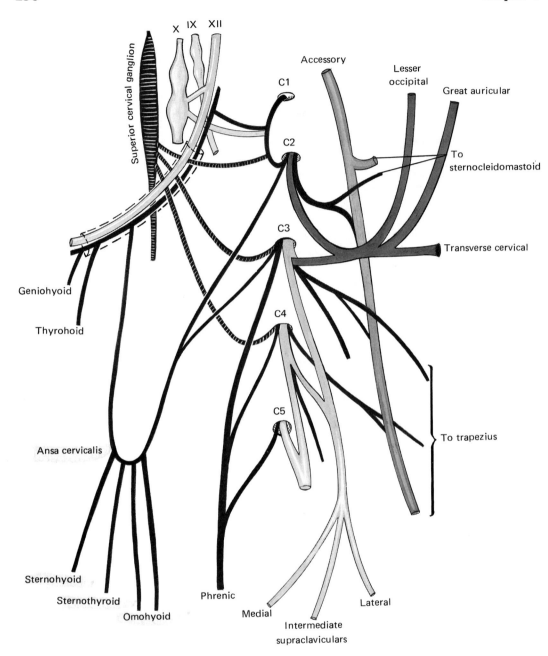

Figure 7.9. Cervical plexus. Note that the cervical sympathetic trunk, vagus nerve, and glossopharyngeal nerve have been cut. The dashed line indicates a segment of the epineurium of the hypoglossal nerve.

glossal, and C2, C3 (inferior root). The superior root of the ansa cervicalis travels for a short distance with the hypoglossal nerve (cranial nerve XII) but does not become a functional part of that nerve. It joins and travels with the hypoglossal nerve opposite the atlas and descends from that nerve as it passes superficial to the external carotid artery. As the superior root leaves the hypoglossal nerve, two filaments (both derived from C1) continue with the hypoglossal nerve for a few millimeters, then branch to supply motor innervation to the thyrohyoid and geniohyoid muscles. The superior root, on the other hand, travels superficial to, embedded within, or just inside the carotid sheath. At the level just below the middle of the neck, it turns posteriorly to form the ansa (loop) in joining with the inferior root which has descended in the neck alongside the carotid sheath. Four branches arise from the ansa cervicalis to supply motor innervation to the sternohyoid, sternothyroid, and both bellies of the omohyoid muscles.

The *phrenic nerve* (C3, C4, C5), the only motor nerve of the diaphragm, also carries sensory fibers (Figs. 7.8, 7.9, 7.13). The nerve passes deep to the prevertebral fascia as it lies on the anterior surface of the anterior scalene muscle. On its way to distribute to the diaphragm, it passes between the subclavian artery and vein and then enters the thorax, where it lies anterior to the root of the lung on the fibrous pericardium. The sensory fibers carried by the phrenic nerve serve the mediastinal pleura and the pericardium of the heart.

The accessory phrenic nerve (C5) is occasionally present. It descends into the thorax lateral to the phrenic nerve and posterior to the subclavian vein to join the phrenic nerve below the first rib. It supplies motor fibers to the diaphragm.

Subclavian Arteries (Fig. 7.10)

The subclavian artery is a short vessel extending as far laterally as the outer border of the first rib. The origins of the right and left subclavian arteries differ in that the left one arises directly from the arch of the aorta, while the right one is one of the terminal branches of the brachiocephalic trunk.

The right subclavian artery originates deep to the sternoclavicular joint, and the left one originates behind the common carotid artery around the third or fourth thoracic vertebra. Both right and left arteries travel superiorly to the root of the neck and posterior to the anterior scalene muscle, emerging into the posterior triangle through the interval between the anterior and middle scalene muscles on their way to the lateral border of the first rib, where each artery becomes known as the axillary artery. This passage, deep to the anterior scalene muscle, permits a convenient division of the subclavian artery into three parts. The first part is from the origin of the vessel to the medial border of the anterior scalene muscle; the second part lies deep to this muscle; while the third part extends from the lateral border of the anterior scalene to the lateral border of the first rib. The branches of the subclavian artery are the vertebral artery, internal thoracic artery, and the thyrocervical trunk from the first part, the costocervical trunk from the second part, and the dorsal scapular artery from the third part.

Vertebral Artery. The vertebral artery takes its origin from the posterosuperior aspect of the first part of the subclavian artery. It ascends behind the anterior scalene muscle, along the transverse process of the seventh cervical vertebra, and enters the foramen transversarium of the sixth cervical vertebra. The artery travels through the foramina transversaria of the upper six cervical vertebrae, enters the suboccipital triangle, from where it traverses the foramen magnum to unite with its contralateral vessel to participate in the formation of the basilar artery. Branches arise from the vertebral artery to supply the spinal

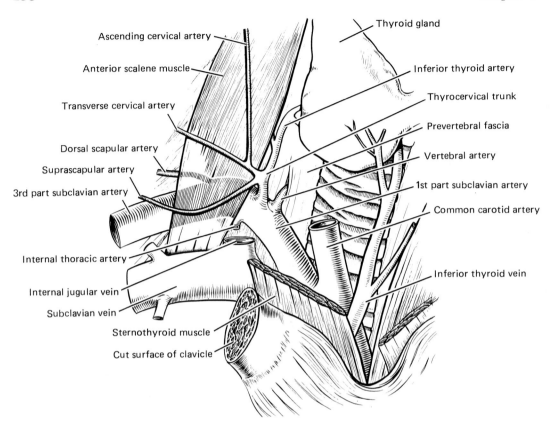

Figure 7.10. Root of the neck. The anterior scalene muscle is made transparent so that the second part of the subclavian artery may be observed deep to it.

cord and deep muscles in the vicinity of the suboccipital triangle. The cranial branches of the vertebral artery will be detailed in the description of the brain and spinal cord.

Internal Thoracic Artery. The internal thoracic artery originates from the inferior aspect of the first part of the subclavian artery. This artery passes directly inferiorly on the internal anterior thoracic wall just lateral to the margin of the sternum to the sixth or seventh rib, where it bifurcates to form the medially-placed superior epigastric and laterally-positioned musculophrenic arteries. Since the internal thoracic artery is a vessel whose distribution is limited to the thorax and abdomen, its branches will not be discussed.

Thyrocervical Trunk. The thyrocervical trunk is a short vessel arising from the superior aspect of the first part of the subclavian artery. Its origin is opposite the point of origin of the internal thoracic artery. This trunk lies just medial to the anterior scalene muscle, where it trifurcates to form three major branches, the suprascapular, transverse cervical, and inferior thyroid arteries. The *suprascapular artery* travels obliquely across the anterior surface of the anterior scalene muscle and deep to the sternocleidomastoid, which it supplies. It passes deep to the inferior belly of the omohyoid to reach the scapular notch. Occasionally, the suprascapular artery is a branch of the third part of the subclavian artery. The *transverse cervical artery* crosses the neck in a fashion similar to, but above, the suprascapular artery. It crosses the floor of the sub-clavian triangle to travel in company with the spinal accessory nerve, to bur-row under the anterior border of the trapezius, supplying it and other muscles in the vicinity. The *inferior thyroid artery* travels superiorly in front of the medial border of the anterior scalene muscle. It then passes deep to the carotid sheath and approaches the inferior aspect of the thyroid gland, which it sup-plies. The inferior thyroid artery has several small branches, including the terminal ascending and descending branches ending in the body of the thyroid gland, as well as muscular branches and the *ascending cervical artery* supply-ing anterior vertebral muscles of the neck.

Costocervical Trunk. The *costocervical* trunk has different origins on the two sides of the body. On the left, it springs from the posterior aspect of the first part of the subclavian artery, while on the right it springs from the posterior aspect of the second part of that artery. This trunk has two terminal branches: the *superior intercostal* and the *deep cervical artery.* The former serves the first and second intercostal spaces, while the deep cervical artery is interposed between the first rib and the transverse process of the seventh cervical verte-bra. The trunk passes between the semispinalis cervicis and semispinalis capitis, supplying these as well as adjacent muscles, finally anastomosing with the occipital and vertebral arteries.

Dorsal Scapular Artery. The dorsal scapular artery is the only branch arising from the third part of the subclavian artery, though quite frequently it is a branch of the second part. The dorsal scapular artery passes among the trunks of the brachial plexus, anterior to the middle scalene muscle, to reach the superior angle of the scapula, where it supplies the muscles in the vicinity.

Subclavian Vein (Fig. 7.10)

The subclavian vein is quite short, since it is the continuation of the axillary vein, and it joins the internal jugular vein to form the large brachiocephalic vein. Thus, the subclavian vein extends from the external border of the first rib to the junction with the internal jugular vein, passing anterior to the anterior scalene muscle which separates it from the subclavian artery. Here it lies in front of the *subclavius muscle,* which originates on the first rib and inserts on the inferior surface of the clavicle. This muscle, innervated by a branch from the brachial plexus complex, acts as a cushion, protecting the underlying ves-sels and nerves.

The main tributary of the subclavian vein is the external jugular vein, though frequently the subclavian may receive the dorsal scapular and anterior jugular veins. The left subclavian vein receives lymph from most of the body via the *thoracic duct,* while lymph from the rest of the body is delivered to the right subclavian vein by the *right lymphatic duct.* These ducts pierce the supe-rior aspects of the subclavian veins, just before these are joined by the internal jugular veins.

Anterior Triangle (Fig. 7.7)

The anterior triangle of the neck is defined by the midline of the neck from the mental symphysis to the jugular notch of the manubrium, the anterior border of the sternocleidomastoid muscle, and the lower border of the mandible. The

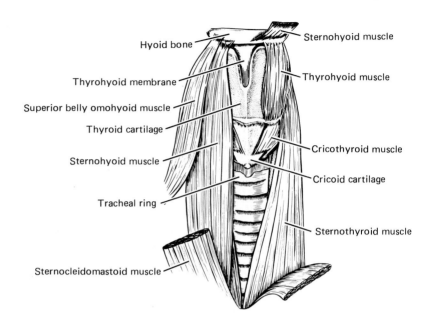

Figure 7.11. Infrahyoid muscles. The thyroid gland has been removed.

subdivisions of the anterior triangle are the submandibular, carotid, muscular, and submental triangles, whose borders have been detailed earlier.

Infrahyoid Muscles (Fig. 7.11)

Four pairs of strap-like muscles represent the infrahyoid muscle group. These are the sternohyoid, sternothyroid, thyrohyoid, and omohyoid. These muscles act as a group to fix and/or depress the hyoid bone during mastication, deglutition, and speech (Table 7.6). The *sternohyoid* is a long, thin muscle originating from the posterior aspect of the sternoclavicular joint region. It ascends to insert onto the inferior border of the the body of the hyoid bone just medial to the insertion of the omohyoid muscle. The *sternothyroid* muscle is wider and shorter than the sternohyoid under which it lies. It originates on the manubrium of the sternum and inserts on the oblique line of the thyroid cartilage.

all muscles accept thyrohyoid is supplied by ansa cervicalis

Strap muscles

TABLE 7.6
The Infrahyoid Muscles

Name	Location	Origin
Sternohyoid	Anterolateral aspect of neck	Posterior aspect of the sternoclavicular joint area
Sternothyroid	Deep to sternohyoid	Manubrium
Thyrohyoid	Deep to sternohyoid	Oblique line of thyroid cartilage
Omohyoid	Posterior and anterior triangles of the neck	Superior border of scapula just medial to scapular notch

The sternothyroid muscle also acts to depress the larynx and/or fix it in position. The *thyrohyoid* muscle lies deep to the sternohyoid. This muscle originates on the oblique line of the lamina of the thyroid cartilage and inserts on the inferior border of the greater cornu and body of the hyoid bone. The thyrohyoid muscle also raises the thyroid cartilage. The *omohyoid* muscle has been treated in this chapter's section on the posterior triangle.

The infrahyoid muscle group receives its nerve supply from the ansa cervicalis (C1, C2, C3), the only exception being the thyrohyoid. This muscle receives fibers from C1 which joins the hypoglossal nerve shortly after exiting its intervertebral foramen. The fibers to the thyrohyoid leave the hypoglossal nerve to innervate this muscle.

Carotid Arteries (Fig. 7.12)

The major blood supply of the head and neck is derived from branches originating from the *common carotid artery*. This vessel is enclosed by the carotid sheath, which is incompletely subdivided into compartments housing the common and internal carotid arteries, the internal jugular vein, and the vagus nerve. The common carotid arteries of the two sides have different origins: the right is a branch of the brachiocephalic trunk, while the left branches directly from the arch of the aorta. Consequently, the right common carotid is contained wholly within the neck, while the left common carotid begins in the upper thorax and enters the neck in the vicinity of the sternoclavicular joint. The right and left common carotids usually bifurcate approximately at the level of the thyroid cartilage (though this is quite variable) into an *external* and an *internal carotid artery*. These are considered "terminal branches," hence the common carotid is said to have no branches in the neck. The common carotid artery is somewhat dilated at its bifurcation, which is known as the *carotid sinus*. This sinus is a modified region of the vessel, richly innervated by branches of the glossopharyngeal nerve which serve to monitor blood pressure. An additional structure, the *carotid body*, is also associated with this region of bifurcation. This small, oval, reddish brown structure lying within the internal carotid artery is innervated by the vagus and glossopharyngeal nerves. The carotid body functions as a chemoreceptor monitoring oxygen tension within the internal carotid artery.

The internal carotid artery has no branches in the neck; instead, it passes through the carotid canal of the temporal bone to enter the cranial cavity. The branches of the internal carotid artery are treated in subsequent chapters.

Insertion	Innervation	Action
Inferior border of hyoid bone	Ansa cervicalis	Depresses and fixes hyoid bone.
Oblique line of thyroid cartilage	Ansa cervicalis	Depresses larynx.
Greater cornu and body of hyoid bone	C1, via the hypoglossal nerve	Depresses and fixes hyoid bone.
Inferior border of body of hyoid bone	Ansa cervicalis	Depresses and fixes hyoid bone.

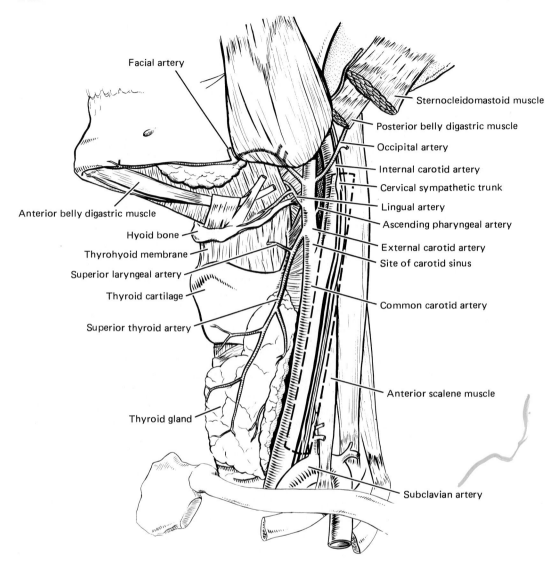

Figure 7.12. Carotid artery in the neck. The dashed outline indicates the relative position of the internal jugular vein.

External Carotid Artery. The external carotid artery has six collateral and two terminal branches.

Branches of the External Carotid Artery

Collateral	**Terminal**
Superior thyroid	Superficial temporal
Ascending pharyngeal	Maxillary
Lingual	
Facial	
Occipital	
Posterior auricular	

Branches of the external carotid artery that supply regions of the neck are treated in this section. However, branches concerned with the superficial and deep face will be discussed in the appropriate chapters.

SUPERIOR THYROID ARTERY. The superior thyroid artery is the first branch of the external carotid artery, arising from its ventral aspect just superior to the bifurcation of the common carotid artery. The superior thyroid artery descends in the neck, accompanied by the same-named vein and the external laryngeal nerve, reaches the superior pole of the thyroid gland, and divides into its terminal branches, some of which anastomose with their counterparts of the other side and with branches of the inferior thyroid artery. The superior thyroid artery has four named branches—the infrahyoid, sternocleidomastoid, superior laryngeal, and cricothyroid arteries—as well as its terminal anterior, posterior, and occasionally lateral branches at the thyroid gland. The *infrahyoid artery* is a small vessel that passes deep to the thyrohyoid muscle, caudal to the body of the hyoid bone, and serves this general area. The *sternocleidomastoid branch* passes ventral to the carotid sheath and supplies the muscle of the same name on its deep surface. To distribute to the larynx, the *superior laryngeal artery* passes superficial to the inferior constrictor muscle and pierces the thyrohyoid membrane accompanied by the internal laryngeal nerve. The *cricothyroid branch* is a small vessel that courses along the cricothyroid ligament supplying the muscle and the vicinity. The terminal branches of the superior thyroid artery are discussed later in this chapter in relation to the thyroid gland.

ASCENDING PHARYNGEAL ARTERY. The ascending pharyngeal artery is the smallest branch of the external carotid artery. It arises on the medial aspect of that artery, shortly after the bifurcation of the common carotid, and ascends between the internal carotid and the pharynx. The ascending pharyngeal artery has unnamed muscular branches to the prevertebral muscles, as well as branches supplying structures in its vicinity. This artery has three named branches: the *pharyngeal*, distributing to some muscles of the pharynx and soft palate; the *meningeal*, entering the cranium via several foramina to vascularize the meninges and bone; and the *inferior tympanic*, supplying the tympanic cavity.

LINGUAL ARTERY. The lingual artery often arises in common with the facial artery becoming then the faciolingual artery. The lingual artery arises near the posterior tip of the greater cornu of the hyoid bone, passes deep to the hypoglossal nerve, then between the middle constrictor and hyoglossus muscles to supply the muscles of the tongue, tonsil, soft palate, epiglottis, floor of the mouth, and sublingual gland. The branches of this artery are described in a later chapter.

FACIAL ARTERY. The facial artery arises just above (or in common with) the lingual artery and ascends deep to the stylohyoid and posterior belly of the digastric muscles to lie in a groove on the posterior aspect of the submandibular gland. The vessel enters the face by crossing the base of the mandible just anterior to the masseter muscle in the groove for the facial artery. Branches of the facial artery in the neck are the ascending palatine, tonsillar, glandular, and submental arteries. Those of the face will be discussed in a later chapter.

The *ascending palatine artery* originates near the tip of the styloid process. It ascends between that process and the superior constrictor muscle, then between the styloglossus and stylopharyngeus muscles, to supply the levator veli palatini, superior constrictor and neighboring muscles, the soft palate, tonsils, and auditory tube. *Glandular branches* distribute as three or four vessels to the submandibular gland to supply it and the adjacent area. The *tonsillar artery* passes between the styloglossus and medial pterygoid muscles and pierces the superior constrictor to supply the palatine tonsil and the posterior tongue. The *submental artery* arises from the facial artery near the anterior border of the masseter. It follows the base of the mandible anteriorly and turns onto the chin at the anterior border of the depressor anguli oris muscle. The artery supplies muscles it encounters along its passage and anastomoses with several arteries in its vicinity.

OCCIPITAL ARTERY. The occipital artery originates on the posterior aspect of the external carotid artery, just opposite the origin of the facial artery. It passes deep to the hypoglossal nerve and posterior belly of the digastric muscle, lodges in the groove for the occipital artery on the medial aspect of the mastoid process, and passes between the splenius capitis and semispinalis capitis muscles to serve the back of the head. Branches of the occipital artery are the sternocleidomastoid, mastoid, auricular, muscular, descending, meningeal, and occipital.

The *sternocleidomastoid* branches supply the same-named muscle as two vessels, an upper and a lower branch. The *mastoid branch* is a small vessel which traverses the mastoid foramen to supply the mastoid air cells and the dura mater in its vicinity. The *auricular branch* vascularizes the back of the auricle. *Muscular branches* of the occipital artery distribute to the digastric, stylohyoid, and splenius capitis muscles. The *descending branch* serves the muscles of the back of the neck. *Meningeal branches* gain entrance to the cranial vault via the condylar and jugular foramina and vascularize the dura and the bones of the posterior cranial fossa. *Occipital branches* of the occipital artery distribute in the company of the greater occipital nerve to serve the muscles and tissues of the scalp. Small branches may pass through the parietal foramen to supply the parietal meninges.

POSTERIOR AURICULAR ARTERY. The posterior auricular artery is a small branch arising deep to the parotid gland, where it passes between the mastoid process and the cartilaginous external auditory tube. It vascularizes the parotid gland as well as the sternocleidomastoid, stylohyoid, and digastric muscles. In addition, the posterior auricular artery has three named branches—the stylomastoid, auricular, and occipital arteries—which are discussed in subsequent chapters.

MAXILLARY AND SUPERFICIAL TEMPORAL ARTERIES. The maxillary and superficial temporal arteries are the two terminal branches of the external carotid artery. The former and its branches are responsible for the vascularization of the deep face, while the latter serves the region of the temple and much of the scalp. These two arteries are discussed in later chapters.

Internal Jugular Vein (Figs. 7.10, 7.12)

The internal jugular vein is the main vessel responsible for collecting blood from the brain, superficial aspects of the face, and the neck. The vessel extends from its dilated origin, the superior bulb housed in the jugular foramen, to its inferior dilation, the inferior bulb terminating in the brachiocephalic vein. The vessel is enclosed in the carotid sheath as it travels the length of the neck, and its tributaries pierce this fascia to deliver their blood to the vessel. The internal jugular vein receives blood from the following tributaries: dural venous sinus drainage from within the cranium; the facial vein from the superficial face; the lingual vein from the tongue and floor of the mouth; pharyngeal, superior and middle thyroid, and occasionally the occipital veins from the neck. The pharyngeal and occipital tributaries are treated presently, while the remaining vessels are discussed in later chapters.

The *pharyngeal veins* arise as small vessels from a plexus of veins, the *pharyngeal plexus,* located on the wall of the pharynx. They empty into the internal jugular vein in the vicinity of the hyoid bone. The *occipital vein* arises from the venous network serving the scalp, perforates the fibers of insertion of the trapezius, and enters the suboccipital triangle. Here it empties its contents into a plexus of veins, tributaries of the vertebral and deep cervical veins. Occasionally, the occipital vein, accompanying the same-named artery, travels along the posterior base of the skull to empty into the internal jugular vein or, less frequently, into the posterior auricular vein.

Thyroid Gland (Figs. 7.10, 7.12)

The thyroid gland is an endocrine organ lying deep to the infrahyoid muscles, situated anteriorly, partly encircling the superior aspect of the trachea, the cricoid cartilage, and the thyroid cartilage. It is composed of two lobes, laterally positioned, and a centrally placed isthmus connecting the right and left lobes. Frequently, a pyramidal lobe is present which extends from the left lobe near its junction with the isthmus occasionally as far up as the body of the hyoid bone. Infrequently, a fibromuscular connection exists between the isthmus of the thyroid gland and the body of the hyoid bone. This is known as the *levator thyroideae.* A similar, nonmuscular structure, the remnant of the *thyroglossal duct,* may appear in this location. As previously noted, this duct may bear accessory thyroid tissue. The gland has its own connective tissue capsule which subdivides the lobes into numerous lobules. In addition, the gland is loosely ensheathed by laminae of the pretracheal layer of the deep cervical fascia. This connective tissue layer is pierced by blood vessels, which then ramify on the external surface of the connective tissue capsule of the gland. They subsequently enter the substance of the gland within the connective tissue septa which subdivides the gland into smaller components. These smaller components are composed of numerous colloid-filled follicles lined by cuboidal cells. The colloid is composed of iodothyroglobulins, which stimulate the rate of cellular oxidation. Additionally, small clumps of parafollicular cells (C cells) have been noted in the thyroid gland. These cells are believed to be responsible for the formation of thyrocalcitonin, a substance that assists in controlling blood calcium levels.

The blood supply of the thyroid gland is exceedingly rich and is derived from the external carotids, the subclavians, and occasionally, the single thyroidea ima artery from the brachiocephalic trunk or from the aortic arch.

Superior Thyroid Artery (Fig. 7.12). The superior thyroid artery is usually the first branch of the external carotid. It passes inferiorly along the lateral edge of the thyrohyoid muscle, gives off branches as detailed earlier in this chapter, and reaches the superior pole of the lateral lobe of the thyroid gland, where it divides. The *anterior branch* follows the superior border of the lateral lobe, distributes to its anterior surface, and anastomoses with the anterior branch of the opposite side across the isthmus. The *posterior branch* follows a similar course on the deep aspect of the lateral lobe, ramifies on that surface, and anastomoses with the inferior thyroid artery, also supplying the parathyroid gland. Occasionally, a lateral branch is present which supplies the lateral aspect of the lateral lobe.

Inferior Thyroid Artery (Fig. 7.10). Branches of the inferior thyroid artery were discussed earlier in the section dealing with the *subclavian artery*. In this section, only its glandular branches are detailed. As this artery reaches the thyroid gland and forms numerous branches vascularizing the gland, the recurrent laryngeal branch of the vagus nerve passes between these branches. The inferior thyroid artery has two main glandular branches; the *inferior* (supplying the inferoposterior aspect of the gland) which anastomoses with the posterior branch of the superior thyroid artery, and the *ascending branch,* which vascularizes the parathyroid glands. The thyroidea ima artery is a small, inconsistent vessel arising either from the brachiocephalic trunk or from the arch of the aorta. It supplies the isthmus of the thyroid.

Venous Drainage. The *superior thyroid vein* is a tributary of the internal jugular vein. Its distribution follows that of the superior thyroid artery, hence it drains the area supplied by that vessel.

The *middle* and *inferior thyroid veins* and, to a certain extent, the superior thyroid veins drain the venous plexus formed on the surface of the thyroid gland. The middle thyroid veins deliver their blood to the internal jugular vein, while the inferior thyroid veins drain into the brachiocephalic veins. Occasionally, the right and left inferior thyroid veins form a single vessel just caudal to the isthmus of the thyroid gland. This is the thyroidea ima vein which joins the left brachiocephalic vein.

Parathyroid Glands
The parathyroid glands are small, oval endocrine glands that lie on the posterior aspect of the lateral lobes of the thyroid gland. Usually, there are two or more on either lobe of the thyroid, the *superior* and *inferior parathyroids.* They are vascularized by branches of the superior and/or inferior thyroid arteries and drained by the middle and inferior thyroid veins. The glands have two major types of cell populations: the principal or chief cells and the oxyphil cells. The former produce parathormone, a substance controlling calcium and phosphorus metabolism. Complete removal of the parathyroids is incompatible with life, since all muscles undergo tetany and death results.

Vagus Nerve (Fig. 7.13)
The vagus or cranial nerve X is the longest cranial nerve in the body, eventually finding its way into the abdominal cavity. It receives detailed treatment in a subsequent chapter, therefore only its cervical branches are treated here. The

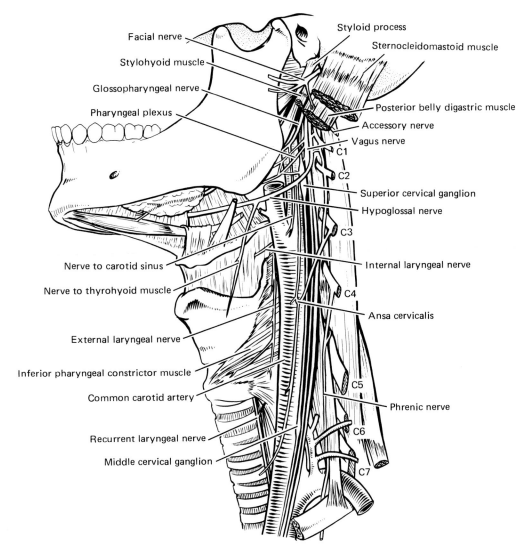

Figure 7.13. Nerve supply to the neck.

nerve enters the neck as it leaves the jugular foramen. Shortly inferior to this foramen, the nerve displays a ganglion, the *nodose* or *inferior ganglion.* The vagus communicates with several other nerves through this ganglion. Branches of the vagus which arise here are *pharyngeal branches,* serving the carotid body, pharynx, and some of the soft palate through the pharyngeal plexus, and the *superior laryngeal nerve,* which bifurcates to form the internal and external laryngeal branches which accompany the medial aspect of the internal carotid artery. The *internal branch* pierces the thyrohyoid membrane in close association with the superior laryngeal branch of the superior thyroid artery to supply the mucous membrane. The *external laryngeal branch* continues inferiorly, accompanied by the superior thyroid artery. It pierces the inferior pharyngeal constrictor muscle, which it supplies in addition to the cricothyroid muscle, and gives branches to the pharyngeal plexus.

Two or three cardiac branches of the vagus are evident in the neck. These are slender filaments which pass deep to the carotid sheath to ramify in the cardiac plexus.

The *recurrent laryngeal branches* of the vagus differ in their recurring locations on the two sides of the body. On the left side, the nerve originates from the vagus at the aortic arch, makes a hairpin loop around the ligamentum arteriosum and ascends into the neck in the tracheoesophageal groove. It comes in close contact with the medial aspect of the lateral lobe of the thyroid gland, passes deep to the inferior constrictor, and gains entrance into the larynx to which it provides sensory and motor innervation. On the right side of the body, the recurrent laryngeal nerve originates from the vagus at the level of the first part of the subclavian artery, around which it recurs, and ascends in the tracheoesophageal groove. Subsequent to this point, the paths taken by the nerves of the two sides are identical. Due to the precarious location of the nerve and intimate association with the thyroid gland, surgical procedures involving that gland must include its isolation and strict protection.

Cervical Sympathetic Trunk (Figs. 7.9, 7.13)

The cervical sympathetic trunk is the cervical continuation of the thoracic sympathetic trunk. It consists of three ganglia connected to each other by short cords. The superiormost of these is the *superior cervical ganglion,* located at the level of the axis and third cervical vertebra. The *middle cervical ganglion,* the smallest of the three, is inconstant and lies at the level of the sixth cervical vertebra. The *inferior cervical ganglion,* located at the level of the seventh cervical vertebra, is often fused with the first (and infrequently with the second and even third) thoracic ganglion, then named the *stellate ganglion.* The cord intervening between the middle and inferior cervical ganglia splits, forming a loop around the subclavian and occasionally the vertebral arteries. The loop around the subclavian artery is constant and is known as the *ansa subclavia.* The cervical sympathetic trunk is embedded in a loose connective tissue layer and positioned between the covering of the prevertebral muscles and the carotid sheath, though often it is located within the deep substance of this structure.

The cervical sympathetic trunk receives no white rami communicantes but does send out gray rami communicantes to each cervical spinal nerve. Preganglionic fibers reach the cervical sympathetic trunk from its thoracic continuation, and these fibers synapse in one of these three cervical sympathetic ganglia. Most of the postganglionic fibers of the head and neck originate from these three ganglia.

Superior Cervical Ganglion. The superior cervical ganglion branches into the internal carotid nerve and the pharyngeal branches. The internal carotid nerve arises from the cephalic portion of the ganglion, reaches the internal carotid artery, around which it forms the *carotid plexus,* and travels into the carotid canal to distribute in the cranial cavity. Communicating branches go to the common and external carotid arteries and distribute to the head. The *pharyngeal branches,* composed of four or more fibers, mingle with branches of cranial nerves IX and X to participate in the formation of the pharyngeal plexus. Other branches also go to some cranial nerves and the cardiac plexus.

Middle Cervical Ganglion. The middle cervical ganglion has three branches which serve cervical spinal nerves, adjacent viscera, and the cardiac plexus.

Inferior Cervical Ganglion. The inferior cervical ganglion has three branches. *Vertebral branches* are supplied to the vertebral artery, forming the vertebral sympathetic plexus which serves the head. The other two branches serve lower cervical spinal nerves and supply fibers to the cardiac plexus.

DEEP PREVERTEBRAL MUSCLES OF THE NECK

There are four deep prevertebral muscles of the neck: the longus colli, longus capitis, rectus capitis anterior, and rectus capitis lateralis. These muscles lie deep to the prevertebral fascia, under the floor of the anterior triangle, and function more or less to flex the head and the neck. These muscles are relatively unimportant; hence, their discussion is not warranted. Information concerning their attachments, innervations, and functions is included in Table 7.7.

CLINICAL CONSIDERATIONS

Clinical involvement of the cervical region is a complex topic, encompassing, among others, congenital malformations, tumors—both benign and malignant—as well as anatomical considerations during surgical procedures, especially those involving the thyroid gland. The intent of this section on clinical considerations is not to detail exhaustively the possible clinical significance of each structure located in this area, but merely to illustrate the importance of sound anatomical bases for clinicians dealing with this complicated region.

Congenital Malformations

During embryonic development of the head and neck, various congenital malformations may occur. Some of these were detailed in Chapter 5 and the reader is referred to that section.

Fascial Layers

Fascial layers play an important role in the localization of infection. However, the spaces between fascial layers occasionally communicate with other regions of the body. One such space, between the two lamina of the prevertebral fascia (or, according to some, between the prevertebral and alar fasciae) is the "danger space" serving as a conduit for the spread of infection from the neck into the thorax.

Muscle Involvements

Torticollis is a condition in which the head is held at an angle, with the ear drawn toward the shoulder of one side. This condition may be either congeni-

TABLE 7.7
Deep Prevertebral Muscles of the Neck

Name	Location	Origin
Longus colli	Anterior surface of vertebral column	Transverse processes of vertebrae C3–T3
Longus capitis	Anterior to longus colli	Transverse processes of vertebrae C3–C6
Rectus capitis anterior	Deep to the longus capitis	Lateral mass and transverse process of the atlas
Rectus capitis lateralis	Just lateral to rectus capitis anterior	Transverse process of atlas

tal or spasmodic. It is believed that congenital torticollis is caused by trauma during birth, where one of the sternocleidomastoids is stretched excessively, causing hemorrhage in the muscle, resulting in fibrous invasion and subsequent shortening of the muscle. Further complications may arise, such as wedge-shaped cervical vertebrae and muscle atrophy. Spasmodic torticollis usually involves the trapezius, sternocleidomastoid, and perhaps other muscles, all of which undergo spasmodic contractions. The position of the head in this condition mimics congenital torticollis. The defect is not in the muscles but is probably related to neurogenic involvement.

Paralysis of the trapezius may occur if deep wounds in the region of the posterior triangle involve the spinal accessory nerve. Such injury limits the movement of the upper limb to the horizontal position during lifting of the arm. In addition, it causes depression of the shoulder on the affected side.

Referred pain in the region of the shoulder may have its origin in pleurisy which is causing irritation of the phrenic nerve. This situation occurs because the phrenic nerve has the same cervical spinal nerve components as the supraclavicular nerves, and signals transmitted via the phrenic nerve may be interpreted as originating in the area of the shoulder served by the supraclaviculars.

Nerve Involvements

During arterial insufficiency of the upper limb, sympathectomy is indicated, whereby the cervical sympathetic trunk is severed. This severing causes Horner's Syndrome, expressed as the inability to sweat, drooping of the upper eyelid, and constriction of the pupil.

Neurocirculatory compression occurs in an individual when the space between the anterior and middle scalene muscles is reduced in size, thus compressing the subclavian artery and brachial plexus traveling through that space. Occasionally, the neurocirculatory compression is due to the presence of a cervical rib or a small slip of muscle, the scalenus minimus, lateral to the anterior scalene. These, both, would reduce the available space. The symptoms involved in this syndrome include drooping of the shoulder, pain, paresthesia,

Insertion	Innervation	Action
Transverse processes of vertebrae C5, C6; bodies of vertebrae C2, C3, and C4; and anterior tubercle of atlas	Ventral primary rami of spinal nerves C2–C7	Flexes and rotates neck and bends neck to one side.
Basilar part of occipital bone	Ventral primary rami of spinal nerves C1–C3	Flexes the head.
Basilar part of occipital bone	Ventral primary rami of spinal nerves C1, C2	Flexes the head.
Jugular process of occipital bone	Ventral primary rami of spinal nerves C1–C2	Bends head to one side.

or even total lack of sensation and reduced circulation in the upper limb of the affected side.

Vascular Involvements

The external jugular vein may be used as a venous manometer, since in a supine patient the venous blood pressure is not high enough to engorge this vessel much above the clavicle. During failure of the right side of the heart, constriction of the superior venae cavae and increased pressure in the thorax induces a pressure buildup in the venous side of the circulatory system, and this is evidenced by engorgement of the external jugular vein. Under severe conditions, the vessel may be filled as high as the base of the mandible. This extremely important sign should be recognized by dental professionals utilizing reclining chairs in their practice; the patient should be referred immediately for possible cardiac care.

The subclavian artery supplies bloodflow to the entire upper extremity via its continuation, the axillary artery. Uncontrollable bleeding in the upper limb may be stopped by applying pressure with a blunt object on the subclavian artery as it crosses the first rib. The pressure should be directed inferoposteriorly, behind the clavicle, just lateral to the clavicular head of origin of the sternocleidomastoid.

Carotid sinus syndrome may result in loss of consciousness due to simple head movements. The syndrome relates to the hypersensitivity of the carotid sinus due to an unknown etiology. Sudden slight pressure changes, such as that occasioned by movement of the head, may result in stimulation of the carotid sinus. Impulses relayed by the sinus reduce blood pressure and slow the pumping action of the heart, thus decreasing blood supply to the brain resulting in sudden loss of consciousness.

Thyroid Gland Involvements

Goiter is an abnormal enlargement of the thyroid gland. Interestingly, the incidence of goiter is greater in females than in males. Occasionally, the enlargement of the thyroid is in an inferior direction, and the condition is referred to as intrathoracic goiter. In this condition, the thyroid physically presses upon the trachea and causes breathing difficulties. Goiter has other serious effects, mainly the overproduction of thyroid hormone. In such a hyperthyroid condition, there is a loss of weight, lack of heat tolerance, diarrhea, muscle weakness accompanied by trembling of the upper extremity, insomnia, and exophthalmos. The last condition could be extremely serious, for severe exophthalmos could damage the cornea due to the inability of the eyelids to accommodate the protruded eye, causing drying out of that structure. Exophthalmos may also stretch and damage the optic nerve to the point of blindness.

Hypothyroidism is a condition caused by a greatly reduced production of thyroid hormone. Although no hormone is produced, excessive amounts of thyroglobulin, which is stored as colloid in the thyroid follicles, greatly enlarges the size of the thyroid gland, causing goiter. The symptoms of hypothyroidism are reduced libido, somnolescence, decreased metabolic rate, decreased heart rate and cardiac output, and myxedema, accumulation of body fluids in the interstitial connective tissues.

Cretinism is a disorder caused by excessive hypothyroid state during early childhood. This condition is characterized by mental retardation and greatly reduced physical stature, especially involving skeletal growth.

Thyroidectomy is a serious procedure. Four major considerations must be kept in mind: parathyroid tetani, external laryngeal nerve, recurrent laryngeal nerve, and thyroid crisis. Since the parathyroid glands are located on the deep surface of the thyroid gland, their presence and vascular supply must be established and the glands must not be extirpated along with the thyroid. Parathyroid removal is not compatible with life, and accidental parathyroidectomy results in parathyroid tetani, whose symptoms are sudden reduction of plasma calcium levels, increased plasma phosphorus levels, and spasmodic muscular contractions, especially in muscles of the larynx, resulting in respiratory obstruction and death.

During thyroidectomy, the external and recurrent laryngeal nerves must be isolated and protected from damage. These two nerves supply the laryngeal musculature and inappropriate handling could damage them resulting in postoperative hoarseness and even loss of speech. Bilateral sectioning of the recurrent laryngeal nerve occasionally may result in dyspnea and, unless surgical intervention ensues, even in death.

A treatment for hyperthyroidism is thyroidectomy. One of the postoperative complications that may arise is known as thyroid storm (thyroid crisis), of which the symptoms are high fever, delirium, cardiac arrhythmia, profuse sweating, vomiting, subsequent dehydration, and if untreated, death.

Superficial Face

CHAPTER 8

SURFACE ANATOMY

The bony structures of the skull are overlaid by muscles, connective tissue, and skin which give a characteristic morphology to the face. The facial skeleton, discussed in Chapter 6, may be palpated easily, since the overlying soft tissue is very thin over much of its surface. The mental protuberance can easily be palpated at the chin as may the body, angle, and ramus of the mandible. The mandibular articulation can be emphasized by repeated opening and closing of the mouth. Proceeding anterosuperiorly from this articulation, the zygomatic arch and zygoma, the prominent portion of the cheek, can be palpated. The zygomatic bone also forms the lateral and part of the inferior rim of the orbit. The rest of the inferior rim is formed by the maxilla, whose inferior extent houses the upper dental arch, evident upon smiling. Immediately superior to the philtrum of the lip is the fleshy and cartilaginous bulb of the nose. The flexible cartilaginous bridge of the nose becomes immobile near the nasal bones, which lead to the root of the nose, positioned between the two orbits. Above the superior rim of the orbit, deep to the eyebrows, is the superciliary ridge of the frontal bone, while the forehead is marked by the frontal eminences. The cranium is covered by the scalp and the face is usually considered to be bounded by the anterior hairline of the scalp, the posterior border of the ramus, and inferior border of the body of the mandible.

SCALP

The scalp is composed of a thick covering of skin and its attending, fibroadipose hypodermis overlying the *epicranius* or *occipitofrontalis muscle* with its intervening *galea aponeurotica*, a thick, fibrous aponeurotic connecting sheet. Deep to this sheet is a fascial cleft containing a loose type of connective tissue often considered the "danger space" of the scalp. This tissue separates the aponeurotic sheet from the *pericranium*, the periosteal covering of the bones constituting the vault of the skull. The pericranium is only loosely attached to the underlying hard tissue, except at the sutures where it is firmly anchored to the intrasutural material.

The vascular and nerve supply of the scalp is tightly bound to the subcutaneous connective tissue, traveling between the muscular-aponeurotic layer and the skin.

153

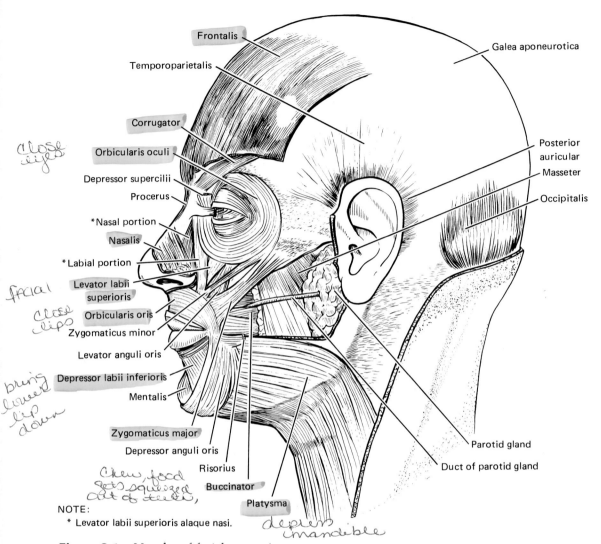

close eyes

facial

close lips

bring lower lip down

chew, food gets squeezed out of teeth,

depress mandible

Figure 8.1. Muscles of facial expression.

NOTE:
* Levator labii superioris alaque nasi.

Muscles (Fig. 8.1; Table 8.1)

Epicranius

The epicranius *muscle* is composed of two bellies, the frontal and the occipital, connected to each other by a tendinous aponeurosis, *galea aponeurotica*, whose collagenous fibers run in an anteroposterior direction. The *frontal belly* is the larger and somewhat fleshier one and is not attached to bone. Its fibers originate from the superficial muscles of the orbit and nose (corrugator, procerus, and orbicularis oculi) and insert into the galea aponeurotica somewhat anterior to the coronal suture. The *occipital belly* originates from bony landmarks—the mastoid process of the temporal bone and the lateral portion of the superior nuchal line of the occipital bone—to insert into the galea aponeurotica.

Temporoparietalis
The temporoparietalis is a muscle of variable size extending between the frontal belly of the epicranius and the anterior and superior auricular muscles of the ear.

The frontal belly of the epicranius and the temporoparietalis are both innervated by the temporal branch of the facial nerve, while the occipital belly receives its innervation via the posterior auricular branch of the same cranial nerve.

These three muscles acting together furrow the forehead, raise the eyebrows, and widen the eyes. The frontal belly acting by itself raises the eyebrow and the temporoparietalis raises the ear.

Vascular Supply (Fig. 8.2)

Arterial supply to the scalp consists of branches from the external and internal carotid arteries. Branches of the external carotid include the *occipital artery*, which suplies the medial aspect of the back of the scalp, the *posterior auricular artery* supplying the area behind and above the ear, and the *superficial temporary artery*, which vascularizes the lateral aspect of the scalp. Two branches of the internal carotid artery are responsible for vascularization of the anterior superior aspect of the scalp, the *supraorbital* and *supratrochlear arteries*. Both arteries leave the orbit and ascend up the forehead, supplying it and the top of the scalp. All of these vessels freely anastomose with each other. Venous drainage accompanies the arteries, and the vessels are named accordingly.

Nerve Supply (Fig. 8.2)

The cutaneous nerves of the scalp follow the main vascular elements. The posterior aspect of the scalp is served by the third occipital and greater occipital nerves. Laterally, the scalp receives its cutaneous innervation via the lesser occipital and auriculotemporal nerves, posterior and anterior to the ear respectively. The region in the vicinity of the temple is supplied by the zygomaticotemporal, while the forehead and midline of the scalp are served by the supraorbital and supratrochlear nerves.

FACE

Muscles (Fig. 8.1; Table 8.1)

The muscles of the face (and scalp) are derived embryologically from hyoid arch mesenchyme which migrates to its final destination. Considering the origin of these muscles, it is not surprising that they receive motor innervation from branches of the facial nerve (cranial nerve VII). These muscles insert into the dermis of the skin. It is important to understand that fascicles of these muscles intermingle with each other, and they tend to act in groups to control the orifices around which they are grouped, such as the orbit, nose, and mouth. It is according to this grouping that they will be examined.

TABLE 8.1
Muscles of the Face and Scalp

Muscle	Location	Origin
Scalp		
Frontalis	Forehead	Procerus, corrugator, orbicularis oculi
Occipitalis	Back of the head	Mastoid process and superior nuchal line
Temporoparietalis	Temple	Temporal fascia
Ear		
Auricularis anterior	Anterior to ear	Temporal fascia
Auricularis superior	Above ear	Temporal fascia
Auricularis posterior	Behind ear	Mastoid process
Nose		
Procerus	Bony bridge of nose	Fascia of nasal bone
Nasalis	Cartilaginous bridge and wing of nose	Maxilla and alar cartilage
Depressor septi	Lateral to the philtrum	Maxilla
Eye		
Orbicularis oculi	Around the orbit	Nasal process of frontal bone, frontal process of maxilla, medial palpebral ligament, and lacrimal bone
Corrugator	Deep to the orbicularis oculi	Medial aspect of superciliary arch
Mouth		
Levator labii superioris	Upper lip	Zygoma and maxilla just above infraorbital foramen
Levator labii superioris alaque nasi	Upper lip and side of nose	Maxilla, frontal process
Levator anguli oris	Corner of mouth	Canine fossa of maxilla
Zygomaticus major	Cheek and corner of mouth	Temporal process of zygoma
Zygomaticus minor	Cheek and corner of mouth	Maxillary process of zygoma
Risorius	Cheek	Masseteric fascia
Depressor labii inferioris	Lower lip	Oblique line of mandible
Depressor anguli oris	Corner of mouth	Oblique line of mandible
Mentalis	Chin	Incisive fossa of mandible
Orbicularis oris	Circumscribes the mouth	Muscles in the vicinity, maxilla, nasal septum, mandible
Buccinator	Cheek	Pterygomandibular raphe, alveolar arches of mandible and maxilla
Neck		
Platysma	Neck and chin	Pectoral and deltoid fascia

Insertion	Innervation (branch of VII)	Action
Galea aponeurotica	Temporal	Wrinkles forehead and raises eyebrow.
Galea aponeurotica	Posterior auricular	Tightens the scalp.
Galea aponeurotica	Temporal	Elevates the ear.
Anterior part of major helix of ear	Temporal	Pulls auricle forward and up.
Superior aspect of ear	Temporal	Pulls auricle up.
Posteroinferior aspect of ear	Posterior auricular	Pulls auricle back.
Dermis above glabella	Buccal	Depresses eyebrows medially.
Dermis of nose across bridge and on bulb	Buccal	Dilates nares.
Septum and ala of nose	Buccal	Constricts nares.
Lateral palpebral raphe, frontalis muscle, corrugator muscle, superior and inferior tarsi	Temporal and zygomatic	Closes the eye.
Dermis covering the supraorbital foramen	Temporal and zygomatic	Forms vertical wrinkles between eyebrows.
Upper lip	Buccal	Elevates upper lip.
Upper lip and alar cartilage	Buccal	Dilates nares and elevates upper lip.
Corner of mouth	Buccal	Lifts corner of mouth.
Corner of the mouth	Buccal	Lifts corner of mouth.
Upper lip medial to corner of mouth	Buccal	Elevates upper lip.
Corner of mouth	Buccal and mandibular	Draws corner of mouth laterally.
Lower lip	Mandibular and buccal	Depresses lower lip.
Corner of mouth	Mandibular and buccal	Depresses corner of mouth.
Dermis of skin	Mandibular and buccal	Wrinkles chin and protrudes lower lip.
Dermis of the lips and surrounding muscles	Buccal and mandibular	Closes, purses, and protrudes lips.
Muscles of the mouth	Buccal	Compresses cheek.
Inferior border of body of mandible, skin of face	Cervical	Depresses mandible, corner of mouth, and lower lip.

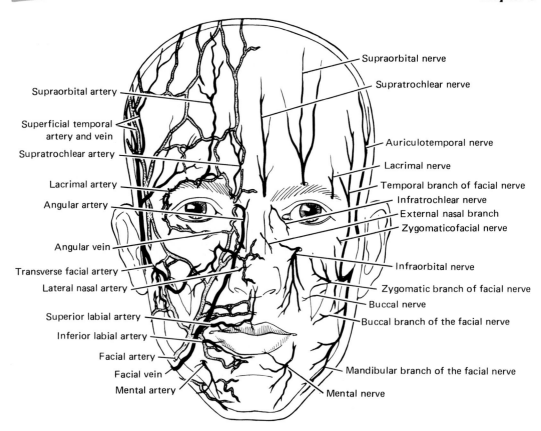

Figure 8.2. Vascular and nerve supply of the superficial face.

Muscles of the Ear and Nose

There are three external muscles of the ear: *auricularis anterior, superior,* and *posterior.* Similarly, there are three muscles of the nose: the *procerus, nasalis,* and *depressor septi.* These two groups of muscles are fairly inconsequential and pertinent information concerning them may be found in Table 8.1.

Muscles Surrounding the Orbit

The three muscles concerned with the orifice of the eye are the orbicularis oculi, corrugator, and the levator palpebrae superioris. The last of this group will be considered in the chapter on the orbit.

Orbicularis Oculi. The orbicularis oculi muscle is composed of two parts, the palpebral portion and the orbital portion. The former originates from the medial palpebral ligament (attached to the medial aspect of the orbit) and inserts into the lateral palpebral raphe (attached to the lateral aspect of the orbit). The orbital portion of the muscle describes an oval around the orbit. The orbicularis oculi is innervated by the temporal and zygomatic branches of the facial nerve and acts to close the eyelid completely. Forceful closure is mediated by the orbital portion, while the palpebral portion is responsible for light closure, as in blinking.

Corrugator. The corrugator (supercillii) muscle is located deep to the supero-medial aspect of the orbicularis oculi, at the medial aspect of the eyebrow. It originates at the medial extent of the supercilliary arch and inserts into the skin of the eyebrow. It is innervated by the temporal and zygomatic branches of the facial nerve; the combined actions of the paired muscles approximate the eyebrows, producing frowns.

Muscles Surrounding the Mouth
The muscles of the mouth act to alter the shape of the orifice. Their fibers of insertion intermingle with each other; therefore, they share a commonality of action and almost always act in concert.

Orbicularis Oris. The orbicularis oris completely encircles the mouth. Its fibers are positioned at various depths and angles in the two lips. Fascicles of this muscle, some of which are derived from those of neighboring muscles—especially the buccinator—freely intermingle with fascicles of other muscles acting on the lips, permitting extensive movability. Many of the fibers of the buccinator cross over each other at the angle of the mouth, so that the upper fibers proceed to the lower lip and the lower fibers to the upper lip. Hence, the origin of the orbicularis oris is quite complex and is usually considered to be from the fibers of the surrounding muscles as well as from the alveolar portion of the maxilla, the septum of the nose, and the area lateral to the incisive fossa of the mandible. Insertion is into the skin and into itself, forming an ellipse around the mouth. The buccal and mandibular branches of the facial nerve innervate this complex muscle, which closes the lips and, during stronger contraction, purses them, as in osculation and whistling.

Risorius. The risorius is a small, horizontally-placed muscle which originates in the masseteric fascia and inserts in the skin of the corner of the mouth. It is innervated by the buccal and mandibular branches of the facial nerve. This is the smiling muscle; it is responsible for drawing the corners of the mouth laterally.

Depressors of the Lip. The *depressor labii inferioris* is quadrangular in shape. It originates on the medial extent of the oblique line of the mandible and inserts into the skin of the lower lip. It acts to depress the lower lip. The *depressor anguli oris (triangularis)* originates on the oblique line of the mandible and inserts into the skin of the corner of the mouth and depresses it, expressing sadness. The *mentalis* is a small muscle of the chin. Its origin is in the incisive fossa of the mandible, and it inserts into the skin of the chin to wrinkle it and also to protrude the lower lip as in drinking. The *platysma* was previously detailed in Chapter 7. All of the muscles of this group, except the platysma, are innervated by the buccal and mandibular branches of the facial nerve.

Elevators of the Lip. Five muscles elevate the lip and corner of the mouth. All of these are innervated by the buccal branch of the facial nerve. The *levator labii superioris alaque nasi* is the most medial of these muscles, and it originates from the frontal process of the maxilla passing inferiorly along the side of the nose. The muscle splits into a medial and a lateral portion to insert into the wing of the nose and into the upper lip. This muscle functions in dilating the nostril and raising the upper lip. The *levator labii superioris* originates from the maxilla and zygoma just inferior to the orbit. Its fibers pass across the infraorbital foramen to insert into the upper lip, lateral to and intermingling with the fibers of the previous muscle. The levator labii superioris elevates and protrudes the upper lip.

The *levator anguli oris* lies deep to the levator labii superioris. It originates below the infraorbital foramen, from the canine fossa of the maxilla, to insert into the corner of the mouth. This muscle elevates the angle of the mouth and assists in the formation of the nasolabial furrow. The *zygomaticus minor,* a slender muscle arising from the maxillary process of the zygomatic bone, inserts just lateral to the insertion of the levator labii superioris muscle. This muscle elevates the upper lip. It also assists in the formation of the nasolabial furrow. The *zygomaticus major* is the lateralmost muscle of this group. It originates on the temporal process of the zygomatic bone and inserts into the corner of the mouth. This muscle elevates the corner of the mouth and pulls it laterally.

Muscle of the Cheek

The *buccinator,* a quadrangular-shaped muscle occupying the space between the mandible and the maxilla, is the primary muscular component of the cheek. It lies deep to the muscles of facial expression and is separated from them by the buccopharyngeal fascia and the buccal fat pad. The parotid duct pierces the substance of this muscle to enter the oral vestibule. The buccinator originates on the maxilla and mandible, specifically on the buccal surfaces of the alveolar processes in the vicinity of the three molars, and from the *pterygomandibular raphe,* a collagenous tendinous inscription attached to the pterygoid hamulus and the mylohyoid line of the mandible. This raphe is interposed between the buccinator and superior pharyngeal constrictor muscles. The buccinator inserts into the fleshy corner of the lip in such a fashion that the upper fascicles and the lower fascicles decussate at the corner of the mouth and insert into the lower and upper lips, respectively, becoming fibers of the orbicularis oris. The highest and lowest fascicles, however, continue without decussation into the upper and lower lips respectively. The buccal branch of the facial nerve innervates this muscle which acts to press the mucosa of the cheek against the teeth, thus aiding in mastication and deglutition. In addition, it assists in forcefully expelling air distending the oral vestibule, as in blowing dust particles off a surface.

Sensory Innervation (Fig. 8.2)

Sensory innervation of the greater part of the face is mediated by the ophthalmic, maxillary, and mandibular divisions of the trigeminal nerve. The region superficial to the angle of the mandible, the posterior aspect of the inferior portion of the ramus, and most of the ear is supplied by the great auricular and, to a lesser extent, the lesser occipital branches of the cervical plexus, as discussed in Chapter 7.

The branches of the trigeminal nerve supplying sensory innervation to the superficial face follow:

Ophthalmic (V_1)	Maxillary (V_2)	Mandibular (V_3)
lacrimal	infraorbital	auriculotemporal
supraorbital	zygomaticofacial	buccal
supratrochlear	zygomaticotemporal	mental
infratrochlear		
external nasal		

Ophthalmic Division

The *lacrimal nerve* leaves the superolateral aspect of the orbit and enters the upper eyelid to distribute to the lateral half of that structure and the conjunctiva of the eye. The frontal nerve bifurcates in the orbit to form the *supraorbital* and *supratrochlear nerves.* The former leaves the orbit via the supraorbital foramen (or notch), while the latter passes superior to the trochlea and leaves the orbit medial to the supraorbital foramen. These two nerves supply sensation to the upper eyelid, the conjunctiva, and the medial half of the forehead and scalp. The *infratrochlear nerve,* a branch of the nasociliary nerve, leaves the orbit by passing between the middle palpebral ligament of the eye and trochlea to innervate the medial half of the eyelids, the medial angle of the eye, and the side of the nose. The *external nasal nerve,* a branch of the anterior ethmoidal branch of the nasociliary nerve leaves the nasal cavity at the distal end of the nasal bone. This nerve provides sensation to the middle of the bridge and part of the ala of the nose.

Maxillary Division

The *infraorbital nerve* is a continuation of the maxillary division of the trigeminal nerve. It enters the face via the infraorbital foramen, where it forms a tuft of nerves which may be categorized into three groups: the inferior palpebral branches serving the skin of the lower eyelid and the conjunctiva, the external nasal branches innervating the side and mobile septum of the nose, and the superior labial branches supplying the upper lip and mucosa of the superior labial vestibule.

The zygomatic branch of the maxillary division of the trigeminal bifurcates to form the *zygomaticotemporal* and *zygomaticofacial nerves.* The former enters the superficial face a little superior to the zygomatic arch and supplies sensation to the region of the temple. The latter emerges in the superficial face by way of the zygomaticofacial foramen to serve the skin over the zygomatic bone.

Mandibular Division

The *auriculotemporal nerve* is a branch of the posterior trunk of the mandibular division. It appears in the superficial face just behind the temporomandibular articulation, where it gives rise to the anterior auricular branches to the anterolateral surface of the ear and superficial temporal branches to the region of the temple up to the coronal suture.

The *buccal nerve* lies on the surface of the buccinator muscle as it emerges from beneath the masseter muscle. The buccal nerve provides sensation to the cheek and, upon piercing the buccinator, supplies sensation to the mucosa of the buccal vestibule and buccal surfaces of the gingivae as far anteriorly as the corner of the mouth.

The *mental nerve* enters the superficial face via the mental foramen of the mandible to serve the chin, lower lip, and the surrounding mucosa of the oral vestibule.

Motor Innervation

Facial Nerve (Figs. 8.2, 11.1)
The facial nerve, the nerve of the second arch, leaves the cranial cavity via the internal acoustic meatus and travels in the temporal bone from where it emerges through the stylomastoid foramen. A *posterior auricular branch* arises from the trunk, passing posterior to the ear on its way to the occipitalis and posterior auricular muscles. The main stem of the facial nerve then supplies fibers to the stylohyoid muscle and the posterior belly of the digastric muscle, prior to entering the deep aspect of the parotid gland. Here, it subdivides into two large divisions, the temporofacial and cervicofacial, forming a loop from which arise the five terminal branches of the parotid plexus supplying motor fibers to the muscles of facial expression (Table 8.2).

The superiormost of these, the *temporal branches,* supply the muscles in the region of the temple and part of the forehead. The *zygomatic branches* fan out to serve muscles in the area of the prominence of the cheek to the lateral angle of the eye. The *buccal branches,* the largest of all, course across the masseter and buccinator muscles to innervate muscles of the upper lip and nose. *Mandibular branches* pass deep to the depressor anguli oris and platysma to supply muscles of the lower lip, while the *cervical branches* pass deep to and innervate the platysma muscle.

Blood Supply (Fig. 8.2)

Arterial Supply
Vascular supply of the superficial face is derived from branches directly or indirectly arising from the external carotid artery, as well as from branches of the ophthalmic artery, a branch of the internal carotid artery. The terminal branches of these vessels form an extensive anastomotic network permeating the superficial aspect of the face. Some of these vessels travel with like-named nerves, and their distribution follows that of their nerve counterparts.

Facial Artery. The facial artery is a branch of the external carotid artery; its cervical branches have been described earlier. This artery crosses the mandible to enter the face just anterior to the masseter muscle, lying in the groove for the facial artery. In the face, the artery travels superficially, just under the cover of the platysma muscle. It passes, via a tortuous path, deep to the zygomaticus major, risorius, and levator anguli oris muscles to the corner of the mouth. Here, it ascends lateral to the nose to terminate as the angular artery at the medial corner of the eye. The branches of the facial artery in the face are the inferior labial, superior labial, lateral nasal, and angular arteries.

The *superior* and *inferior labial arteries* arise near the corner of the mouth and, traveling deep to the depressor anguli oris muscle, pierce the orbicularis

TABLE 8.2
Branches of the Facial Nerve in the Superficial Face

Branches	Muscles innervated
Temporal	Auricularis anterior; auricularis superior; frontalis; orbicularis oculi; corrugator
Zygomatic	Orbicularis oculi; corrugator
Buccal	Procerus; nasalis; depressor septi; zygomaticus major; zygomaticus minor; levator labii superioris; levator anguli oris; levator labii superioris alaque nasi; risorius; orbicularis oris; buccinator
Mandibular	Depressor anguli oris; depressor labii inferioris; orbicularis oris; mentalis; risorius
Cervical	Platysma

oris to supply the upper and lower lips respectively. The superior also provides small branches to the wing (ala) and bulb of the nose. The *lateral nasal artery* arises near the wing of the nose to supply that structure and the bridge of the nose. The *angular artery* is the terminal continuation of the facial artery, supplying the tissues in the vicinity of the medial corner of the eye.

Superficial Temporal Artery. The superficial temporal artery, one of the terminal branches of the external carotid artery, arises near the level of the earlobe. The vessel branches profusely at its cranialmost aspect to supply the region superficial to the zygomatic arch as far medially as the lateral corner of the eye as well as the temple and the lateral aspect of the scalp. The *transverse facial artery,* a branch of the superficial temporal, accompanies and supplies the parotid duct in its path across the masseter muscle. In addition, it sends branches to the parotid gland and other soft tissues in the vicinity.

The rest of the arterial supply of the superficial face is derived from either the maxillary artery, a terminal branch of the external carotid artery, or from the ophthalmic artery, a branch of the internal carotid artery.

Branches of the Maxillary Artery. The *maxillary artery,* lying deep to the ramus of the mandible in the infratemporal fossa, provides vascularization of the face through some of its branches. Only those serving the superficial face are described here, while its other branches are treated in subsequent chapters. The branches of the maxillary artery supplying the superficial face are the infraorbital, buccal, and mental arteries. The *infraorbital artery,* a branch of the third or pterygopalatine portion of the maxillary artery, passes through the infraorbital fissure to lie in the floor of the orbit. It travels in the infraorbital canal and enters the superficial face via the infraorbital foramen to distribute to the lower eyelid, the upper lip, and the area between these two structures. The *buccal artery,* a branch of the second or pterygoid portion of the maxillary artery, makes its appearance on the face on the superficial surface of the buccinator muscle to supply it, the connective tissue of the cheek, and the mucosa of the buccal vestibule. The *mental artery* arises from the inferior alveolar branch of the maxillary artery. The mental artery enters the face via the mental foramen to supply the soft tissues of the chin.

Branches of the Ophthalmic Artery. Branches of the ophthalmic artery supplying the face are the zygomaticofacial, supraorbital, supratrochlear, and dorsal nasal arteries.

The *zygomaticofacial artery* is derived from the lacrimal branch of the ophthalmic artery. It enters the face via the zygomaticofacial foramen to supply the region of the face superficial to the zygomatic bone. The *supraorbital* and *supratrochlear arteries* both arise in the orbit. The former enters the face via the supraorbital foramen (or notch), while the latter makes its appearance medial to the supraorbital notch. These vessels supply the forehead and the scalp. The *dorsal nasal artery,* a terminal branch of the ophthalmic artery, leaves the orbit at its medial corner to supply the dorsum of the nose.

Venous Drainage

Venous drainage of the superficial face is via the supraorbital, posterior auricular, retromandibular, buccal, infraorbital, submental, and superior and inferior labial veins, all of which accompany like-named arteries. Two additional collecting veins, the facial and superficial temporal, empty into the internal and external jugular veins respectively.

Facial Vein. The facial vein serves as the principal venous vessel of the superficial face. It begins in the medial corner of the eye as the angular vein, passes inferiorly following the course of the facial artery deep to the zygomaticus major and zygomaticus minor muscles, where it parts company with the artery to empty into the internal jugular vein. The facial vein communicates with the pterygoid plexus of veins as well as with the ophthalmic veins, both of which present possible passageways to the cavernous sinus due to lack of directional valves.

Superficial Temporal Vein. The superficial temporal vein follows the course of the same-named artery to drain the scalp, temple, and part of the forehead and ear. One of its tributaries is the transverse facial vein, which follows the path of the transverse facial artery.

CLINICAL CONSIDERATIONS ═══════════════════════════════════════

Scalp

Bleeding in the scalp is extremely difficult to stop and is quite dangerous. The blood supply is extensive and the vessels pass through fibrous septa of the superficial fascia which mechanically inhibit vessel contraction. Hemorrhage in this region has a tendency to be contained in the loose connective tissue, the subaponeurotic layer, deep to the galea aponeurotica. Further, infection may result in a localized abscess which, having no outlet to the surface, may enter the valveless emissary veins of this region, also known as the "danger zone of the scalp," and travel to the diploë and/or the dural venous sinuses. Such infection may result in osteomyelitis, thrombosis, and possibly death.

Face

Danger Area of the Face

The area bordered by the upper lip, lateral aspect of the nose, and lateral corner of the eye superior to the supraorbital ridge represents the danger area of the face. Squeezing pimples and tampering with boils in this region should be avoided, since the area may be drained by the ophthalmic vein which leads directly into the cavernous sinus of the cranial fossa. Infection may enter the cavernous sinus via this route resulting in thrombosis, cerebral edema, and possibly death.

Bell's Palsy

Damage to the facial nerve (or its accidental analgesia during dental procedures) results in paralysis of the muscles of the affected side. Damage may occur during surgical involvement of the parotid gland, infection of the middle ear, knife wounds, or at birth during forceps delivery. Paralysis of the facial muscles results in ptosis of the eye (lower eyelid drooping), depression of the corner of the mouth with accompanying oozing of saliva, speech disorder (especially involving labial sounds), lack of muscle tone, and a sagging, distorted face.

Trigeminal Neuralgia

Trigeminal neuralgia (tic douloureux), an extremely painful, debilitating condition involving pain fibers of the trigeminal nerve, is due to an unknown etiology though often associated with dental carious lesions. The pain is often excruciating and is experienced over the face, teeth, gingivae, nasal and paranasal cavities, as well as the external ear canal. These are the areas served by the maxillary and mandibular divisions, though infrequently the area served by the ophthalmic division of the trigeminal nerve may be affected. Treatment varies from alcohol injection into the trigeminal division affected to sectioning of the trigeminal nerve between the pons and the ganglion.

CHAPTER 9

Cranial Fossa

The *cranial fossa,* or the cavity inside the skull, is occupied by the brain and its associated meninges. This chapter will discuss the dural lining, its venous sinuses, and cranial nerves which exit the skull. The osteology of this region is presented in Chapter 6.

DURA MATER

The brain is surrounded by three layers of meninges: a tough, fibrous outer *dura mater* and two delicate layers, the innermost *pia mater* and the middle, web-like, *arachnoid.* The latter two layers are discussed further in Chapter 17, while the dura mater is described here. The dura is a thick, collagenous, coarse investment that does not follow the contours of the brain. It consists of two layers: the one in intimate contact with the bones of the skull is the vascular *periosteal layer* and the other, in intimate contact with the arachnoid, is the *meningeal layer.* These two layers adhere closely to one another, except in regions occupied by veins and venous sinuses.

The *periosteal layer* is quite vascular and is attached to the underlying bone via collagenous, Sharpey's fibers. These attachments are particularly notable at the suture lines, where the dura is firmly bound to the intrasuture materials. The periosteal layer of the dura covers the meningeal arteries which groove the inner surface of the cranial vault.

Dural Reflections (Figs. 9.1, 9.2)

The meningeal layer of the dura is folded in certain areas, forming incomplete subdivisions of the cranial cavity. These dural reflections are interposed between various parts of the brain, providing it with additional support and protection. The two major folds are the tentorium cerebelli and the falx cerebri, while the three minor ones are the falx cerebelli, the diaphragma sella, and the covering of the trigeminal cave.

Tentorium Cerebelli

The tentorium cerebelli is a horizontally positioned reflection of the meningeal dura that lies between the cerebellum, which it covers, and the occipital region of the cerebral hemispheres, which it supports. The anterior margin of the tentorium cerebelli is free and concave and assists in the formation of an oval opening, the tentorial incisure, whose anterior extent is limited by the dorsum sellae of the sphenoid bone. The attachments of the tentorium cere-

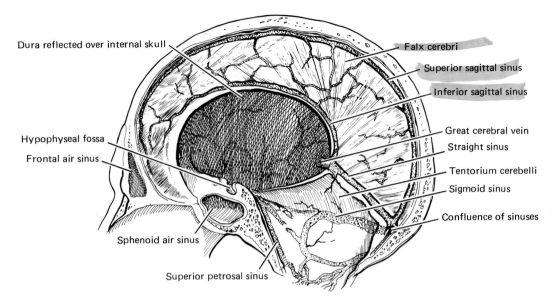

Figure 9.1. Dural reflections (midsagittal view).

belli, which fix this structure and make it taut, are as follows: anteriorly, it is
fixed to the anterior and posterior clinoid processes of the sphenoid bone; laterally, it attaches to the superior edge of the petrous temporal bone; and posteriorly, it is fixed to the periosteal dura attached to the lips of the groove for the
transverse sinus of the occipital bone, thus participating in the formation of
that sinus.

Falx Cerebri

The falx cerebri is a sickle-shaped structure. Its inferior edge is free and forms
an arc interposed between the two cerebral hemispheres. Anteriorly, the falx
cerebri attaches to the crista galli of the ethmoid bone; superiorly, it is fixed to
the periosteal dura along the lips of the groove for the superior sagittal sinus,
thus participating in the formation of that sinus; posteriorly, the falx cerebri is
attached to the periosteal dura of the occipital bone, assisting in the formation
of the inferior aspect of the superior sagittal sinus; inferiorly, it joins to the
tentorium cerebelli, and these two meningeal reflections of the dura form the
straight sinus at their line of intersection. The rest of the inferior aspect of the
falx cerebri is not attached, and this free inferior margin contains the inferior
sagittal sinus.

Falx Cerebelli

The falx cerebelli, a small meningeal reflection, subdivides the cerebellar fossa
into right and left halves. It is attached to the inferior surface of the tentorium
cerebelli and is interposed between the two cerebellar hemispheres. The attachments of the falx cerebelli are posteriorly, the periosteal dura of the region
of the internal occipital crest, containing the occipital sinus; and superiorly,
the inferior surface of the tentorium cerebelli. Its anterior edge is free, except
at the anterior terminus, where it is attached on either side of the foramen
magnum.

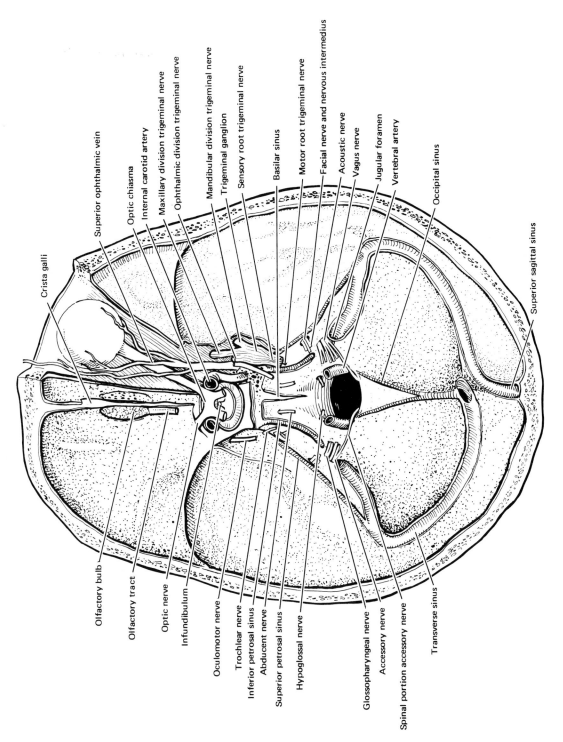

Figure 9.2. Dural venous sinuses and cranial nerves in the floor of the cranial cavity. Observe that the orbital plate of the frontal bone has been removed as has a portion of the dura from the middle cranial fossa.

Diaphragma Sella

The diaphragma sella is an incomplete covering composed of meningeal dura that acts as a membraneous lid over the sella turcica of the sphenoid bone. The sella turcica houses the pituitary gland. The diaphragma sella is perforated in the middle, permitting the infundibulum and accompanying vessels of the pituitary gland to pass through it.

Covering of the Trigeminal Cave

The trigeminal ganglion sits on the periosteal (dural) lining in the trigeminal impression on the apex of the petrous portion of the temporal bone. The ganglion is covered by a meningeal reflection, thus transforming the depression into a cave, known as *Meckel's*, or the *trigeminal cave.*

Blood Supply of the Dura Mater

The dura mater receives its principal vascularization via the anterior, middle, accessory, and posterior meningeal arteries. The *anterior meningeal artery,* derived from the anterior ethmoidal branch of the ophthalmic artery, serves the dura of the anterior cranial fossa.

The *middle meningeal artery* is the largest of the meningeal vessels supplying the dura. It is a branch of the mandibular (or first part) of the maxillary artery and enters the cranial cavity via the foramen spinosum of the sphenoid bone. It grooves the lateral wall of the cranial cavity and divides into branches, forming an arboreal distribution. This vessel and its branches serve the dural lining of the parietal, sphenoid, temporal, and occipital bones. Some of its branches also vascularize the trigeminal ganglion and roots of the trigeminal nerve.

The *accessory meningeal artery,* also a branch of the maxillary artery, gains entry to the cranial fossa through the foramen ovale to vascularize the dura of the trigeminal cave and the trigeminal ganglion.

The *posterior meningeal arteries,* branches of the ascending pharyngeal and occipital arteries, enter the cranial fossa via the jugular foramen, hypoglossal canal, foramen lacerum, and mastoid foramen. An additional posterior meningeal artery arises from the vertebral artery after that vessel has passed through the foramen magnum. All of these small vessels supply the dura of the infratentorial space of the posterior cranial fossa.

Venous drainage of the dura mater is by the anterior, posterior, and middle meningeal veins which have distributions similar to the corresponding arteries. The anterior meningeal vein empties into dural sinuses of the anterior cranial fossa, the posterior meningeal veins empty into the posterior dural venous sinuses, while the middle meningeal vein delivers its blood into the sphenoparietal sinus and the pterygoid venous plexus.

Venous Sinuses of the Dura (Figs. 9.1, 9.2, 9.3)

The dural venous sinuses are large spaces in comparison to their slender venous tributaries, such as the emissary veins and those which drain the brain and the diploë of the skull. Since the sinuses are endothelially lined spaces between reflections of taut dura mater, their walls are rigid and possess no valves. The sinuses deliver their blood either directly or indirectly via other

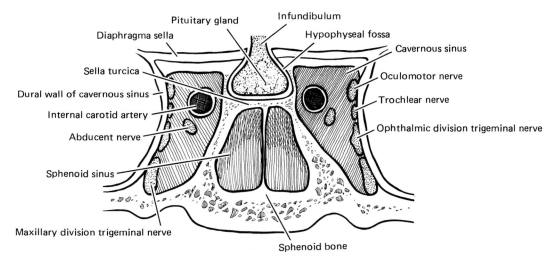

Figure 9.3. Cavernous sinus. Schematic diagram illustrating structures within the sinus and its walls.

dural venous sinuses to the *superior bulb of the internal jugular vein* situated in the jugular foramen. The dural sinuses are named: superior sagittal, inferior sagittal, straight, occipital, confluence of sinuses, transverse, petrosquamous, sigmoid, cavernous, intercavernous, sphenoparietal, superior petrosal, inferior petrosal, and basilar.

The *superior sagittal sinus,* located in the superior aspect of the falx cerebri, begins as a narrow channel just anterior to the crista galli at the foramen cecum, where it may receive a small emissary vein from the nasal cavity. This sinus receives several of the superior cerebral, dural, diploic, and emissary veins, as well as communications from the *lacunae lateralis,* situated on either side of the superior sagittal sinus which leaves a depression in the parietal bone. The superior sagittal sinus enlarges in diameter as it passes posteriorly toward its termination to empty into the right transverse sinus.

The *inferior sagittal sinus* occupies the free, inferior margin of the falx cerebri and, draining posteriorly, empties into the straight sinus along with the great cerebral vein. The *straight sinus* occupies the line of intersection between the falx cerebri and tentorium cerebelli. It receives the great cerebral vein, superior cerebellar veins, and the inferior sagittal sinus and delivers its blood to the left transverse sinus. Occasionally, the superior sagittal sinus empties into the left transverse sinus and the straight sinus then terminates in the right transverse sinus.

The *occipital sinus* lies in the space between the periosteal and meningeal dura of the falx cerebelli. It empties into the confluence of sinuses. The *confluence of sinuses* is a region receiving several of the sinuses into the large dilated space located at the internal occipital protuberance. The superior sagittal, straight, and occipital sinuses empty into the confluence, which is then drained by the right and left transverse sinuses.

The *transverse sinus* occupies the dural space at the attached perimeter of the tentorium cerebelli. The sinus of the right side usually receives blood from the superior sagittal, while the one on the left usually drains the straight sinus. The *petrosquamous sinus* is located at the fusion of the temporal squama and its petrous portion. This sinus, the superior petrosal sinus and the diploic, emissary, inferior cerebral, and inferior cerebellar veins also empty into the transverse sinus. The transverse sinus continues anteriorly as the *sigmoid sinus,* which grooves the temporal, parietal, and occipital bones and empties into the superior jugular bulb of the internal jugular vein.

The *cavernous sinus* is a labyrinthine space, covered by the meningeal layer of the dura mater, lying against the body of the sphenoid bone just lateral to the sella turcica. This sinus receives blood from the orbit, via the inferior and superior ophthalmic veins, from the pterygoid plexus of veins via emissary veins, and from the brain via cerebral veins. The sphenoparietal sinus and intercavernous sinuses also empty into the cavernous sinus. This large sinus is drained by the superior and inferior petrosal sinuses, delivering the blood to the superior jugular bulb of the internal jugular vein. Two structures pass through the cavernous sinus, each separately isolated from the bloodstream by endothelially-lined fibrous sheaths. These are the internal carotid artery and the abducent nerve. Additionally, several nerves are embedded in the lateral wall of the cavernous sinus, these are, from superior to inferior, the oculomotor and trochlear nerves and the ophthalmic and maxillary divisions of the trigeminal nerve. The two *intercavernous sinuses* are termed the *anterior* and *posterior intercavernous sinuses,* passing anterior and posterior to the infundibulum, respectively. These connect the right and left cavernous sinuses, thus forming a ring-shaped circular sinus.

The *sphenoparietal sinus* is a small sinus passing along the inferoposterior ridge of the lesser wing of the sphenoid. It receives small venous contributions from the surrounding dura and empties into the cavernous sinus.

The *superior petrosal sinus* assists in draining the cavernous sinus, and empties into the transverse sinus. It passes along the superior border of the petrous portion of the temporal bone. Along its course, it also receives cerebellar, inferior cerebral, and tympanic veins.

The *inferior petrosal sinus* also drains the cavernous sinus and empties directly into the superior jugular bulb. It travels in the inferior petrosal sulcus, a depression created at the juncture of the occipital clivus and petrous temporal bones. The internal auditory veins, cerebellar veins, as well as smaller veins of the brainstem join the inferior petrosal sinus.

The *basilar plexus* interconnects the two inferior petrosal sinuses. The plexus lies on the basilar portion of the occipital bone and receives blood from the vertebral plexus of veins.

DIPLOIC AND EMISSARY VEINS

Diploic Veins

The diploic veins are located between the two compact layers of bone that form the vault of the skull. They travel in the diploë and, in adults, communicate with each other, the meningeal veins, veins of the scalp, and the dural sinuses. There are four diploic veins: the frontal, draining into the superior sagittal sinus; the anterior temporal, serving mostly the frontal bone, emptying into the sphenoparietal sinus; the posterior temporal, responsible for draining the parietal diploë and emptying into the transverse sinus; and the occipital, which serves the occipital bone delivering blood to the confluence of sinuses directly or to the transverse sinus.

Emissary Veins

The emissary veins, as their collective name implies, serve to connect the veins of the external aspect of the skull with the dural venous sinuses. Some emissary veins are small and, as such, inconstant. Since these vessels do not possess valves, blood flow through them responds to pressures within the system. Consequently, they are possible passageways of infection in an extra-to intracranial direction.

The mastoid emissary vein links the occipital vein with the transverse sinus via the mastoid foramen. The parietal emissary vein interconnects the veins draining the scalp with the superior sagittal sinus by the way of the parietal foramen. The deep cervical veins are united with the transverse sinus by the condyloid emissary vein, which passes through the condyloid foramen. The venous drainage of the nasal cavity is connected with the superior sagittal sinus via the emissary vein of the foramen cecum. The internal jugular vein is interlinked with the cavernous sinus via the emissary veins of the carotid canal and the foramen of Vesalius. The pterygoid plexus of veins is united with the cavernous sinus via the emissary veins of the foramen lacerum and foramen ovale. The vertebral vein is connected to the transverse sinus by emissary veins of the hypoglossal canal.

CRANIAL NERVES (Fig. 9.2)

The 12 cranial nerves emanating from the brain leave the cranial cavity via foramina located in the cranial fossa. During removal of the brain from the cranial cavity, the connections between the brain and the cranial nerves are severed, and these detached nerves may be observed on the floor of the internal base of the skull.

The anteriormost nerve structure is the *olfactory tract* and *bulb*, lying just lateral to the crista galli on the cribriform plate of the ethmoid bone. The *olfactory nerve*, or cranial nerve I, passes through the perforations of the cribriform plate to enter the bulb.

The *optic nerve*, or cranial nerve II, passes through the optic foramen to the retina of the eye. It emerges from the optic chiasma, which rests on the chiasmatic groove of the sphenoid bone just anterior to the infundibulum of the hypophysis.

The *oculomotor nerve*, or cranial nerve III, passes through the dura in the vicinity of the cavernous sinus on its way to the orbit via the superior orbital fissure.

The *trochlear nerve*, or cranial nerve IV, the smallest of the cranial nerves, courses along the free margin of the tentorium cerebelli. It pierces the dura at the posterior clinoid process to pass forward in the lateral wall of the cavernous sinus, eventually to traverse the superior orbital fissure on its way to the orbit.

The *trigeminal nerve,* or cranial nerve V, the largest of the cranial nerves composed of two roots, is evident just inferior and posterior to the small trochlear nerve. The roots enter the trigeminal cave deep to the dural cover, where the sensory portion displays its sensory ganglion, while the motor portion passes deep to that structure. The *trigeminal (semilunar) ganglion* trifurcates into *ophthalmic, maxillary,* and *mandibular divisions,* which leave the cranial cavity via the superior orbital fissure, the foramen rotundum, and the foramen ovale, respectively. The motor root accompanies the mandibular division and, subsequent to passing through the foramen ovale, merges with it.

The *abducent nerve,* or cranial nerve VI, is noted piercing the dura medial and inferior to the root of the trigeminal nerve. It passes through the cavernous sinus to exit the cranial vault and enter the orbit via the superior orbital fissure.

The two roots of the *facial nerve,* or cranial nerve VII, and the *acoustic nerve,* or cranial nerve VIII accompany each other into the internal acoustic meatus, under the canopy of the tentorium cerebelli.

The *glossopharyngeal nerve,* or cranial nerve IX, the *vagus nerve,* or cranial nerve X, and the *spinal accessory nerve,* or cranial nerve XI, all leave the cranial cavity via the jugular foramen. The spinal accessory nerve is composed of a spinal portion ascending through the foramen magnum and a cranial portion with which it unites in the cranial cavity.

The *hypoglossal nerve,* or cranial nerve XII, exits the internal base of the skull via the hypoglossal foramen.

The cranial nerves and their distributions are discussed in chapters relevant to their locations. Specific information concerning the individual cranial nerves is detailed in Chapter 18.

CHAPTER 10

Orbit and Ear

ORBIT

The orbit contains the organ of sight, its associated muscles, nerves and vessels, along with some accessory structures, all of which are embedded in periorbital fat. The bulb of the eye and its associated structures function in unison to receive light rays through the cornea and lens of the eye, so that the rays may be focused on the posterior wall of the bulb. Here the retina, with its specialized cells, stimulated by the light, transmits impulses to the brain for processing into a visual image.

The eye develops from three sources. The retina and optic nerve are outgrowths of the forebrain and are first observable at about four weeks of development. The lens and some of the accessory structures in the anterior portion of the eye are derived from surface ectoderm of the head. Associated structures within the orb, as well as its tunics, are derived from adjacent mesenchyme.

Bony Orbit (Fig. 10.1; Tables 10.1, 10.2)

The bony orbit, lined by periorbita (periosteum), is conical in shape, with its base located on the superior face, its apex directed posteriorly. The "flattened" cone possesses medial and lateral walls along with a roof and floor. The medial walls lie nearly parallel to each other on either side of the midline-located ethmoid bone. The lateral walls are directed posteromedially, so that if continued, they would converge near the middle of the skull. For this reason, all structures entering the orbit from its apex are directed laterally from the midline. The attachments of two specific ocular muscles correct for this lateral divergence.

Chapter 6 discusses the bony orbit, so the reader may wish to review that section for details.

Anterior Anatomy (Fig. 10.2)

Eyelid

The eyeball is covered anteriorly by the eyelids, which protect it from injury. The skin of the eyelids covers the circularly-oriented orbicularis oculi muscle, while internally the lids are lined with the conjunctiva, a mucous membrane that reflects onto the anterior portion of the sclera. In addition, the upper lid possesses the *levator palpebrae superioris* muscle, which makes the upper lid larger than the lower lid. Everting the lid permits observation of the *tarsal glands* deep to the conjunctiva. These glands secrete an oily substance that assists in sealing the margins of the lids when the lids are closed and prevents

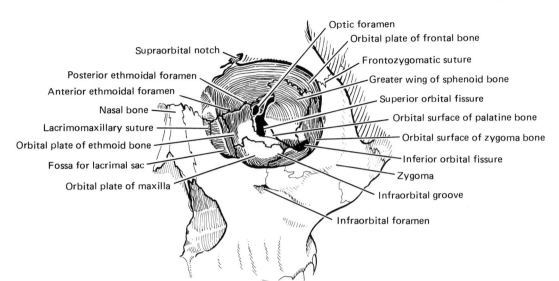

Optic foramen
Orbital plate of frontal bone
Supraorbital notch
Frontozygomatic suture
Posterior ethmoidal foramen
Greater wing of sphenoid bone
Anterior ethmoidal foramen
Superior orbital fissure
Nasal bone
Orbital surface of palatine bone
Lacrimomaxillary suture
Orbital surface of zygoma bone
Orbital plate of ethmoid bone
Inferior orbital fissure
Fossa for lacrimal sac
Zygoma
Orbital plate of maxilla
Infraorbital groove
Infraorbital foramen

Figure 10.1. Bony orbit.

overflow of tears when the lids are open. These glands, along with the *ciliary glands*, modified sudoriferous glands located in the margin, open via small pores onto the margin adjacent to the eyelashes. The eyelashes, arranged in rows of two or three, curve upward and downward on the upper and lower lids respectively.

The opened margins form an elliptical *palpebral fissure* narrowing laterally into an acute lateral palpebral commissure (lateral canthus) and medially into a larger medial palpebral commissure (medial canthus) possessing an enlarged triangular lacus lacrimalis with its caruncula.

TABLE 10.1
Bones of the Orbit

Region	Bones						
	Maxilla	*Frontal*	*Ethmoid*	*Lacrimal*	*Zygoma*	*Sphenoid*	*Palatine*
Apex						Lesser wing, body	
Floor	Orbital plate				Orbital process		Orbital process
Roof		Orbital plate				Lesser wing	
Medial wall	Frontal process		Orbital lamina	Orbital surface		Body	
Lateral wall					Orbital process	Greater wing (orbital surface)	
Base	Orbital rim	Orbital rim			Orbital rim		

Lacrimal Apparatus (Fig. 10.2)

The *lacrimal (tear) gland* is located in the lacrimal fossa at the anterosupero-lateral aspect of the orbit. The gland secretes fluid which is emptied into the conjunctival sac of the bulb of the eye. Each time the cornea dries, the lids, acting as windshield wipers, move the fluid over the sclera and cornea. The fluid moves medially to the lacrimal ducts, which begin as *puncta* (tiny orifices) at the lateral aspects of the lacus lacrimalis on the medial margins of the lids. The fluid passes from here to the *lacrimal sac* located in the groove mostly within the lacrimal bone. The sac represents the upper dilated portion of the *nasolacrimal duct,* which opens into the nasal cavity at the inferior nasal meatus.

Orb Anatomy (Fig. 10.3)

The bulb of the eye is almost spherical, except for its anterior portion which bulges away from the surface in the region of the eyelids. This anteriorly directed surface projection is the cornea. The transparent cornea represents a segment of a sphere occupying the anterior one-sixth of the bulb, while the remaining opaque bulb represents a more complete segment of a different-sized sphere. The anterior pole of the curvature of the cornea is nearly parallel with the posterior pole of the curvature of the remaining bulb, forming the optical axis. Due to the lateral divergence of the orbit cone, the optical axis and

TABLE 10.2
Communications of the Orbit

Openings communicating with the orbit*	Bones of the Orbit						
	Maxilla	*Frontal*	*Ethmoid*	*Lacrimal*	*Zygoma*	*Sphenoid*	*Palatine*
Optic foramen						x	
Superior orbital fissure		x				x	
Inferior orbital fissure	x				x	x	x
Infraorbital canal	x						
Anterior ethmoidal foramen		x	x				
Nasolacrimal sulcus	x			x			
Posterior ethmoidal foramen		x	x				
Supraorbital foramen		x					
Zygomatico-orbital foramen					x		

* When more than one bone is indicated, the opening is at the junction of two or more bones, or in the case of foramina, at a suture.

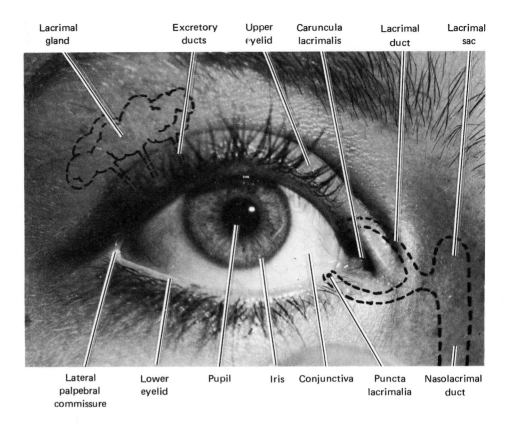

| Lacrimal gland | Excretory ducts | Upper eyelid | Caruncula lacrimalis | Lacrimal duct | Lacrimal sac |

| Lateral palpebral commissure | Lower eyelid | Pupil | Iris | Conjunctiva | Puncta lacrimalia | Nasolacrimal duct |

Figure 10.2. External anatomy of the eye.

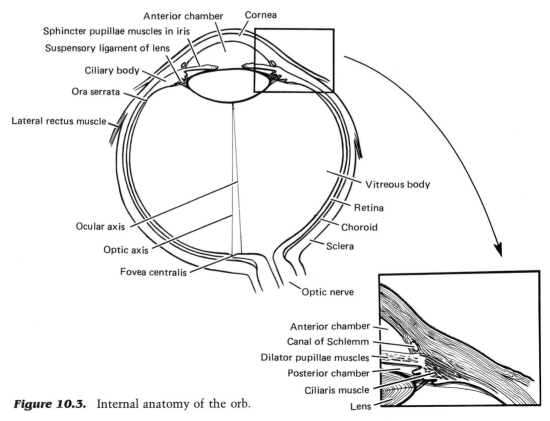

Figure 10.3. Internal anatomy of the orb.

the orbital axis do not coincide. The optic nerve (cranial nerve II) enters the posterior wall of the orb at the orbital axis about 3 mm to the nasal side of the optical axis, represented by the *macula.*

Tunics (Fig. 10.3)

The bulb of the eye is composed of three separate layers fabricated into one wall. The outer covering is the sclera and its modified anteriorly placed cornea. The middle or intermediate tunic is the pigmented, vascular coat composed of the choroid, ciliary body, and iris. The innermost tunic is the nervous component or retina.

The *sclera* is a tough fibrous layer comprising the outer wall of the bulb. It is white and very smooth, except where the extrinsic muscles insert into it. Its posterior portion is pierced by the optic nerve, while anteriorly it is covered by the conjunctiva. The anterior portion of the sclera, or the white of the eye, gives way to the transparent, anteriorly bulging *cornea.*

The *choroid,* the posteriorly located portion of the intermediate tunic, is a vascular, darkly pigmented layer closely adhering to the sclera and the retina. It is pierced by the optic nerve posteriorly.

The *ciliary body,* an intermediate zone between the choroid and the iris portions of the vascular tunic, extends from the most anteriorly located parts of the retina to the iris. Contained within the ciliary body, which juts away from the wall, is the ciliary muscle. Attached to the body are the suspensory ligaments of the lens. The involuntary (smooth) ciliary muscle receives its innervation via parasympathetic fibers originating in the oculomotor nerve. Contractions of this muscle reduce the tension on the suspensory ligament of the lens, permitting the lens to become more convex, thereby accommodating the eye to focus on objects nearby.

The *iris* is the most anteriorly placed portion of the intermediate tunic. The circular disc, imparted with color from a deep pigmented layer, possesses two separately arranged layers of smooth muscle whose contractions, when stimulated by autonomic nerves, alter the diameter of the hole in the center of the disk known as the *pupil.* The iris is continuous with the ciliary body and is connected to the cornea at its periphery. Its location, between the lens and the cornea, separates this space into an anterior chamber in front of it and a posterior chamber behind it. A watery fluid, the *aqueous humor,* is secreted into the posterior chamber of the eye by the ciliary body. This fluid passes from this chamber into the anterior chamber through ^he pupil lying upon the anterior surface of the lens. It exits the anterior chamber by draining into the canal of Schlemm located at the junction of the iris and cornea.

The *internal tunic* is composed of the nervous layer of the retina, posteriorly, and the nonnervous pars ciliaris and pars iridica retinae, anteriorly. Posteriorly, the nervous retina fans out from the optic nerve, where it is thickest, to near the ciliary body, where it ends in an irregular margin, the *ora serrata.* Though the nervous portion ends here, a remaining membrane passes over the ciliary body and the iris as the pigmented pars ciliaris and pars iridica retinae.

The nervous retina is composed of ten layers, the outer layer being the pigmented layer next to which lie the specialized receptors of light, the *rods* and *cones.* The rods are more numerous than the cones, except in the area of the *macula* and its centrally depressed *fovea centralis,* where the cones are concentrated making vision most acute. There are no rods or cones located in the optic disk which marks the exit of the optic nerve and entrance of the artery of the retina. This disk represents the only spot on the retina insensitive to light and is thus known as the *blind spot.*

Space does not permit the discussion of the individual layers of the retina. Further information may be gained from any standard histology textbook.

Refractive Media (Fig. 10.3)

The refractive media of the eye include (in order from anterior to posterior) the cornea, aqueous humor, lens, zonula ciliaris, and the vitreous body. The cornea and the aqueous humor have been discussed. The lens, a biconvex body which develops from surface ectoderm, is composed of several transparent layers covered by a capsule and retained in position by suspensory ligaments attached to the ciliary body. The transparent zonula ciliaris, ribbon-like fibrils radiating out from the ciliary body to the lens, imparts refractive capability. Filling the concavity behind the lens and the posterior chamber is the semigelatinous vitreous body, which is the most posterior light-refracting structure.

Muscles of the Eye (Figs. 10.3, 10.4, 10.5; Table 10.3)

Extrinsic Muscles

There are seven extrinsic muscles of the eye: the levator palpebrae superioris, the superior, inferior, medial, and lateral recti muscles, and the superior and inferior oblique muscles.

The *levator palpebrae superioris* originates on the inferior surface of the lesser wing of the sphenoid bone and inserts into the upper lid. As previously described, it functions to elevate the upper lid. The four *recti muscles— lateral, medial, superior,* and *inferior*—originate from a common tendinous ring surrounding the optic foramen. Each of these four muscles passes into the orbit and inserts into the sclera of the orb, a few millimeters posterior to the cornea in the position indicated by their names. These muscles function to pull the orb in the direction of the muscle insertion. Again, because of the lateral divergence of all structures entering the orbit, the resultant action of the superior and inferior recti muscles are complicated by a slight rotation and medialward deviation.

The *superior oblique muscle* arises from the body of the sphenoid bone immediately above the superior rectus muscle and passes anteriorly to end in a tendinous pully attached to the *trochlear fovea* of the frontal bone. From here, the tendon turns laterally beneath the superior rectus muscle to insert into the sclera between the superior and lateral rectus muscles. Contraction of this muscle directs the eye downward and laterally.

The *inferior oblique muscle* arises from the orbital surface of the maxilla lateral to the lacrimal groove. The muscle passes between the orbital floor and the inferior rectus to be inserted in the sclera between the lateral rectus and superior oblique muscles. The inferior oblique muscle functions to direct the eye upward and lateralward.

The levator palpebrae superioris and the superior, inferior, and medial recti, as well as the inferior oblique muscles are all innervated by branches of the oculomotor nerve. The superior oblique muscle is innervated by the trochlear nerve, the sole function of this nerve. Innervation to the lateral rectus muscle is provided by the abducent nerve, another cranial nerve which serves only a single function.

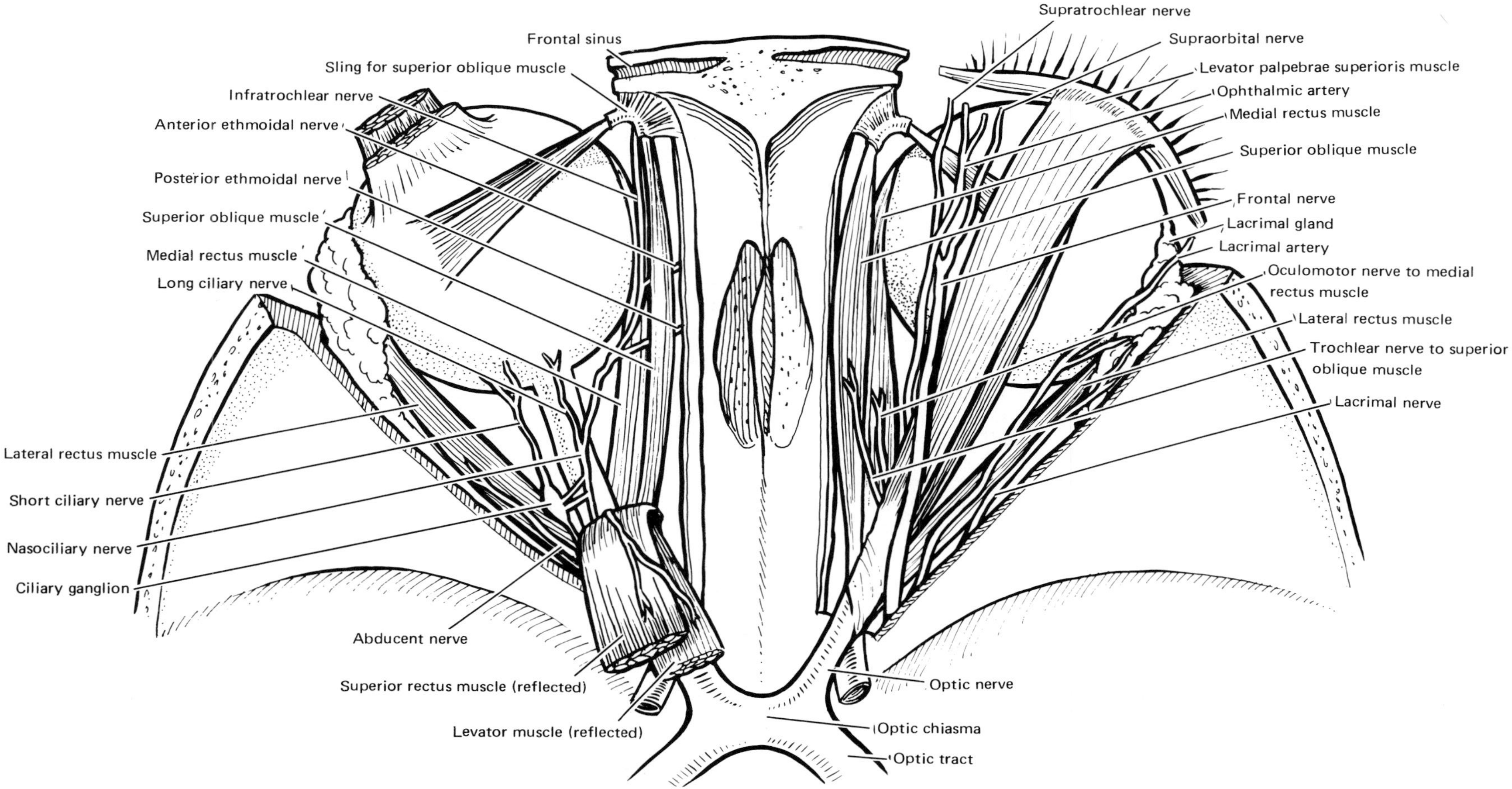

Figure 10.4. Structures within the orbit. Observe that the orbital plate of the frontal bone has been removed as has the periorbital fascia and fat. The right side represents a superficial dissection while the left side is a deeper view.

Supratrochlear nerve

Supraorbital nerve

Levator palpebrae superioris muscle

Ophthalmic artery

Medial rectus muscle

Superior oblique muscle

Frontal nerve

Lacrimal gland

Lacrimal artery

Oculomotor nerve to medial rectus muscle

Lateral rectus muscle

Trochlear nerve to superior oblique muscle

Lacrimal nerve

Optic nerve

Optic chiasma

Optic tract

Frontal sinus

Sling for superior oblique muscle

Infratrochlear nerve

Anterior ethmoidal nerve

Posterior ethmoidal nerve

Superior oblique muscle

Medial rectus muscle

Long ciliary nerve

Lateral rectus muscle

Short ciliary nerve

Nasociliary nerve

Ciliary ganglion

Abducent nerve

Superior rectus muscle (reflected)

Levator muscle (reflected)

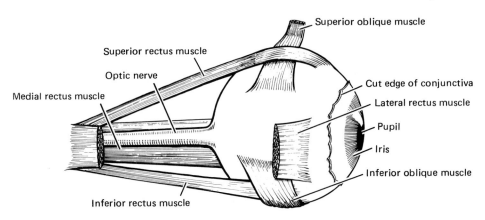

Figure 10.5. External muscles of the eye.

Intrinsic Muscles (Fig. 10.3)

The three intrinsic muscles of the eye are all involuntary. The *ciliary muscle,* which functions in accommodation, was described with the choroid layer. The two remaining intrinsic muscles, both located within the iris, are the sphincter pupillae and dilatator pupillae.

The *sphincter pupillae muscles* are arranged in a circular fashion in the iris around the pupil. Their contraction constricts the pupil. The *dilatator pupillae muscles* are arranged in a radiating band from near the margin of the pupil to the outer walls of the deep surface of the iris. Contractions of this muscle group produce a dilation of the pupil. Both of these muscle groups are innervated by fibers of the autonomic system. The sphincter muscle group is supplied by parasympathetic fibers originating in the oculomotor nerve. The dilator muscle group is innervated by the sympathetic system, whose postganglionic cell bodies are located in the superior cervical ganglion.

Nerves of the Orbit (Fig. 10.4)

The orbit possesses nerve components from six cranial nerves: the optic, oculomotor, trochlear, trigeminal, abducent, and secretomotor fibers from the facial. In addition, sympathetic fibers also serve the orbit.

Optic Nerve

The optic nerve consists of the axons of the ganglionic layer of the retina passing to the brain from the bulb through the optic foramen and to the optic chiasma. Here certain of the fibers cross over to the contralateral side to enter the optic tract to the brain, while other fibers remain on the ipsilateral side to enter the optic tract. Chapter 18 discusses this nerve in more detail.

Oculomotor Nerve

The oculomotor nerve enters the orbit through the superior orbital fissure, where it divides into superior and inferior divisions to innervate the intrinsic ciliary and sphincter muscles and all of the extrinsic muscles except the lateral rectus and the superior oblique. The superior division sends branches to the

TABLE 10.3
Muscles of the Eye

Muscle	Origin	Insertion	Innervation	Action*
Levator palpebrae superioris	Orbit roof	Upper eyelid, tarsal plate	Oculomotor	Elevates eyelid.
Extrinsic:				
Recti				
Superior	Common tendinous ring surrounding the optic foramen	Superior sclera anterior to equator	Oculomotor	Elevates cornea slightly medialward.
Inferior		Inferior sclera anterior to equator	Oculomotor	Depresses cornea slightly medialward.
Medial		Medial sclera anterior to equator	Oculomotor	Rotates cornea medially.
Lateral		Lateral sclera anterior to equator	Abducent	Rotates cornea laterally.
Obliques				
Superior	Orbit roof	Trochlea to posterosuperior quadrant of sclera	Trochlear	Rotates cornea inferolaterally.
Inferior	Orbit floor	Sclera, posteroinferior to superior oblique	Oculomotor	Rotates cornea superolaterally.
Intrinsic:				
Ciliary	Located in ciliary body adjacent to iris and attached to suspensory ligament of lens		Oculomotor via ciliary ganglion, short ciliary nerves	Releases pressure on side ligament of lens permitting it to accommodate.
Pupillae				
Sphincter	Circular band in iris surrounding the pupil		Oculomotor via ciliary ganglion and short ciliary nerves	Constricts pupil.
Dilatator	Radiating out in deep layers of iris from pupil		Sympathetic from superior cervical ganglion via long and short ciliary nerves	Dilates pupil.

* Actions described are assuming each muscle is acting alone.

levator palpebrae superioris and the superior rectus, while the inferior division innervates the medial and inferior recti and the inferior oblique muscles. This division also supplies parasympathetic motor fibers to the ciliary ganglion, a parasympathetic terminal ganglion located about 1 cm from the apex of the orbit between the optic nerve and the lateral rectus muscle. Preganglionic parasympathetic fibers synapse on postganglionic cell bodies within the ganglion. The axons of these cell bodies reach the orb via the *short ciliary nerves,* to be distributed to the ciliary and sphincter muscles.

Trochlear Nerve

The trochlear nerve enters the orbit through the superior orbital fissure on its way to the superior oblique muscle, the only muscle it serves.

Trigeminal Nerve

The *ophthalmic division* of the trigeminal nerve enters the orbit through the superior orbital fissure as three branches: the lacrimal, frontal, and nasociliary, all serving sensory function only.

The smallest, the *lacrimal,* runs laterally, superior to the lateral rectus, on its way to supply the lacrimal gland and adjacent conjunctiva with sensory innervation. This nerve often communicates with a secretomotor postganglionic parasympathetic fiber for the lacrimal gland from the pterygopalatine ganglion. Preganglionic fibers reach the ganglion from the facial nerve, while the postganglionic fibers are distributed to the lacrimal nerve via zygomaticotemporal branches of the maxillary division of the trigeminal nerve.

The *frontal nerve* is the largest nerve. It courses forward above the levator palpebrae superioris muscle. Midway in the orbit, it divides into a medial supratrochlear and a lateral supraorbital nerve. The *supratrochlear nerve* pierces the orbital fascia and supplies the conjunctiva, lid, and skin over the medial part of the forehead. The *supraorbital nerve* exits the orbit through the supraorbital notch or foramen to supply the frontal sinus, forehead, and scalp.

The *nasociliary nerve* crosses over the optic nerve on an oblique course to the anterior ethmoidal foramen. It communicates with the ciliary ganglion, where sensory fibers may pass through the ganglion without synapsing on their way to the orb via the short ciliary nerves. Other branches, termed *long ciliary nerves* (sensory), pass to the orb directly. Branches enter the anterior and posterior ethmoidal foramina. Just prior to entering the anterior ethmoidal foramen, the *infratrochlear nerve* arises to pass to the medial angle of the eye, supplying the skin of the lids and side of the nose. The *anterior* and *posterior ethmoidal nerves* serve the ethmoidal and frontal sinuses. *Internal* and *external nasal branches,* derived from the anterior ethmoidal nerve, supply the mucous membranes of the anterior septum and the skin over the ala of the nose, respectively.

The maxillary division of the trigeminal nerve enters the floor of the orbit through the inferior orbital fissure. It is not discussed here, since its only contribution to the orbit is a few periosteal branches.

Abducent Nerve

The abducent nerve enters the orbit through the superior orbital fissure passing laterally to innervate the lateral rectus muscle.

Sympathetic Nerves

Postganglionic sympathetic fibers whose cell bodies are located in the superior cervical ganglion find their way into the orbit as communications to several cranial nerves from the carotid plexus, traveling to their destination via these routes or via the arteries of the orbit. Those destined for the dilatator pupillae muscles reach the orb either by long ciliary nerves or by passing, with sensory branches from the nasociliary, through the ganglion and the short ciliary nerves.

Vascular Supply (Fig. 10.4)

The *ophthalmic artery* enters the orbit through the optic canal and divides into two groups. The orbital group serves some of the accessory structures to the orb, and the ocular group serves the extrinsic muscles and the orb proper, including the retina, ciliary body, and the intrinsic muscles.

Superior and *inferior ophthalmic veins* drain the structures of the orbit and empty their contents into the cavernous sinus. A branch of the inferior ophthalmic vein also empties into the pterygoid venous plexus.

CLINICAL CONSIDERATIONS

Abnormal protrusion of the eyeball, exophthalmos, may occur in hyperthyroidism or in an aneurysm of an orbital artery. Changes in the length dimension of the optical axis will cause images to be focused anterior to the retina (myopia) or posterior to the retina (hyperopia).

Sudden jolts absorbed in the orbit may detach the retina thus requiring surgery.

Cataract is a condition in which the lens loses its transparency and becomes milky, causing blurred vision. Modern techniques now permit surgical placement of plastic lenses.

Glaucoma refers to a condition resulting from increased pressure in the anterior chamber of the eye due to more aqueous humor being produced than is being drained off. Over a prolonged period, the increased pressure can damage the retina causing blindness. Drugs may be employed to reduce the production of the humor.

EAR

Development

The organ of hearing and balance begins its development shortly after that of the eye. It develops from a thickening of the hindbrain to form the mechanism for balance and the cochlea for hearing, both of which make up the internal ear and eventually become surrounded by the petrous portion of the temporal bone.

The middle ear and auditory tube develop from the first pharyngeal pouch, as described in Chapter 5. Interposed between the endodermal lining of the auditory tube and the ectodermal lining of the pharyngeal groove is the closing plate, which persists as the *tympanum* (eardrum) (Fig. 5.4).

It is within this middle ear cavity that the bony ossicles develop. By way of review, the *malleus* (hammer) and its muscle the *tensor tympani* develop from first arch mesoderm, as does the *incus* (anvil). The *stapes* (stirrup) and its muscle, the *stapedius,* develop from second arch mesoderm. In keeping with the rule that structures developing within an arch are innervated by the nerve of that arch, it then follows that the tensor tympani muscle is innervated by the trigeminal nerve, while the stapedius muscle is innervated by the facial nerve.

External Ear (Fig. 10.6)

The external ear comprised of the pinna and the external auditory meatus, develop from the first pharyngeal groove and tubercles of tissue from arches I and II around the groove.

Several muscles develop from the second arch in the vicinity of the ear, all of which are innervated by the facial nerve. They are the extrinsic muscle group, including the anterior, superior, and posterior auricular muscles, and an

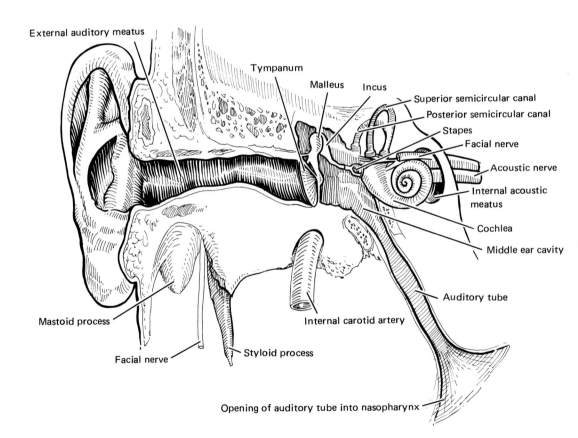

Figure 10.6. The ear.

intrinsic group including some six small, insignificant, vestigial muscles which are not described here.

Nerve Supply

Sensory innervation to the pinna and the external auditory meatus is broad and overlapping. It includes the great auricular, auricular branch of the vagus, auriculotemporal branch of the trigeminal, and the lesser occipital nerves.

Middle Ear (Fig. 10.6; Table 10.4)

The middle ear or tympanic cavity is a mucous membrane-lined, air-filled space within the temporal bone that communicates with the mastoid air cells through a small opening and with the nasopharynx via the cartilaginous auditory tube (Fig. 4.20). It is through the latter communication that atmospheric pressure is equalized on either side of the tympanum.

The rostral end of the tympanic cavity contains the bony ossicles. On the lateral wall, attached to the tympanum by several ligaments, is the malleus and its muscle, the tensor tympani. The stapes and the stapedius muscle are attached by the ligaments to the medial wall, where the footplate of the stapes impinges upon the *fenestra vestibuli* (oval window) of the cochlea. Interposed between the malleus and the stapes is the incus, which articulates with both. Located inferior to the oval window is the *fenestra cochleae* (round window) covered by a membrane, the secondary tympanic membrane.

Vessels and Nerves

Many vessels supply the structures of the middle ear. These vessels arise from several sources, which include the tympanic branches from the maxillary, the stylomastoid branch of the posterior auricular, and many small branches from the pharyngeal, middle meningeal, and the internal carotid arteries. Venous drainage follows the arteries to become tributaries of the superior petrosal sinus and the pterygoid plexus of veins.

The *tympanic plexus* of nerves located in the middle ear is derived from

TABLE 10.4
Bony Ossicles and Their Associations

Ossicle	Attachments		Ligaments	Muscle	Nerve
	Lateral	*Medial*			
Malleus (Hammer)	Tympanum	Incus	Anterior Superior Lateral	Tensor Tympani	Chorda tympani crosses manubrium
Incus (Anvil)	Malleus	Stapes	Posterior Superior		
Stapes (Stirrup)	Incus	Oval window of the cochlea	Annular ligament of base	Stapedius	

the glossopharyngeal nerve and sympathetic fibers which serve the mucous membranes. In addition, the cranial portion of the facial nerve enters the bony medial wall of the cavity on its way to the stylomastoid foramen, where it will exit the skull. While there it gives off a motor branch to the stapedius as well as to the chorda tympani, which passes over the tympanic membrane and across the malleus to exit the cavity.

Inner Ear (Fig. 10.6)

The inner ear, entirely embedded in the petrous temporal bone, lies medial to the middle ear. It consists of a bony and a membranous labyrinth. The *bony labyrinth* is composed of the vestibule, semicircular canals, and the cochlea, filled with fluid (perilymph). Suspended within the perilymph is the *membranous labyrinth* containing its own endolymph.

The *vestibule,* containing the oval window, occupies a central position in the bony labyrinth. Projecting from it, posteriorly and superiorly, are the three *semicircular canals,* arranged so that each canal and its dilated ampulla lies at right angles to the other two. Projecting anteriorly from the vestibule is the *cochlea,* a bony structure turned upon itself two and one-half times around a central core termed the *modiolus,* giving it the appearance of a snail's shell. The lateral wall contains the round window.

The membranous labyrinth is composed of the semicircular ducts, the cochlear duct, and two sacs, the utricle and the saccule. The utricle occupies the vestibule, while the saccule lies anteroinferior to it. The endolymph from the semicircular ducts is received in the utricle. Endolymph from the cochlear duct is received into the saccule via the small ductus reuniens. A small endolymphatic duct ending in a blind pouch projects posteriorly with communications from the saccule and utricle. The cochlear duct separates the cochlea into the scala vestibuli superiorly and scala tympani inferiorly. These two scalae are in communication near the summit of the cochlea through a tiny pore called the *helicotrema.* The cochlear duct, composed of a spiral membranous tube, houses the *spiral organ of Corti* in its basilar membrane. The spiral organ receives peripheral nerve endings from that portion of the acoustic nerve responsible for receiving sensations and transmitting them to the brain for processing into what we perceive as sounds.

Nerves

The acoustic nerve (cranial nerve VIII), in company with the facial nerve (cranial nerve VII), enters the internal auditory meatus of the temporal bone. Shortly thereafter, the facial nerve departs from the acoustic nerve to enter the facial canal. Remembering that it supplies the stapedius with motor fibers and that it gives rise to the chorda tympani is sufficient at this point. On the other hand, the acoustic nerve is the nerve that conveys impulses from both the vestibular (balance) and auditory (hearing) mechanisms. The acoustic nerve consists of two separate sets of fibers: the vestibular nerve for balance and the cochlear for hearing. After entering the meatus as a single nerve, the two separate and enter the membranous labyrinth to terminate as special endings at the receptor sites.

For additional information regarding the stato-acoustic system, refer to Gray's Anatomy for a more thorough discussion of its anatomy and function.

CLINICAL CONSIDERATIONS

The auditory tube permits the spread of infection from the nasal cavity into the middle ear cavity. This condition *(otis media)* resulting from acute infection may rupture the eardrum and/or it may pass into the mastoid air cells. Antibiotics are used to circumvent and treat this condition. Occasionally, the stapes becomes immobilized due to bony deposits around the oval window. This condition, *otosclerosis,* is correctable by surgical procedures. These two situations, if left untreated, will most assuredly result in deafness. Acoustic nerve destruction will also lead to deafness, as will some drugs and other factors, including intense noise of high frequency over a prolonged period of time.

CHAPTER 11

Parotid Bed

SUPERFICIAL ANATOMY AND BOUNDARIES (Fig. 11.1)

The space lying between the ramus of the mandible, the external acoustic meatus, and the mastoid and styloid processes of the temporal bone is the *parotid bed.* The medial extent of this bed is at the posterior belly of the digastric muscle and the muscles of the styloid process. Inferiorly, the bed is bounded by the superoanterior border of the sternocleidomastoid muscle. This rather irregularly shaped area houses the parotid gland, which is molded into this space thus assisting in filling out the contour of the jaw/neck/ear junction.

Representatives of two cranial nerves—the facial and trigeminal—pass through the substance of the gland to reach their destinations in and about the head and neck. Similarly, the external carotid artery and some of its branches course through the gland as do some of the tributaries forming the external jugular vein.

PAROTID GLAND (Figs. 11.1, 11.2, 11.3)

The parotid gland is the largest of the three major salivary glands and is enclosed within a capsule which is part of the deep cervical fascia. It is located on the lateral aspect of the face in the parotid bed. Since the gland is molded into an irregular space, it is also irregular in shape. The superficial aspect of the gland extends superiorly over the masseter muscle to the zygomatic arch, where an accessory portion of the gland may be detached from the main substance. Inferiorly, it is mostly confined to the region between the mastoid process, the sternocleidomastoid muscle, and the angle of the mandible, where it extends over the posterior aspect of the masseter muscle. Medially, the gland extends into the deeper portions of the parotid bed to the styloid process and its attached musculature. Here, a wedge-shaped portion of the gland may intervene between the medial and lateral pterygoid muscles for a short distance. Often glandular lobes extend into other spaces adjacent to the parotid bed. One such lobe passes between the ramus of the mandible and the medial pterygoid muscle above its insertion, while others pass between the external auditory meatus and the temporomandibular joint and between the external carotid artery and the superior constrictor muscle of the pharynx.

Emanating from the anterior aspect of the superficial portion of the gland is the *parotid duct (Stenson's duct),* which passes anteriorly, superficial to the masseter muscle, to dive medially into the buccal fat pad, where it pierces the buccinator muscle on its way to the oral vestibule. It delivers the parotid salivary secretions at the opening of the parotid papilla opposite the second maxillary molar.

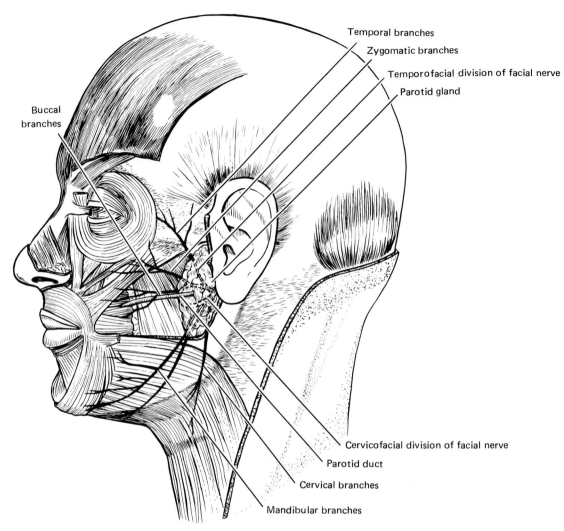

Temporal branches
Zygomatic branches
Temporofacial division of facial nerve
Parotid gland
Buccal branches
Cervicofacial division of facial nerve
Parotid duct
Cervical branches
Mandibular branches

Figure 11.1. Parotid gland and facial nerve.

Relationships

Since the parotid gland is irregular in shape, possessing many finger-like projections radiating in several directions from the parotid bed, the gland associates with or engulfs many of the structures passing through this region. Those structures associated with the superficial aspect of the gland include branches of the great auricular nerve from the cervical plexus that provide sensory innervation to the region and small lymph nodes which drain the superficial area. Structures associated with the deep aspect of the gland, provided it sends projections medial to the styloid process, include the external and internal carotid arteries, internal jugular vein, and both the vagus and glossopharyngeal nerves.

Several structures pass through the gland. The external carotid artery enters the substance of the gland, and it is there that several of its branches arise, including the posterior auricular, maxillary, and superficial temporal arteries. The retromandibular vein, as well as the veins uniting to form it, also pass through the gland.

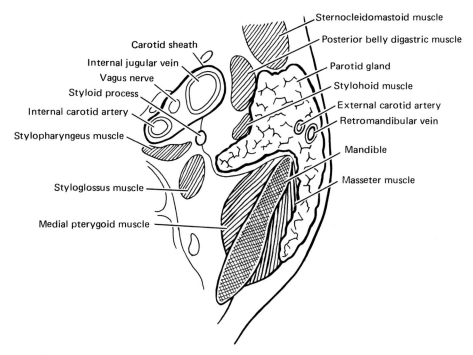

Figure 11.2. Cross section through parotid bed.

The facial nerve, or cranial nerve VII, exits the stylomastoid foramen and enters the substance of the gland. In the gland, the facial nerve forms a plexus before exiting to innervate the muscles of facial expression. The *auriculotemporal nerve,* a branch of the mandibular division of the trigeminal nerve or cranial nerve V, enters the substance of the gland from its deep aspect along the neck of the mandible and emerges from the gland just inferior to the root of the zygomatic arch. While within the gland, it will communicate with the facial nerve and distribute fibers to the gland. These functions are considered in the next section and in the section in this chapter on the facial nerve.

The structures entering the parotid gland exit from its posterior, superior, inferior, and anterior surfaces. The posterior auricular artery exits from the posterior aspect of the gland. The superficial temporal artery and vein, auriculotemporal nerve, and temporal branches of the facial nerve may be observed at the superior margin of the gland. Inferiorly, the retromandibular vein exits the parotid gland just prior to joining the posterior auricular vein to form the external jugular vein. Emanating from the entire facial margin of the gland are the terminal branches of the facial nerve, which are grouped into the five major branches: the *temporal, zygomatic, buccal, mandibular,* and *cervical branches.*

Vascularization, Lymphatics, and Innervation

The posterior auricular artery, arising from the external carotid artery within the substance of the gland, provides branches which vascularize the gland. Additional small glandular branches from the superficial temporal and transverse facial arteries also supply the gland. Venous drainage is via the tributaries passing through the gland which empty into the external jugular vein.

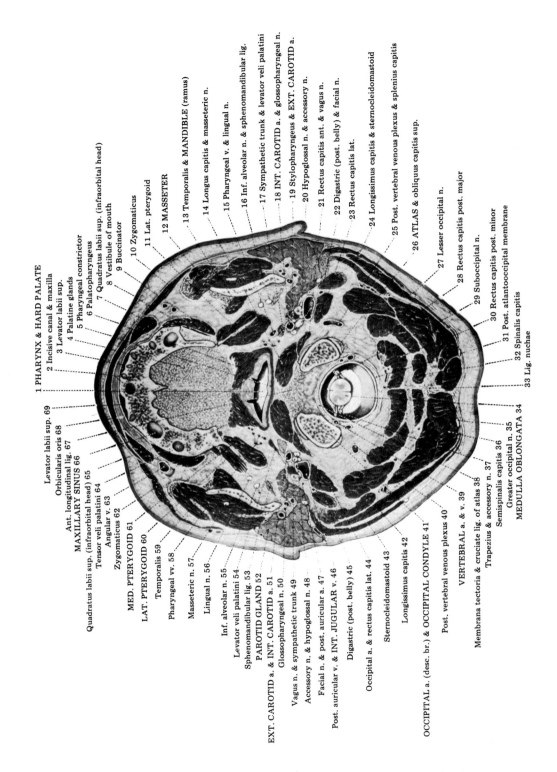

Figure 11.3. The head in cross-section. Observe the extent of the parotid gland in and about the structures deep to the parotid bed. (From B. L. Carter, J. Morehead, S. M. Wolpert, S. B. Hammershlag, H. J. Griffith and P. C. Kahn *Cross-sectional Anatomy*, 1st ed., New York, Appleton-Century-Crofts, 1977.)

Lymph nodes located superficially and within the substance of the gland drain the lymphatics into the *superficial* and *deep cervical lymph nodes.* A more detailed discussion of the lymphatic system of the head and neck is found in Chapter 20.

Innervation of the parotid gland is of sensory and autonomic function. General sensation is provided by branches of the *great auricular nerve* as it ramifies over the surface of the gland. The sympathetic component of the autonomic system reaches the gland via postganglionic sympathetic fibers of the carotid plexus, which travel on the external carotid artery and its branches in the gland. Sympathetic innervation to the parotid gland mediates vasoconstriction within the gland.

Parasympathetic innervation is distributed to the gland by the auriculotemporal nerve, though the parasympathetic fibers do not arise within the trigeminal complex. Preganglionic parasympathetic fibers from the glossopharyngeal nerve, or cranial nerve IX, pass from its tympanic branch to the otic ganglion, where they synapse on postganglionic cell bodies. Fibers from here then join the auriculotemporal branch of the mandibular division of the trigeminal nerve to be distributed to the gland effecting secretomotor functions.

CAROTID ARTERIES (Figs. 11.2, 11.3, 11.4)

The internal and external carotid arteries arise in the neck from a bifurcation of the common carotid artery at the level of the superior border of the thyroid cartilage. The internal carotid artery then ascends in the neck, providing no branches until it enters the carotid canal of the petrous portion of the temporal bone. In its ascent deep to the parotid gland, the digastric muscle, and the muscles attached to the styloid process, this artery is contained within the carotid sheath in company with the internal jugular vein and the vagus nerve.

The external carotid artery, in contrast, supplies many of the structures of the neck and face. Those branches supplying the neck are described in Chapter 7. Branches originating from the external carotid artery inferior to the parotid bed, such as the lingual and facial arteries, are discussed in appropriate chapters. Several arteries either originate in or are in close association with the parotid bed and are best described at this point. These arteries are the ascending pharyngeal, occipital, posterior auricular, maxillary, and the superficial temporal.

The *ascending pharyngeal artery* arises from the external carotid near its origin and ascends between the pharynx and the internal carotid artery. Through its several named branches, it supplies some of the prevertebral muscles, a portion of the tympanic cavity, and portions of the soft palate. Pharyngeal branches supply the stylopharyngeus and the pharyngeal constrictor muscles before the artery terminates as meningeal branches upon entering the jugular foramen.

The *occipital artery* originates from the posterior aspect of the external carotid artery just prior to its diving deep to the posterior belly of the digastric muscle. The occipital courses under the cover of the digastric and stylohyoid muscles, which it supplies with muscular branches, as it passes posteriorly to groove the mastoid process of the temporal bone. This artery supplies the sternocleidomastoid muscle, auricle, posterior neck musculature, and men-

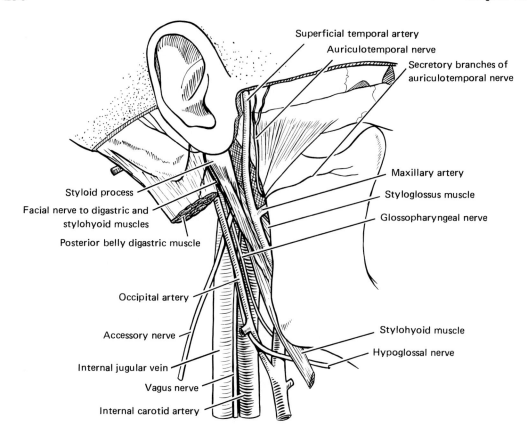

Figure 11.4. Structures deep to the parotid bed.

inges through its named branches, while the terminal branches serve the scalp and its musculature.

The internal and external carotid arteries become separated from their close association in the parotid bed as they pass deep and superficial, respectively, to the styloid process. The superficial position places the external carotid within the substance of the gland and, while there, the posterior auricular artery arises as do the two terminal arteries of the external carotid, the maxillary and superficial temporal.

The *posterior auricular artery* arises near the apex of the styloid process and, passing through the parotid gland which it supplies, sends branches to the digastric, stylohyoid, and sternocleidomastoid muscles. Named branches include the *stylomastoid artery,* which enters the like-named foramen to supply the tympanic cavity; the *auricular artery* passing to the posterior aspect of the ear; and the *occipital artery,* which supplies the scalp and occipitalis muscle.

The *maxillary artery* arises from the external carotid artery as it nears the deep aspect of the neck of the mandible, while within the gland, branches named the *deep auricular* and *anterior tympanic* pass posteriorly to the ear and tympanic cavity. The artery then passes anteriorly between the ramus of the mandible and the sphenomandibular ligament, where it exits the substance of the gland to enter the deep face. Its branches and distribution are presented in Chapter 12.

The smaller, terminal *superficial temporal artery* exits the parotid gland to become superficial as it crosses the zygomatic arch posterior to the mandible, in company with the auriculotemporal nerve. While within the parotid gland, the artery sends unnamed branches to the gland, the temporomandibular joint, and the masseter muscle. Also originating while within the gland is the *transverse facial artery,* which exits the gland between the zygomatic arch and the parotid duct. Its distribution is discussed in Chapter 8.

Other named branches arising from the superficial temporal artery include the middle temporal; zygomaticoorbital; anterior auricular; and the terminal, frontal and parietal branches. These branches freely anastomose with arteries distributing to these same areas.

FACIAL NERVE (Fig. 11.1)

The facial nerve is treated in detail in Chapter 18; however, since the nerve is in intimate association with the parotid bed and gland, its relationship and distribution to the structures in this area are discussed here.

The *facial nerve* exits from the cranial cavity at the stylomastoid foramen located in the temporal bone just posterior to the styloid process. Upon exiting, it communicates with the glossopharyngeal and vagus nerves and with the great auricular nerve of the cervical plexus. The auriculotemporal nerve from the mandibular division of the trigeminal nerve communicates with the facial nerve after it has entered the substance of the parotid gland. Presumably, this communication provides general sensory fibers from the trigeminal nerve to the facial nerve for distribution to the face. Branches arising from the facial nerve as it passes through this area include the posterior auricular, digastric, stylohyoid, and the parotid plexus with its terminals.

The *posterior auricular nerve* arises near the stylomastoid foramen and ascends behind the ear. This branch supplies motor innervation to the auricular and occipital muscles. The *digastric* and *stylohoid* branches provide motor innervation to the like-named muscles as each branch arises near that muscle. Upon entering the substance of the parotid gland, the facial nerve terminates into two communicating branches often forming a loop within the gland. The superior is the temporofacial branch, while the cervicofacial branch is the inferior portion of the nerve. Arising from this *parotid plexus* are the five major nerve branches emanating from the facial aspect of the parotid gland, which ramify over the superficial face as the temporal, zygomatic, buccal, mandibular, and cervical branches serving the muscles of facial expression with motor innervation. The specific distribution of these branches is described in Chapter 8.

STRUCTURES DEEP TO THE PAROTID BED (Fig. 11.4)

Muscles and Ligament

Technically, there are no muscles within the parotid bed. However, several muscles yet to be described are in close association with and/or form the boundaries of the bed and are, therefore, best described here.

The *masseter muscle,* which is attached to the lateral aspect of the ramus of the mandible is in intimate association with the parotid gland. However, since it is one of the muscles of mastication, a discussion of it is deferred to Chapter 12.

The *digastric muscle,* it will be recalled, serves to form the boundaries of several of the subtriangles in the anterior triangle of the neck. It also assists in forming the medial boundary of the parotid bed and is comprised of two separate bellies united by an intermediate tendon at the hyoid bone. The posterior belly, the only portion associated with the parotid bed, arises from the mastoid notch on the temporal bone and passes anteroinferiorly to the hyoid bone. It is about this bone that the intermediate tendon unites the two bellies, as the tendon perforates the stylohyoid muscle near its insertion on the hyoid bone. The posterior belly of the digastric muscle is innervated by a branch of the facial nerve which enters its deep surface at about midbelly. With its anterior component, the posterior belly functions to fix the hyoid bone. Specifically, the posterior belly pulls the hyoid bone posteriorly. A more thorough discussion of both bellies will be presented in Chapter 15 on the submandibular region.

The *stylohyoid muscle,* another muscle forming the medial boundary of the parotid bed, arises from the posterior and lateral aspects of the styloid process of the temporal bone. The origin of this muscle places it anterior to the posterior belly of the digastric. The two muscles are rather closely associated, since the stylohyoid also passes anteroinferiorly to insert on the body of the hyoid bone. The muscle is perforated, as described previously, by the digastric tendon. The stylohyoid muscle is innervated by a branch of the facial nerve, which passes very close by, on its way to the parotid gland. This muscle, not unlike the posterior belly of the digastric, assists in fixing the hyoid bone by pulling it posteriorly and superiorly.

Associated with the stylohyoid muscle and the styloid process is a ligamentous band, the *stylohyoid ligament,* suspended between the tip of the styloid process and the lesser cornu of the hyoid bone. This ligament, formed by a thickening of the deep parotid fascia, assists in separating the parotid and submandibular glands, as does the similarly formed stylomandibular ligament, described as an accessory ligament to the temporomandibular joint.

Two other muscles arise from the styloid process in addition to the stylohyoid muscle. These are the styloglossus and stylopharyngeus muscles. Though a more complete discussion regarding these two muscles is presented in subsequent chapters, a brief discussion is warranted here.

The *styloglossus muscle* arises from the styloid process and inserts into the side of the tongue. This muscle is innervated by the hypoglossal nerve (cranial nerve XII) and functions to draw the tongue superiorly and posteriorly.

The *stylopharyngeus muscle* arises from the styloid process and inserts into the lateral wall of the pharynx between the superior and medial pharyngeal constrictor muscles. The glossopharyngeal nerve (cranial nerve IX) innervates this muscle.

Arteries and Nerves

Immediately deep to the muscles originating on the styloid process are the last four cranial nerves, the internal carotid artery, and the internal jugular vein. The glossopharyngeal, vagus, and spinal accessory nerves exit the skull through the jugular foramen, while the hypoglossal nerve exits the skull via the hypoglossal canal. As these nerves descend to the structures they will innervate, they may be observed passing on the lateral surface of the internal carotid artery and internal jugular vein. These two vessels and the vagus nerve are housed in the carotid sheath. The laterally-placed internal jugular vein, originating at the jugular foramen, descends to enter the subclavian vein at the root of the neck. The internal carotid artery ascends within the sheath to enter the carotid canal in the petrous portion of the temporal bone.

CLINICAL CONSIDERATIONS

There is some evidence that the facial nerve may supply parasympathetic innervation to the parotid gland in addition to that from the glossopharyngeal nerve. This subject is treated in Chapter 18.

Occasionally, the stylohyoid ligament becomes cartilaginous and/or ossifies and thus appears as a radiopaque structure in a radiograph. Apparently, this condition has no pathologic consequence.

Mumps, a viral infection of the parotid gland which causes profuse swelling of the gland, impinges upon the auriculotemporal and great auricular nerves causing much pain as the gland is pressured during mastication.

Tumors of the parotid gland may be excised but with extreme care, since any damage to the facial nerve will result in at least partial facial paralysis. Total destruction of the facial nerve results in complete facial paralysis (Bell's palsy).

Occasionally, calculus accumulations occur in the parotid duct, thereby obstructing salivary flow. Radiological examination upon injecting radiopaque dye into the parotid duct opening *(sialography)* identifies the region which may be relieved surgically.

CHAPTER 12

Deep Face

The region to be described in this chapter is considered the deep face. It encompasses the structures deep to the mandible, including three of the muscles of mastication. The fourth muscle of mastication, the masseter muscle, lies superficial to the mandible, but it is described here for the sake of continuity. The normal functioning of this muscle group, a part of the stomatognathic system, is essential for good oral health.

Located within the deep face are certain sensory branches of the maxillary and mandibular divisions of the trigeminal nerve which transmit sensory innervation from the teeth and associated structures of the upper and lower jaws, respectively. In addition, the mandibular division provides sensory innervation to the temporomandibular joint, another component of the stomatognathic system. The motor root of the trigeminal nerve unites with the mandibular division just outside the skull for distribution to the muscles of mastication and the few additional muscles developed within the first branchial arch mesoderm. The vascular supply to this region similarly serves some of the oral cavity and teeth, in addition to supplying the temporomandibular joint, some parts of the ear, and the muscles of mastication.

A thorough understanding of this region of anatomy is of paramount importance to the dental professional, if that person is to comprehend the complexities of the stomatognathic system in normal and pathologic functions. It is imperative that a person diagnosing and treating inadequate anaesthesia, malocclusion, the maladies of pain, and the spread of infection in and about the oral cavity "know her or his anatomy."

DESCRIPTIONS AND BOUNDARIES

Temporal Fossa (Fig. 6.5)

The side of the head anterior and superior to the ear is commonly called the *temple*. The skin, fascia, and portions of the extrinsic muscles of the ear in this region overlie the deeper fan-shaped temporalis muscle attached to the bones of the *temporal fossa*. This fossa is bounded by the superior temporal line, superiorly, while its inferior boundary is arbitrarily designated to be the zygomatic arch, even though the temporalis muscle extends inferiorly below the arch into the infratemporal fossa. The floor of the temporal fossa is formed by the bones of the side of the head—portions of the frontal, sphenoid, temporal, and parietal bones. The superiormost extent of the origin of the temporalis muscle marks these bones with the temporal lines. These lines begin at the zygomatic process of the frontal bone and arch posteriorly over the parietal bone before descending to the temporal bone and blending into the zygomatic process of this bone.

Infratemporal Fossa (Fig. 6.6; Table 12.1)

The region inferior to the zygomatic arch and deep to the mandible is termed the *infratemporal fossa*. This irregular space, posterior to the maxilla which forms its anterior wall, is bounded laterally by the ramus and coronoid process of the mandible, while its medial extent is the lateral pterygoid plate of the sphenoid bone. Superiorly, the fossa is limited by the infratemporal surface of the greater wing of the sphenoid bone and the very antero-inferiormost portion of the temporal squama. The bony ridge extending across these two bones is known as the *infratemporal crest*, delineating the superiormost extent of the roof of the fossa. Inferiorly, the infratemporal fossa has no boundary but extends into the neck lateral to the pharynx.

Communications

The infratemporal fossa communicates with the temporal fossa as the temporalis muscle descends from its origin in the temporal fossa to be inserted onto the coronoid process of the mandible. Nerves and vessels supplying the temporalis muscle pass from the infratemporal fossa to the temporal fossa to pierce the deep surface of this muscle. Two foramina open onto its roof on the medial aspect of the infratemporal region of the greater wing of the sphenoid. The larger of the two, the foramen ovale, transmits the mandibular division of the trigeminal nerve exiting from the cranial vault and the accessory meningeal artery proceeding to the cranium. The smaller foramen, the foramen spinosum, lies between the foramen ovale and the spine of the sphenoid. It transmits the middle meningeal artery and the recurrent meningeal nerve from the fossa into the cranium.

The fossa communicates with the orbit at its most superoanterior aspect via the inferior orbital fissure between the maxilla and the greater wing of the sphenoid. Through this fissure pass the maxillary division of the trigeminal nerve, on its way to the floor of the orbit, as well as the zygomatic branch which arises from it. The cleft between the maxilla and the lateral pterygoid plate is the pterygomaxillary fissure communicating with the pterygopalatine fossa, medially. It is through this fissure that the maxillary artery distributes to the fossa, eventually to reach the nasal cavity via the sphenopalatine foramen. The posterior superior alveolar nerve, arising from the maxillary nerve as the latter nerve traverses the pterygopalatine fossa, utilizes the pterygomaxillary fissure as an exit on its way to the tuberosity of the maxilla.

MUSCLES AND FASCIA

The muscles of mastication (Table 12.2), all of which are developed in first branchial arch mesoderm, are located within the confines of the deep face, with the exception of the masseter muscle previously described as lateral to the mandible. These muscles, excepting the masseter, originate on the deep bony aspect of the temporal and infratemporal fossae and insert upon the me-

TABLE 12.1
Boundaries, Communications, and Contents of Infratemporal Fossa

Region	Boundary	Communications	Contents
Superior	Infratemporal surface of greater wing of sphenoid and infratemporal crest plus small part of temporal	Cranial cavity via foramen ovale, foramen spinosum; temporal fossa	Temporalis muscle (inferior portion) Medial pterygoid muscle Lateral pterygoid muscle Maxillary artery and branches Pterygoid plexus of veins Chorda tympani nerve Otic ganglion Mandibular nerve and branches Posterior superior alveolar nerve
Inferior	Continuous with submandibular region		
Medial	Lateral pterygoid plate of sphenoid	Pterygopalatine fossa via pterygomaxillary fissure	
Lateral	Ramus and coronoid process of mandible		
Anterior	Posterior aspect of maxilla to the inferior orbital fissure	Orbit via inferior orbital fissure	
Posterior	Continuous with structures about the styloid process		

dial aspect of the mandible. The masseter, in contrast, originates on the zygomatic arch and inserts upon the lateral aspect of the mandible. This group of muscles, the temporalis, medial pterygoid, lateral pterygoid, and masseter are covered by their epimysia, which become the fascia encircling the *masticator compartment.* The masticator compartment contains the four muscles of mastication and the ramus of the mandible (Fig. 12.1). The *temporal fascia* spans from the superior temporal line over the temporalis muscle to attach to the zygomatic arch on both its medial and lateral surfaces. The *parotideomasseteric fascia,* attached cranially to the zygomatic arch, splits to encompass the parotid gland as it passes on the lateral surface of the masseter muscle to become continuous with the deep cervical fascia about the suprahyoid muscles. The *masseteric fascia* covers the masseter muscle and encircles the ramus of the mandible, inferiorly, where it becomes continuous with the *pterygoid fascia.*

Both the lateral and medial pterygoid muscles are enclosed by the pterygoid fascia. However, the fascia is much thicker covering the inferior aspect of the medial pterygoid muscle, where it becomes continuous with the cervical and masseteric fascia as well as with the stylomandibular ligament. Where the pterygoid fascia reflects over the superior portion of the medial pterygoid muscle, it splits to encompass the lateral pterygoid muscle as well and is attached to the bony origin of that muscle and to the spine of the sphenoid bone. The latter attachment is much thickened, forming the *sphenomandibular ligament* from the spine of the sphenoid bone to the lingula of the mandible (Fig. 13.2). The thickened portion of the pterygoid fascia, located between the two pterygoid muscles spanning between the spine of the sphenoid and the lateral pterygoid plate, is known as the *pterygospinous ligament.* Occasionally this ligament is ossified. When that is the case, a pterygospinous foramen is present

TABLE 12.2
Muscles of Mastication

Muscle	Origin	Insertion
Masseter	Superficial: tendinous aponeurosis from zygomatic process of maxilla and anterior two-thirds of inferior border of zygomatic arch Deep: medial aspect and inferior border of posterior one-third of zygomatic arch	Lateral aspect of ramus and angle of mandible as far anteriorly as the last molar tooth, as far superiorly as base of coronoid process
Temporalis	Inferior temporal line and bones of the temporal fossa	As a tendon on coronoid process and anterior border of ramus of mandible as far inferiorly and anteriorly as third molar
Medial (internal) pterygoid	Pterygoid fossa and medial surface of lateral pterygoid plate; one slip from lateral portion of pyramidal process of palatine bone and adjacent maxillary tuberosity	Medial surface of mandibular ramus as far superiorly as the sphenomandibular ligament, inferiorly to mylohyoid groove
Lateral (external) pterygoid	Superior head: greater wing of sphenoid and infratemporal crest Inferior head: lateral surface of lateral pterygoid plate	Superior head: articular capsule of TMJ—the disk and the superior portion of mandibular neck Inferior head: anterior surface of mandibular neck

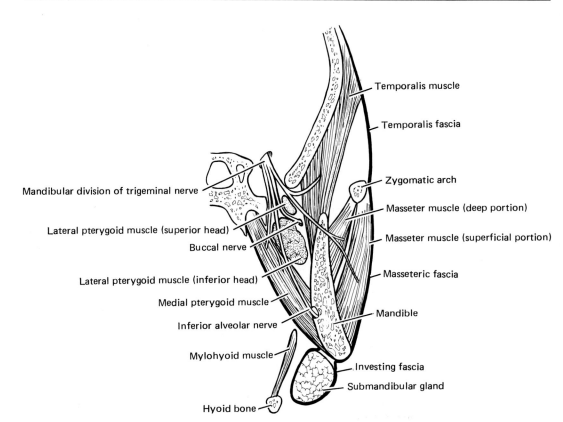

Figure 12.1. Muscles of mastication and their fascia.

Vascularization	Innervation	Function
Masseteric branch from maxillary artery	Masseteric branch from mandibular division of trigeminal nerve	Powerful elevator of jaw
Anterior and posterior deep temporal arteries from maxillary artery. These anastomose with middle temporal from superficial temporal artery.	Anterior and posterior deep temporal nerves of the mandibular division of the trigeminal nerve	Primarily an elevator of mandible. Some fibers (post and middle) act as retractor.
Branch from maxillary artery	Medial pterygoid nerve from trunk of mandibular division of the trigeminal nerve	Primarily, elevator of mandible
Branch from maxillary artery	Lateral pterygoid nerve from mandibular division of trigeminal nerve	Superior head: mandibular stabilizer Inferior head: jaw depressor and slight protruder; initiates jaw opening

between the ligament and the skull for the transmission of branches of the mandibular nerve to the muscles. The fascia possesses an interval, near the neck of the mandible, for the passage of the maxillary vessels to the infratemporal fossa. Lying between the temporalis and over much of the surface of the pterygoid muscles is the *venous pterygoid plexus,* connecting many of the venous tributaries both inside and outside the cranial cavity, face, deep face, orbit, and nasal cavity.

Temporalis (Figs. 12.1, 12.2)

The *temporalis* is a fan-shaped muscle originating on the bones of the broad temporal fossa. Specifically, the site of origin extends inferiorly from the inferior temporal line over the entire temporal fossa, including parts of the parietal, and most of the squama of the temporal bones, and the greater wing of the sphenoid including its infratemporal crest and the temporal surface of the frontal bone. Occasionally, some fibers arise from the posterior temporal surface of the frontal process of the zygoma. The muscle bundles converge to insert as a tendon on the coronoid process of the mandible and down along its anterior surface and the anterior border of the ramus as far anteriorly as the third molar. The anterior fibers of this muscle are directed in a vertical plane from origin to insertion, the middle fibers in an oblique plane, and the posterior fibers in an almost horizontal plane.

The muscle is primarily an elevator of the mandible; however, because of the directional alignments of the muscle fibers, the posterior and middle portions of the muscle are reported to act also in retracting the mandible.

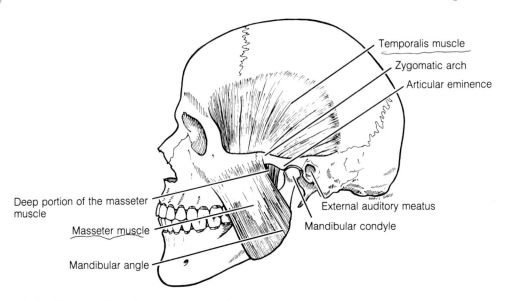

Figure 12.2. Temporalis and masseter muscles.

The temporalis muscle is innervated by anterior and posterior deep temporal nerves from the mandibular division of the trigeminal nerve. The nerves enter the muscle from its deep aspect in the temporal fossa.

Vascularization is supplied to the temporalis muscle via branches of the superficial temporal and maxillary arteries. Arising from the former is the middle temporal artery, which enters the muscle on its superficial aspect. Anterior and posterior deep temporal arteries, arising from the maxillary artery, accompany the like-named nerves and enter the deep aspect of the muscle, where they anastomose with the middle temporal artery.

Masseter (Figs. 12.1, 12.2)

The shape of the posterior region of the jaw is due to the quadrangular form of the *masseter muscle* overlying the angle and ramus of the mandible. The masseter muscle, as previously described, is the only muscle of mastication that lies outside the anatomical confines of the deep face, since it originates on the zygomatic arch and inserts into the lateral surface of the mandible. This muscle possesses, from its origin, a superficial portion and a smaller deep portion. The superficial portion arises, via a tendinous aponeurosis, from the zygomatic process of the maxilla and the anterior two-thirds of the inferior border of the zygomatic arch. The smaller, deep portion arises from the inferior border of the posterior one-third of the zygomatic arch and from along its entire medial aspect. It is reported that the origin of the superficial portion is limited posteriorly by the zygomaticotemporal suture. The origin of the deep portion is limited posteriorly by the anterior slope of the articular eminence of the zygomatic arch. The fibers of the superficial and deep portions of the muscle fuse to become inserted on the mandible, broadly covering the angle, along with some of the ramus and the body, as far anteriorly as the region directly below the last molar. Some fibers derived from the deeper portion insert as far superiorly as the base of the coronoid process. It is in this region that fibers of the temporalis

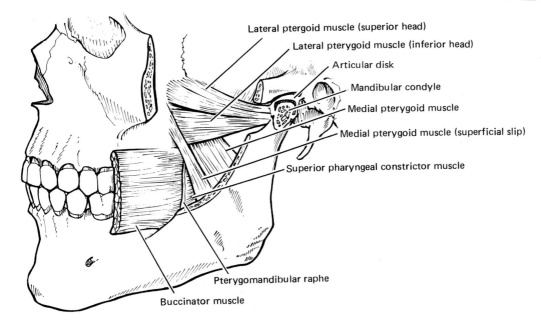

Figure 12.3. Pterygoid muscles (lateral view). Note the insertion of the lateral pterygoid muscle into the head of the mandible and into the disk.

muscle, arising from the inner surface of the zygomatic arch, may be fused with those of the deep portion of the masseter, then termed the *zygomatic-omandibularis muscle.*

The masseter muscle functions as a powerful elevator of the jaw. The superficial fibers act to direct a powerful force on the molars, while the deep fibers, more vertically directed, effect a retractive force, especially in closing the jaws.

The muscle is innervated by the *masseteric nerve* derived from the mandibular division of the trigeminal nerve. This motor nerve enters the muscle on its deep aspect adjacent to the mandibular notch, through which it gains access from its origin in the deep face.

Vascular supply to the muscle is provided by the masseteric branch of the maxillary artery. The artery and vein accompany the nerve in its path to the muscle.

Medial Pterygoid (Figs. 12.1, 12.3, 12.4, 12.5, 12.6)

The medial (internal) pterygoid muscle, originating in the deepest aspect of the deep face, inserts onto the medial aspect of the mandible about the ramus and angle. Thus, it is anatomically and functionally a counterpart to the masseter muscle. The specific sites of origin are the pyramidal process of the palatine bone in the pterygoid fossa and the medial surface of the lateral pterygoid plate. This area of origin is broad in that it extends to the tensor veli palatini muscle. An additional anterior muscular slip arises from the lateral portion of the pyramidal process and the adjacent region of the maxillary tuberosity. While the main mass of the muscle lies deep to the lateral pterygoid muscle, the additional anterior slip lies superficial to that muscle.

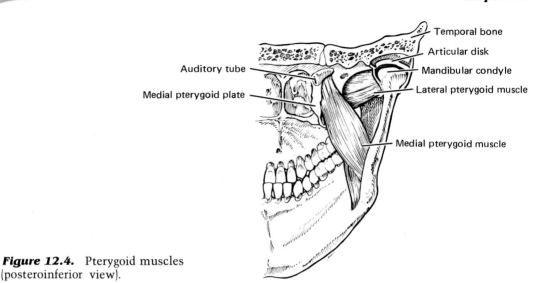

Figure 12.4. Pterygoid muscles (posteroinferior view).

The medial pterygoid muscle is directed inferiorly, posteriorly, and laterally to be inserted onto the medial surface of the ramus of the mandible. The insertion site lies between the mandibular angle, mylohyoid groove, and the mandibular foramen. The sphenomandibular ligament marks the superiormost extent of the insertion. Occasionally, a tendinous inscription denotes the meeting of the fibers of the masseter and medial pterygoid muscles at the inferior border of the angle of the mandible. This arrangement is referred to as the *pterygomasseteric sling.*

The medial pterygoid muscle functions primarily as an elevator of the mandible. The fibers are directed in an oblique fashion; however, the force is more pronounced in a vertical direction. The insertions of the masseter and medial pterygoid muscles, suspending the angle of the mandible between them, form the *mandibular sling,* about which these muscles act synergistically utilizing the temporomandibular joint as a guide.

The medial pterygoid muscle receives its motor innervation from a likenamed nerve branching from the mandibular division of the trigeminal nerve and entering the deep surface of the muscle. The muscle is vascularized by a branch of the maxillary artery.

Lateral Pterygoid (Figs. 12.3, 12.4, 12.5)

The lateral (external) pterygoid muscle is a short muscle filling the remainder of the infratemporal fossa and covering much of the medial pterygoid muscle. This muscle possesses two heads of origin. The smaller, superior head originates from the infratemporal region of the greater wing of the sphenoid bone as far laterally as the infratemporal crest. The larger, inferior head originates from the lateral surface of the lateral pterygoid plate.

The fibers of the superior head course posteriorly and laterally in an almost horizontal direction from the infratemporal crest. Fibers of the inferior head are directed posteriorly, laterally, and slightly superiorly on their way to the mandible. Though the two heads of origin are separated from each other,

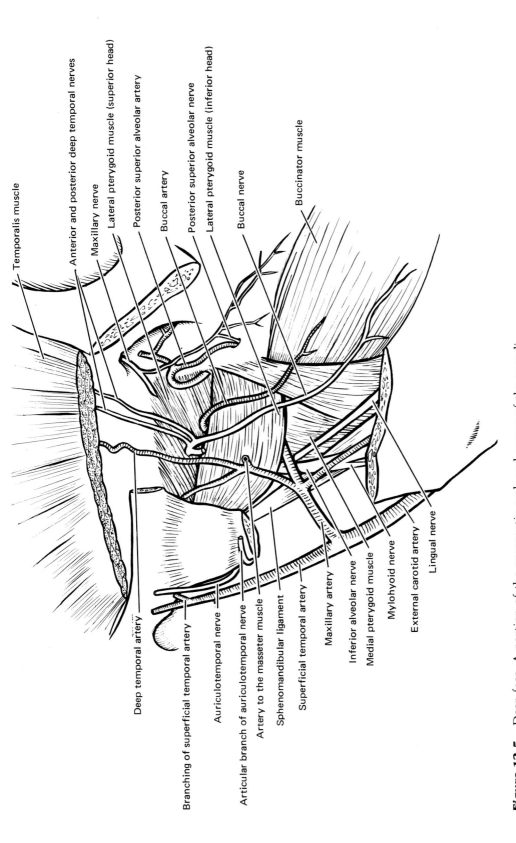

Temporalis muscle

Anterior and posterior deep temporal nerves

Maxillary nerve

Lateral pterygoid muscle (superior head)

Posterior superior alveolar artery

Buccal artery

Posterior superior alveolar nerve

Lateral pterygoid muscle (inferior head)

Buccal nerve

Buccinator muscle

Deep temporal artery

Branching of superficial temporal artery

Auriculotemporal nerve

Articular branch of auriculotemporal nerve

Artery to the masseter muscle

Sphenomandibular ligament

Superficial temporal artery

Maxillary artery

Inferior alveolar nerve

Medial pterygoid muscle

Mylohyoid nerve

External carotid artery

Lingual nerve

Figure 12.5. Deep face. A portion of the zygomatic arch and ramus of the mandible have been cut away to reveal the deep structures. Note the maxillary artery diving beneath the lateral pterygoid muscle.

209

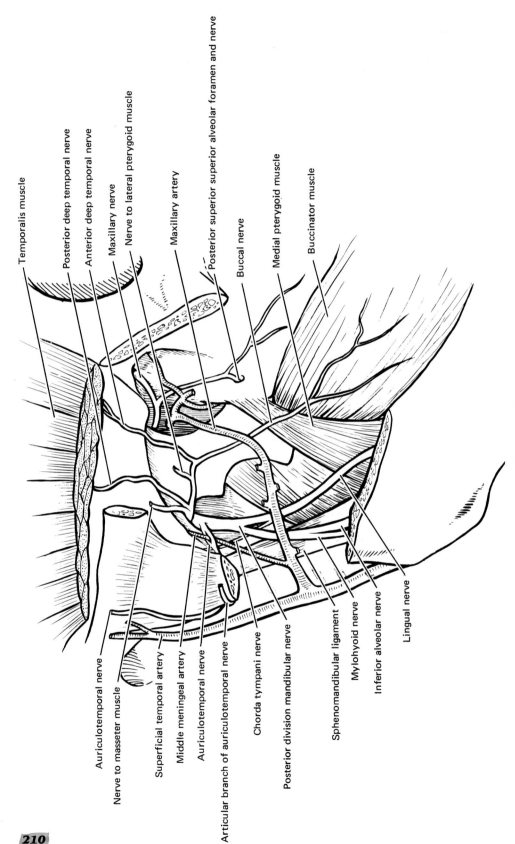

Temporalis muscle

Posterior deep temporal nerve

Anterior deep temporal nerve

Maxillary nerve

Nerve to lateral pterygoid muscle

Maxillary artery

Posterior superior superior alveolar foramen and nerve

Buccal nerve

Medial pterygoid muscle

Buccinator muscle

Auriculotemporal nerve

Nerve to masseter muscle

Superficial temporal artery

Middle meningeal artery

Auriculotemporal nerve

Articular branch of auriculotemporal nerve

Chorda tympani nerve

Posterior division mandibular nerve

Sphenomandibular ligament

Mylohyoid nerve

Inferior alveolar nerve

Lingual nerve

Figure 12.6. Arteries and nerves of the deep face. The lateral pterygoid muscle has been removed to reveal the mandibular division of the trigeminal nerve.

their fibers converge as they approach the site of insertion on and about the mandible. The superior head inserts into the articular capsule of the temporomandibular joint, the anterior border of the articular disk, and the superior part of the mandibular neck. The inferior head inserts along the anterior surface of the mandibular neck. Recent evidence indicates that the two heads remain separated even at the insertion site, perform different functions, and may be separately innervated.

The lateral pterygoid muscle is described classically as the "jaw opener," which protrudes the mandible and moves the mandible from side to side when functioning unilaterally. Recent evidence supporting the concept of the lateral pterygoid muscle being two separate muscles, with the superior head attached to the articular capsule and disk, is reported to function in stabilizing the mandibular condyle, while the inferior head is reported to function in pulling the mandible and disk forward and down, effecting jaw opening.

The lateral pterygoid muscle is innervated by a branch entering its deep surface from either the anterior division separately or as a branch of the buccal nerve from the mandibular division of the trigeminal nerve. Vascular supply is provided by a branch from the maxillary artery as it passes either superficial or deep to the muscle. Prolongations of the buccal fat pad fill in the spaces between the muscles of mastication deep to the mandible.

VASCULAR SUPPLY (Figs. 12.5, 12.6) ══════════════════════════════

The vascular supply to the entire region of the deep face is provided by branches of the maxillary artery along with a small contribution from the middle temporal artery to the superior surface of the temporalis muscle.

Maxillary Artery

The maxillary artery, the larger one of two terminals of the external carotid artery, arises from that artery deep to the neck of the mandible embedded within the substance of the parotid gland. The artery immediately turns anteriorly, passing between the mandibular ramus and the sphenomandibular ligament on its way to the pterygopalatine fossa, where it subsequently divides into terminal branches. Along its course to the fossa, it provides branches to the ear, temporomandibular joint, meninges, muscles of mastication, teeth and supporting structures of the mandible, buccinator muscle, cheek, and mucous membrane of the mouth. Terminals, branching from the artery while it is within the pterygopalatine fossa, serve the teeth and supporting tissues of the maxilla, the nasal cavity, and the palate. The major terminal enters the floor of the orbit as the infraorbital artery, which eventually exits upon the face.

The discussion which follows is confined mostly to descriptions of the artery and its branches supplying the structures of the deep face. Excluding a few exceptions, the terminal branches have been or will be detailed in the appropriate chapters.

The maxillary artery is described as consisting of three segments as it courses through the mandibular, pterygoid, and pterygopalatine regions.

Mandibular Portion

The mandibular portion runs behind the mandible between the ramus and the sphenomandibular ligament. Branches arising from this portion include the deep auricular and anterior tympanic (described in Chapter 13). Arising also from this portion are the *middle* and *accessory meningeal arteries*. Both of these arteries ascend to enter the skull via the foramen spinosum and foramen ovale, respectively. The distributions of these arteries is described in Chapter 9. Another artery arising from this portion of the maxillary artery, the *inferior alveolar artery,* descends to enter the mandibular foramen. The *mylohyoid artery* arises from the inferior alveolar artery just prior to the latter's entering the foramen. The mylohyoid artery courses along the mylohyoid groove to the mylohyoid muscle, which it supplies. Within the mandibular canal, the inferior alveolar artery supplies the bone, teeth, and adjacent supporting structures as far anteriorly as the first premolar tooth, where it divides into an incisive branch and a mental branch. The *incisive branch* continues on to vascularize the anterior teeth and supporting structures. The *mental branch* exits the mandible through the mental foramen to anastomose with the inferior labial and submental arteries vascularizing the area of the chin.

Occasionally, a *lingual artery* may arise from the inferior alveolar artery near its origin from the mandibular portion of the maxillary artery. When present, this artery will descend to assist in vascularizing the mucous membrane of the mouth.

Pterygoid Portion

Branches arising from the pterygoid segment of the maxillary artery are responsible for vascularizing the muscles of mastication and the buccinator muscle. The course of this portion of the artery is not constant, since it may pass either superficial or deep to the lateral pterygoid muscle.

The *masseteric artery,* arising from this portion of the maxillary artery, passes through the mandibular notch to enter the masseter muscle. The *anterior* and *posterior deep temporal arteries* accompany the like-named nerves to enter the deep surface of the temporalis muscle, anastomosing with the middle temporal branch of the superficial temporal artery. The short *pterygoid arteries* arise from this portion to vascularize the medial and lateral pterygoid muscles. The *buccal artery* accompanies the buccal nerve as it passes to and enters the buccinator muscle. Though the nerve does not innervate this muscle, the buccal artery vascularizes it, as well as the adjacent skin and mucous membrane of the mouth. This artery anastomoses with the facial and infraorbital arteries.

Pterygopalatine Portion

This portion of the maxillary artery enters the pterygopalatine fossa via the pterygomaxillary fissure. As the vessel enters the fossa to terminate into several arteries, the *posterior superior alveolar artery* arises from it and descends over the maxillary tuberosity to enter the posterior superior alveolar foramen with the like-named nerve. The artery vascularizes the molar and premolar teeth, adjacent supporting tissues, and the maxillary sinus.

The remaining arteries of this portion will be described in Chapters 14 and 16.

Pterygoid Plexus and Maxillary Vein

The pterygoid plexus of veins is a massive network of venous channels lying on and about the surfaces of the lateral and medial pterygoid muscles and extending into the spaces of the deep face within the infratemporal fossa. The plexus receives venous tributaries from vessels corresponding to the named arteries branching from the maxillary artery. This plexus is in direct or indirect communication with a vast area, including the cranial cavity and cavernous sinus, the nasal cavity, orbit, paranasal sinuses, facial vein, deep facial veins, and angular veins.

The *maxillary vein* is the short venous trunk which accompanies the maxillary artery as it lies behind the mandible. This vein serves to connect the pterygoid plexus with the superficial temporal vein, thus forming the retromandibular vein.

INNERVATION (Figs. 12.5, 12.6)

Most of the sensory innervation and all of the motor innervation to the structures constituting the deep face are supplied by branches of the mandibular division of the trigeminal nerve.

Trigeminal Nerve

Mandibular Division

The mandibular division of the trigeminal nerve exits the cranium via the foramen ovale. Motor and sensory roots pass individually through the foramen before uniting into a trunk within the infratemporal fossa. The trunk is very short, and it divides into two major divisions. The anterior division is mostly motor with some sensory branches, while the posterior division is mainly sensory with some motor branches.

Two branches arise from the trunk: the meningeal branch and the medial pterygoid nerve. The *meningeal branch* reenters the cranial cavity through the foramen spinosum in company with the middle meningeal artery. Within the cranial cavity, it provides sensory innervation to the dura mater. The *medial pterygoid nerve* arises from the medial aspect of the trunk, passing through the adjacent otic ganglion on its way to the medial pterygoid muscle. Two small branches arise from the medial pterygoid nerve close to its origin and are named the *nerve to the tensor tympani* and the *nerve to the tensor veli palatini*. The former passes to the auditory tube and on to the same-named muscle in the middle ear cavity. The latter nerve enters the tensor veli palatini muscle near its origin.

The *anterior division of the mandibular nerve* provides motor innervation to all the remaining muscles of mastication. This division also contains a sensory component for the skin and mucous membrane of the cheek. Arising from this division are the masseteric, deep temporal, lateral pterygoid, and buccal nerves.

The *masseteric nerve* passes superior to the lateral pterygoid muscle then laterally to the mandibular notch, sending a twig to the temporomandibular joint (TMJ) before gaining access to the deep portions of the masseter muscle. The *deep temporal nerves,* usually an anterior and posterior (sometimes an intermediate also), ascend between the two heads of the lateral pterygoid muscle to enter the deep surface of the temporalis muscle. Occasionally, these nerves may arise from either the masseteric or buccal nerves. The *lateral pterygoid nerve* enters the deep surface of the muscle lying over it. The *buccal nerve* passes between the two heads of the lateral pterygoid muscle and continues anteriorly beyond the border of the masseter muscle as it forms a plexus on the surface of the buccinator muscle. Here it freely communicates with the facial nerve, sending sensory branches with the facial nerve to supply the skin over the cheek. The nerve then pierces the muscle to provide sensory innervation to the mucous membrane of the cheek and adjacent gingiva.

The *posterior division of the mandibular nerve* is mostly sensory, possessing but one motor nerve to the mylohyoid muscle. Arising from this division are the auriculotemporal, lingual, and inferior alveolar nerves.

The *auriculotemporal nerve* arises from the posterior division of the mandibular nerve, usually as two roots that join after encircling the middle meningeal artery just before that artery enters the foramen spinosum. The auriculotemporal nerve then courses deep to the lateral pterygoid muscle as it passes posteriorly undercover of the parotid gland. The nerve then surfaces between the auricula and the temporomandibular joint below the zygomatic arch. It subsequently passes superficial to the zygomatic arch, along with the superficial temporal artery, to be distributed to the side of the head.

Near its origin, the auriculotemporal nerve receives communications from the otic ganglion. These are postganglionic parasympathetic fibers to be distributed to the parotid gland via the auriculotemporal nerve. As the nerve passes through the gland, these fibers will leave it to provide secretomotor innervation to the gland. The preganglionic fibers are a part of the glossopharyngeal nerve and reach the otic ganglion via the lesser petrosal nerve.

The auriculotemporal nerve communicates also with the facial nerve within the substance of the parotid gland. These sensory fibers are communicated to the facial nerve for further distribution over the face.

As the auriculotemporal nerve passes by the ear and the temporomandibular joint, it provides the *anterior auricular branches* to the skin of the anterior portion of the ear and the external acoustic meatus and *articular branches* to the joint. Superior to the zygomatic arch, the nerve branches into *superficial temporal nerves* which distribute to the skin of the side of the head.

The *lingual nerve* arises deep to the lateral pterygoid muscle and descends to pass superficially over the medial pterygoid muscle as it courses anteriorly to enter the submandibular region. The lingual nerve is joined by the chorda tympani nerve while it is under the cover of the lateral pterygoid muscle. The *chorda tympani nerve,* a branch of the facial nerve, makes its appearance in the deep face at the spine of the sphenoid. The nerve carries special sensory fibers for taste and preganglionic parasympathetic fibers destined for the submandibular ganglion.

The lingual nerve provides general sensation to the anterior two-thirds of the tongue, adjacent areas of the mouth, and the lingual gingiva. Special sensory taste fibers from the chorda tympani are distributed to the anterior two-thirds of the tongue. Preganglionic parasympathetic fibers leave the nerve at the submandibular ganglion, where they synapse on postganglionic parasympathetic cell bodies whose secretomotor fibers are distributed to the submandibular, sublingual, and minor salivary glands in the floor of the mouth. Details of the pathway followed by the lingual nerve are outlined more precisely in Chapter 15.

The *inferior alveolar nerve* originates deep to the lateral pterygoid muscle and lateral to the lingual nerve. This nerve passes between the sphenomandibular ligament and the ramus of the mandible to enter the mandibular foramen. Inside the mandibular canal, the nerve distributes to the mandibular teeth, supporting structures, and gingiva.

A branch, the *mental nerve,* emerges from the mental foramen to provide sensory innervation to the skin of the chin and lower lip. *Incisive branches* continue anteriorly in the mandibular canal to innervate the canine and incisor teeth, supporting structures, and gingiva. Just before the inferior alveolar nerve enters the mandibular foramen, it gives off the *mylohyoid nerve,* the only motor component of the posterior division. This motor nerve courses along the groove for the mylohyoid nerve before it enters the mylohyoid muscle. Upon crossing its superficial surface, the nerve provides motor innervation to the anterior belly of the digastric muscle.

Maxillary Division
A small contribution from the maxillary division of the trigeminal nerve is observed in the deep face. As the maxillary nerve passes through the pterygopalatine fossa, a small branch arises from it and passes laterally into the deep face via the pterygomaxillary fissure. This *posterior superior alveolar nerve* descends over the maxillary tuberosity to enter the posterior superior alveolar foramen, while some twigs continue on to innervate the gingiva and mucous membranes of the cheek. Those fibers entering the foramen distribute to the maxillary sinus, teeth, supporting structures, and gingiva as far anteriorly as the first molar, where a dental plexus is formed with the middle and anterior superior alveolar nerves, innervating the remaining maxillary sinus, teeth, supporting structures, and gingiva.

MASTICATION

Though it is not within the scope of this text to detail the precise timing and coordination of events in the process of mastication, a generalized description is warranted. The reader wishing more detail is referred to the Selected References at the end of this book.

The complex process of mastication involves many muscle groups besides the group commonly known as the "muscles of mastication." The process may be initiated consciously; however, the total movements and the rhythmic activity is controlled by complex neural circuitry within the central nervous system. The exact process varies among individuals, but once the pattern is established, it remains fairly constant within an individual. This is not to imply that the process is static; indeed it is altered, since changes within the stomatognathic system are constant and dynamic throughout life.

The process begins with ingestion or the cutting of food by the anterior teeth and continues as the food is maneuvered by the muscles within the cheek and the tongue to approximate the food between the premolars and molars. The muscles of mastication then act to elevate the mandible (masseter, temporalis, medial pterygoid), move it from side to side (elevators of contralateral side and ipsilateral internal pterygoid), depress it (lateral pterygoid, digastric, mylohyoid, and geniohyoid), protrude it (external pterygoid), and retrude it (part of temporalis) effecting a grinding action in a coordinated pattern. More information regarding the muscles involved in the exact movement patterns may be found in Chapter 13 on the temporomandibular joint.

The forces applied to the bolus of food are carefully monitored by special receptors (proprioception) located within the periodontal ligaments and the muscles themselves, preventing the possible self-destruction of the stomatognathic system.

The process of mastication prepares the food for deglutition by reducing the ingested bolus to approximately 2–5 mm in diameter. Chewing also serves to bring the food in contact with saliva in the mouth and stimulates the secretion of digestive juices within the digestive system.

CHAPTER 13

Temporomandibular Joint

The *temporomandibular joint (TMJ)* is the site of articulation between the mandible and the skull, specifically the area about the *articular eminence of the temporal bone.* This bilateral joint functions to open and close the jaws and to approximate the teeth of each jaw during mastication. The articulation consists of parts of the bony mandible and temporal bones which are covered by cartilage and surrounded by several ligaments. Interposed between the two bones is a fibrous articular disk, compartmentalizing the joint into two separate synovial-lined cavities. Several pairs of muscles attached to the mandible produce the movements necessary to suckle, ingest, and masticate food, swallow, yawn, and produce speech.

Interrelationships of the stomatognathic system in occlusion, neuromuscular function, and temporomandibular articulation are of paramount importance to the dental professional, since treatment of any component affects the functioning of this entire system.

JOINT ANATOMY

The anatomy of the temporomandibular joint structure is depicted in Figures 3.4, 6.2, 6.5, 6.6, 6.7, and 6.11. These illustrations show the relationship between the mandible and the temporal bone.

Mandible (Fig. 6.11)

The mandible possesses two articular surfaces, a condyle (head) located on the superior extremity of each of the bilateral condylar processes. Each condyle articulates with a meniscus (disk) which is interposed between it and the temporal bone. The condyles, which are characteristically "football-shaped" measure about 20 mm through the long medial-lateral axis and 10 mm through the anterior-posterior axis. The condyles are directed at an oblique angle to each other and to the frontal plane, so that if the planes of the long axes were continued they would meet at the foramen magnum. The long axis is also at right angles to the ramus of the mandible. Anteriorly, the condyle is strongly convex, while posteriorly, the convexity is reduced to medial and lateral slopes. This resembles (from a lateral view) the profile of an anteriorly tilted clenched fist. It is important to remember, however, that individual variations do exist in the shape, form, and size of the mandibular condyle, variations which may

217

be due to any one or a combination of factors including heredity and environmental adaptation.

Temporal Bone (Figs. 6.5, 6.6)

The site of articulation on the temporal bone is on the inferior surface of the zygomatic process. The specific location is situated on the posterior slope of the *articular tubercle.* The term "articular tubercle," as it applies here, is being replaced with the term "articular eminence" by those specializing in the study of the temporomandibular articulation. Though the new term has not as yet been adopted universally, the following terms and their definitions are of broad use and will be adopted in this text. The *articular eminence* is defined as the strongly convex bony elevation on the root of the zygomatic process representing the anteriormost boundary of the articular or glenoid fossa. The *articular tubercle* is the bony "knob" on the lateral aspect of the articular eminence, where the fibrous capsule and temporomandibular ligament attach. It would appear in the dried skull that, lying immediately anterior to the external auditory meatus, the mandibular condyle articulates within the glenoid fossa between the bony articular eminence and the postglenoid process. Close observation of the glenoid (mandibular) fossa reveals a rather thin bony roof separating it from the middle cranial fossa. This fact, coupled with the knowledge of the biconcave anatomy of the disk, simply does not support the conclusion that the glenoid fossa functions as the stress-bearing articulation. Indeed, radiographic evidence indicates articulation about the eminence.

Disk (Fig. 13.1)

The *articular disk (meniscus)* is a compact, dense and fibrous connective tissue plate, oval in shape and contoured to fit between the mandibular condyle and the articular eminence of the temporal bone. Its inferior surface is concavely contoured to fit the convexly shaped condyle of the mandible. Superiorly, its surface is concavo-convex. The convex portion conforms to the concave glenoid fossa posteriorly, while anteriorly the disk becomes concave to fit the convex posterior aspect of the articular eminence. The disk is thickest at its periphery and thinnest at the stress-bearing area of the joint. Peripherally, the disk becomes less dense as it merges into the surrounding capsule. Occasionally, the disk is perforated at its center, where it is thinnest.

Articular Coverings

The coverings of the articular surfaces of the condyle and articular eminence are composed of dense collagenous connective tissue. The heaviest stress-bearing areas are fibrocartilaginous, as the meniscus may become in later life. These structures are avascular; however, they are bathed in synovial fluid, which provides the cellular coverings with nourishment as well as lubrication. Peripheral regions of the disk are very vascular, while the central, stress-bearing portion is void of blood vessels.

Capsule (Figs. 13.1, 13.2)

The capsule encloses the entire articulating region of the temporal bone, disk, and mandibular condyle. Superiorly, it is attached to the circumference of the

External
auditory
meatus   Temporomandibular
ligament   Articular
tubercle   Coronoid process
of mandible

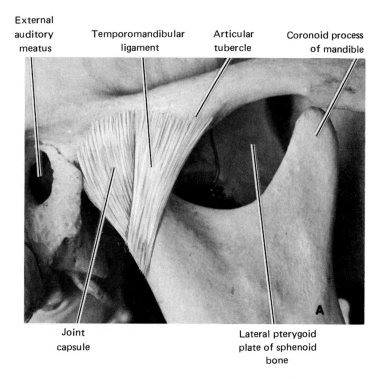

Joint
capsule   Lateral pterygoid
plate of sphenoid
bone

Joint
capsule   Superior synovial
compartment   Articular
disk   Temporomandibular
ligament

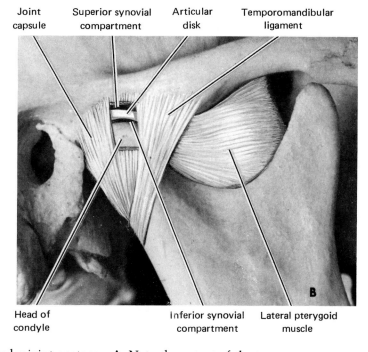

Head of
condyle   inferior synovial
compartment   Lateral pterygoid
muscle

Figure 13.1. Temporomandibular joint anatomy. **A.** Note the extent of the capsule model and the differentiated lateral ligament (temporomandibular ligament). **B.** Observe the capsule model has been cut away to reveal the disk and its relationship to the articulating surfaces of the joint.

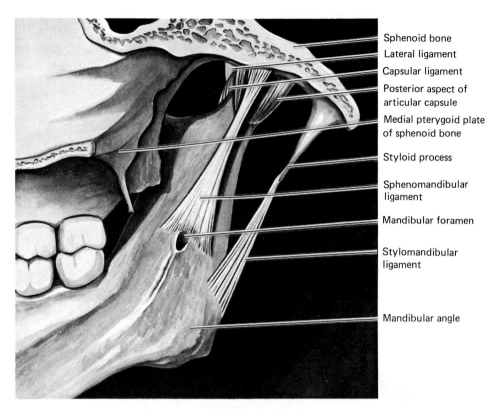

Sphenoid bone
Lateral ligament
Capsular ligament
Posterior aspect of
articular capsule
Medial pterygoid plate
of sphenoid bone

Styloid process

Sphenomandibular
ligament

Mandibular foramen

Stylomandibular
ligament

Mandibular angle

Figure 13.2. Accessory ligaments of the temporomandibular joint. Drawn from a medial view.

glenoid fossa and anteriorly around the articular eminence. Inferiorly, the capsule is attached to the mandibular neck. The placement of the disk between the two articulating bones and its peripheral attachments to the walls of the capsule causes the capsule to be divided into separate compartments. The larger, superior compartment between the disk and temporal bone permits some freedom of movement between the disk and articular eminence. Anteriorly, the capsule and disk are tightly fused, permitting the insertion of some fibers of the lateral pterygoid muscle into the disk. Medially and laterally, the capsule and disk are attached to the condyle margins, thus necessitating associated simultaneous movement of the condyle and disk. The inferior compartment encloses the entire neck of the mandible and is more firmly attached to the disk. This attachment prohibits excessive movement between the disk and condyle.

Innervation and Vascularization

The joint capsule is heavily endowed with sensory endings from the mandibular division of the trigeminal nerve, most of which are supplied from branches of the auriculotemporal nerve. Additional branches supplying the joint are derived from the masseteric branch of the mandibular nerve. Vascular supply to the joint is provided by branches of the superficial temporal and maxillary arteries as they pass by the joint.

Ligaments (Figs. 13.1, 13.2)

Reinforcements of the joint capsule along its medial and lateral margins by bundles of collagenous fibers are responsible for naming the medial portion the *capsular ligament* and the more pronounced lateral portion the *lateral ligament.*

The lateral ligament, or *temporomandibular ligament,* possesses two separate bands of fibers, whose directions are oblique to each other. The superficial layer, which is more extensive, arises as a broad band from the lateral surface of the articular eminence at the articular tubercle. The ligament narrows as it passes obliquely inferior and posterior to be inserted on the posterior aspect of the mandibular neck just inferior to the lateral aspect of the condyle.

The smaller, medially-situated ligament arises from the crest of the articular tubercle. It passes almost horizontally to insert into the lateral aspect of the condyle and the disk. The capsular and lateral ligaments permit free movement in the anteroinferior plane but check mediolateral movements of the joint. The superficial portion of the larger lateral ligament prevents lateral movement, while the deeper fibers prevent posterior displacement of the condyle. It is interesting that a similar arrangement does not exist on the medial side of the condyle with the capsular ligament. This difference can be understood by recognizing that the bilateral temporomandibular joints are connected through the mandible, and, therefore, that the articulations do not function independently but rather as a single unit.

Two additional ligaments are considered accessory to the temporomandibular articulation. The *sphenomandibular ligament,* a remnant of Meckel's cartilage, is a flat band that spans the space between the spine of the sphenoid bone and the lingula at the mandibular foramen. The *stylomandibular ligament,* another accessory ligament, is a specialization of the deep cervical fascia. This ligament extends as a thin band from the apex of the styloid process of the temporal bone to the posterior border of the angle and ramus of the mandible.

The exact functions of these two accessory ligaments is not fully understood as they relate to the temporomandibular articulation. The sphenomandibular ligament assists in limiting lateral mandibular movement, while the stylomandibular ligament apparently assists in limiting the anterior extent of protrusion of the mandible.

TYPES OF MOVEMENT

The joint just described is composed essentially of two convex structures opposed to each other with an intermediate articular disk placed between them. Considering the anatomy of the disk, it becomes clear that movement within the temporomandibular joint is basically of two types.

Ginglymus (hinge) movement is possible between the condyles of the mandible and the inferior surface of the disk. The other movement possible within the joint is a gliding motion. This becomes possible as the superior surface of the articular disk slides down at the articular eminence. The mandibular/disk movement is *rotatory* and that of the disk/temporal bone is *translatory.* Functionally, movements of the joint are translated as mandibular locations away from the resting position, such as opening, closing, protrusion, retrusion, and lateral rotation.

The *resting position* is defined as having the head in the anatomical position (in an upright posture). This places the masticatory musculature at rest, permitting a small free-way space to exist between the teeth of the upper and lower jaws but having the lips touching. It is in this attitude that the mandibular condyles are positioned so that the anterosuperior articulating surfaces are opposite the posterior slopes of the articular eminence of the temporal bone, with the disk between the bones.

Opening the jaws involves the translatory (gliding) movement of the disk and condyle down the slope of the articular eminence coupled with rotatory (hinge) movement of the mandibular condyles against the disk. The translatory phase effects a slight antero-inferior movement as the mandible slides down the eminence. The hinge action phase (condyles rotating) produces a center of suspension in the ramus. Thus, the posterior portion of the angle of the mandible moves slightly posterior, while the body moves inferiorly to open the jaw. The lateral pterygoid muscles initiate the action, followed by the digastric, geniohyoid, and mylohyoid muscles depressing the mandible. This assumes that the hyoid bone has been fixed by the infrahyoid musculature.

Closing the jaws is more involved. First the mandible is protruded as the condyles and disk slide down and forward on the articular eminence. This is followed by fixing the condyles and elevating the mandible coupled with depression/retraction. The lateral pterygoid muscle assisted by the medial pterygoid muscles protrude the mandible, while the masseter and temporalis muscles elevate it. Retrusion is performed by the deep portion of the masseter and some fibers of the temporalis muscles.

Mandibular protrusion, or jutting the mandible forward, is accomplished by contracting the lateral pterygoids, which causes the disk and condyles to slide forward and down the articular eminence. Retrusion, in contrast, returns the mandible to a position posterior to the resting position. This action is accomplished by portions of the temporalis muscles.

Lateral rotation—that is, a lateral rotatory motion on one side—is accomplished by the condyle and disk of the opposite side sliding inferiorly and anteriorly on the articular eminence while moving medially. The result of this active process effects a passive lateral rotation on the opposite side. The lateral pterygoid muscle of the side opposite the lateral rotation effects the movement.

It must be pointed out that the entire masticatory and accessory musculatures are involved in producing any one or combinations of these movements. Space limitations do not permit an extensive discussion of the muscles involved in the entire masticatory process. Generally, the information presented here is in agreement with published research in regard to muscle function for specific and separate actions of the temporomandibular joint. The process of ingesting and masticating food is a very intricate one involving the entire stomatognathic complex under voluntary and involuntary control of the nervous system. It should be clear from this brief description that the double temporomandibular joint is not controlled by one or a pair of muscles at any one time. Rather, all muscles affecting movement are synchronized and function in unison as prime movers, synergists, antagonists, fixers, sling balancers, and so on. There is considerable disagreement concerning the actions of muscles in pro-

TABLE 13.1
Muscles Acting on the Temporomandibular Joint

Muscles	Function				
	Opening	*Closing*	*Protrusion*	*Retrusion*	*Lateral Shift*
Muscles of mastication					
Masseter		+	+	√	√
Temporalis[1]		+ A, M, P		+ M, P	√ + P (Ipsilateral)
Medial pterygoid		+	+	√	√
Lateral pterygoid	+		+		+
Suprahyoid muscles					
Digastric	√	√	√	√	√
Mylohyoid	√	√	√	√	√
Geniohyoid	√	√	√	√	√
Stylohyoid[2]					

CODE: + Major Activity   √ Minor Activity
[1]Fibers of temporalis are coded: A—anterior, M—middle, P—posterior.
[2]The stylohyoid, though not connected to the mandible, does assist in fixing the hyoid bone.

ducing the various movements at the temporomandibular articulation. The major difficulties in resolving this dilemma arise from the duality of the joint, its interrelated multiple movements, its complex movements from particular points in space, and associated organs and musculatures in and about the oral apparatus. A table of muscular activity effecting temporomandibular joint function is presented in this chapter. It must be emphasized, however, that this table is grossly oversimplified and attempts to present merely a synopsis of muscle function in a very general manner (Table 13.1). The reader seeking more information on the subject of the temporomandibular joint is referred to material cited in the Selected References at the end of this book.

CLINICAL CONSIDERATIONS

Alterations in any one or a combination of the functioning components of the stomatognathic system—that is, teeth, periodontal ligament, TMJ, and the muscles of mastication—eventually result in temporomandibular joint dysfunction syndrome. Changes in the free-way dimensions (normally 2–4 mm) of the rest position imposed by occlusal changes, disease, muscle spasms, nervous tension, restorative prostheses, and so on may develop into TMJ dysfunction syndrome.

Temporomandibular problems, often difficult to diagnose, may result from a number of joint pathologies as well, including trauma, arthritis, and some general diseases.

Etiological studies have demonstrated a definite relationship between dental status and the prevalence of TMJ dysfunction syndrome.

Dislocation of the mandible may occur in an anterior direction only as the condyles slide down unchecked along the slope of the articular eminence to pass anteriorly into the infratemporal fossa. This condition may result from muscle spasm or from a convulsive yawn.

CHAPTER 14

Pterygopalatine Fossa, Nasal Cavity, and Paranasal Sinuses

PTERYGOPALATINE FOSSA

The pterygopalatine fossa, a small, pyramid-shaped space, is situated between the maxilla, sphenoid, and palatine bones. It communicates via canals, fissures, and foramina with various regions of the skull. The contents of the pterygopalatine fossa include the terminal portion of the maxillary artery, the pterygopalatine ganglion, the maxillary division of the trigeminal nerve, and branches of these structures. The osteology of this region is detailed in Chapter 6, where its communications with other regions are noted.

Maxillary Artery

The third, or *pterygopalatine portion,* of the maxillary artery enters the pterygopalatine fossa from the infratemporal fossa via the pterygomaxillary fissure. Branches of the pterygopalatine portion of the maxillary artery are the posterior superior alveolar, infraorbital, greater palatine, pharyngeal, and sphenopalatine arteries, as well as the artery of the pterygoid canal.

The *posterior superior alveolar artery* branches from the maxillary artery as that vessel enters the pterygomaxillary fissure. It travels on the maxillary tuberosity and enters the posterior superior alveolar foramen in conjunction with the like-named nerve. The vessel ramifies within the maxilla to vascularize the maxillary sinus, molars, and premolars, as well as the neighboring gingiva.

The *infraorbital artery,* a continuation of the maxillary artery, enters the orbit by the inferior orbital fissure, lies in the infraorbital groove, leaves the orbit via the infraorbital canal, and enters the face through the infraorbital foramen. Branches of the infraorbital artery are the *orbital branches,* serving the lacrimal gland and the inferior oblique and inferior rectus muscles; *anterior superior alveolar branches,* which vascularize the anterior teeth and the maxillary sinus; and the facial branches, discussed in Chapter 8.

The *greater palatine artery* and its branch, the *lesser palatine artery,* pass through the pterygopalatine canal and gain entrance to the palate via the *greater palatine* and *lesser palatine foramina,* respectively, to vascularize the soft and hard palates as well as associated structures. The *pharyngeal branch* passes dorsally, through the *pharyngeal canal,* to vascularize the auditory tube, sphenoidal sinus, and portions of the pharynx. The *sphenopalatine artery* leaves the pterygopalatine fossa via the *sphenopalatine foramen* on its medial wall to enter the nasal fossa. The distribution of this vessel and its branches is discussed later in this chapter. The small *artery* of the *pterygoid canal* passes through the posterior wall of the pterygopalatine fossa via the pterygoid canal. It supplies part of the auditory tube, pharynx, middle ear, and sphenoidal sinus.

Maxillary Nerve

The *maxillary division* of the *trigeminal nerve* enters the pterygopalatine fossa at its posterior boundary via the *foramen rotundum.* While in the fossa, it gives off the *zygomatic nerve,* which, passing into the orbit through the inferior orbital fissure, will bifurcate to form the zygomaticotemporal and zygomatico-facial nerves. The *posterior superior alveolar nerves* also branch from the maxillary nerve, exit the fossa via the pterygomaxillary fissure, and enter the maxillary tuberosity to serve the maxillary sinus, molars, and adjacent gingiva and cheek. The maxillary nerve then enters the orbit by way of the inferior orbital fissure and is referred to as the *infraorbital nerve.* While in the pterygopalatine fossa, the maxillary nerve communicates with the *pterygopalatine ganglion* via two small trunks, the *pterygopalatine nerves,* previously known as the sensory roots of the pterygopalatine ganglion. However these nerves do not bear a functional relationship with the ganglion. Postganglionic parasympathetic fibers derived from the ganglion ride along and distribute with branches of the maxillary division of the trigeminal nerve. These branches, which appear to arise from the ganglion are described here and, in more detail, in Chapter 18.

Orbital branches are slender nerves which supply the periosteum of the orbit and ethmoidal and sphenoidal sinuses. The *greater palatine nerve* and its branches, the *lesser palatine* and *posterior inferior nasal branches,* descend through the pterygopalatine canal to supply regions of the palate, gingiva, tonsil, and lateral wall of the nasal fossa. The *posterior superior nasal branches* leave the pterygopalatine fossa via the sphenopalatine foramen to serve the posterior aspect of the nasal fossa and part of the ethmoidal sinus. Its *nasopalatine branch* grooves the vomer bone in its path to the incisive foramen of the anterior hard palate, which it supplies. The *pharyngeal nerve* traverses the *pharyngeal canal* to innervate part of the nasopharynx.

Pterygopalatine Ganglion (Fig. 14.1)

The pterygopalatine ganglion appears to be functionally associated with the maxillary division of the trigeminal nerve, since it is suspended by the pterygopalatine nerves within the fossa. It is, however, a parasympathetic ganglion of the facial nerve (cranial nerve VII). This ganglion receives its parasympathetic, preganglionic root, whose fibers synapse within this structure, by way of the pterygoid canal which opens onto the posterior wall of the fossa. Postsynaptic, parasympathetic fibers leave the ganglion and distribute with branches of the maxillary division of cranial nerve V. These fibers are secretomotor in function. They provide parasympathetic flow to the lacrimal gland and mucosal glands of the nasal fossa, palate, and pharynx.

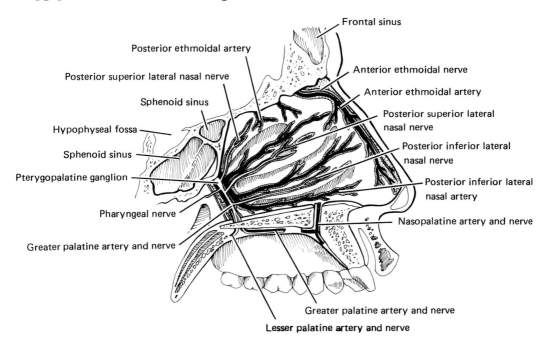

Figure 14.1. Pterygopalatine ganglion and associated nerves and arteries.

EXTERNAL NOSE

General Morphology (Fig. 14.2)

The external nose is triangular in shape. The base of the nose is located between the two orbits, and its distal portion overhangs the upper lip. Its skeleton is both bony and cartilaginous and is covered by integument. The skin is movable over the bony and superior part of the cartilaginous support but is intimately attached to the cartilage comprising the bulb of the nose. The region of the nose between the two orbits is known as the *root,* from which the bony bridge extends along the dorsum, inferiorly, to terminate in the movable bulbous apex. The inferior surface of the apex contains the two oval openings, the *nares,* leading into the internal nose. The two nares are separated by a midline *columna* (columella), the inferior part of the nasal septum.

The lateral aspect of the naris is formed by the *ala,* or wing, of the nose. The skin of the nose follows the contours of the nares and enters the internal nose for a short distance to form a junction with the mucous membrane lining the cavity. Short, thick, bristle-like hairs, *vibrissae,* protrude from skin rich in sebaceous glands, to strain particulate matter from the inhaled air.

Skeleton

The skeleton of the nose is both bony and cartilaginous. The bony root is composed of the nasal bones, which articulate with each other, the maxillae, frontal, and ethmoid bones.

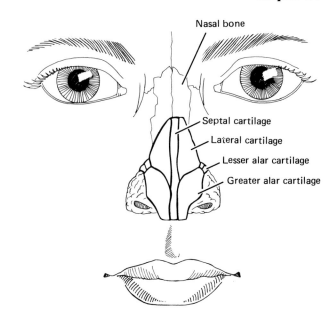

Figure 14.2. Skeleton of the nose.

The cartilaginous framework of the external nose is composed of five large, principal cartilages and a variable number of smaller cartilages. The principal cartilages are the median nasal septal and the paired lateral nasal and greater alar cartilages. The smaller ones are the vomeronasal, lesser alar, and accessory cartilages.

The *median nasal septal cartilage* is a quadrangular plate of hyaline cartilage that articulates with the nasal bone and the lateral and greater alar cartilages superoanteriorly; the perpendicular plate of the ethmoid bone posteriorly; and the vomer, anterior nasal spine, and vomeronasal cartilage, inferiorly. It separates the nasal cavity into right and left halves. The *lateral nasal cartilage* forms the part of the dorsum of the nose. It is a triangular plate of hyaline cartilage whose base articulates with the nasal and maxillary bones superolaterally, the median septal cartilage medially, and the lesser and greater alar cartilages, inferiorly. The *greater alar cartilage* is a C-shaped hyaline cartilage forming the lateral and medial walls of the nostril of the same side so that the nares present a constant opening. It is connected to the lesser alar and lateral nasal cartilages, superiorly, and the median nasal septal cartilage medially and inferiorly.

The muscles, vascular supply, and nerve supply of the nose are discussed in Chapter 8.

INTERNAL NOSE

The internal nose is the nasal cavity and the structures surrounding it. The osteology of this region is described in Chapter 6.

Nasal Cavity (Figs. 14.1, 14.3)

The *median nasal septum*, consisting of bony and cartilaginous components, subdivides the *nasal cavity* into a right and left *nasal fossa*. Each nasal fossa

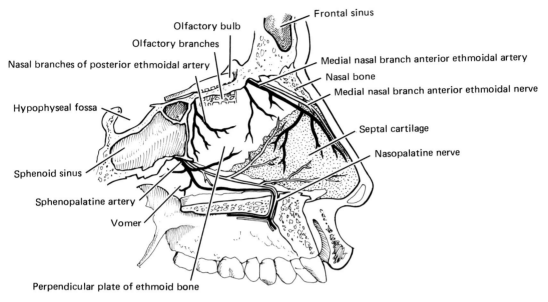

Figure 14.3. Arterial and nerve supply of the median nasal septum.

has anterior and posterior apertures, the *naris* and *choana*, respectively. In addition, each possesses four outpocketings termed the *paranasal* or *accessory sinuses*; a medial and lateral wall; a floor and a roof. The entrance into the nasal fossa immediately superior to the naris is a bilateral area of that cavity ringed by the greater alar cartilage. It is termed the *vestibule*. The vestibule is lined by skin possessing vibrissae and sebaceous glands. The superiormost portion of the nasal fossa, specialized for olfaction, is the olfactory region, while the larger, inferior portion is the respiratory region.

Medial Wall
The medial wall of the nasal fossa is composed of the vomer, the perpendicular plate of the ethmoid, and the median nasal septal cartilage. The entire median nasal septum is lined by mucoperiosteum. Frequently, this septum deviates to one side, infringing upon the nasal fossa of that side. Associated with the anteroinferior aspect of the septum is the vestigial Jacobson's organ lying upon the vomeronasal cartilage. This structure, olfactory in nature, is well developed in some lower animals.

Lateral Wall
The lateral wall of the nasal fossa differs from the medial wall. Instead of being relatively smooth, it presents three scrolled laminae of bone which jut medially into the nasal fossa. These *turbinate bones*, covered by mucoperiosteum are referred to as the *superior, middle,* and *inferior nasal conchae.*

Inferior and lateral, under the cover of the projecting concha, is the correspondingly named meatus. Superior to the *superior meatus*, just anterior to the body of the sphenoid bone, is the *sphenoethmoidal recess* containing the *ostium* (opening) *of the sphenoidal sinus.* A region of another sinus, the posterior ethmoidal air cells, opens below the superior concha into the anterior region of the superior meatus.

The middle nasal concha overlies the *middle meatus* and covers the lateral wall of that meatus, from which there is a marked, rounded projection formed by the middle ethmoidal air cells of the ethmoidal air sinus. This rounded projection is known as the *ethmoidal bulla,* inferior to which is a thin, arched ledge of bone, the *uncinate process of the ethmoid.* Located between the bulla and the uncinate process is an arch-shaped opening, the *semilunar hiatus,* connecting the ethmoidal infundibulum with the middle meatus. The anterior ethmoidal air cells, the maxillary sinus, and, frequently, the frontonasal duct from the frontal sinus open into the ethmoidal infundibulum.

The inferior nasal concha, usually the largest of the three conchae, is a separate bone, while the middle and superior conchae are projections of the ethmoid bone. The inferior concha overhangs the inferior meatus, whose inferior extent is formed by the floor of the nasal cavity. The *nasolacrimal duct* opens into the anterosuperior aspect of the inferior meatus.

Floor and Roof

The floor of the nasal fossa is formed by the horizontal process of the palatine bone and the palatine process of the maxilla. The *incisive canal,* transmitting the nasopalatine nerve and vessels, perforates the mucous membrane of the anteromedial aspect of the floor adjacent to the septum, leading into the *incisive foramen.* The contained nerves and vessels serve the anterior hard palate. The roof of the nasal fossa is concave cranially, and its bony vault is composed of the cribriform plate of the ethmoid bone as well as parts of the sphenoid, palatine, vomer, frontal, and nasal bones.

The mucous membrane lining the nasal fossa may be classified into two categories: a pink to red, richly vascularized respiratory muscosa lining most of the nasal fossa and moistening the inhaled air, and a yellowish-brown olfactory mucosa, located superiorly.

Paranasal Sinuses (Fig. 6.10)

The maxillae, frontal, ethmoid, and sphenoid bones contain hollow cavities, the paranasal sinuses, lined by respiratory mucosa. These cavities, as described earlier, communicate with the nasal fossae via small ostia. The function of these sinuses is not known, though it has been suggested that they act as resonators during speech and decrease the weight of the head. The latter explanation is not reasonable, since the weight of bone marrow and cancellous bone which would occupy this space is negligible. The capacity of these sinuses as resonators during speech is also questionable, since they are present in animals which very seldom vocalize. Further, in the human body, blocked or fluid-filled sinuses do not impair speech production to any great extent. The sinuses develop postnatally, though the anlagen of the sphenoidal, maxillary, and ethmoidal sinuses are present at birth. The mucous membrane lining the sinuses is continuous with that of the nasal fossae via the various ostia of the sinuses into the fossa. These openings and the chambers with which they are associated are listed in Table 14.1. The ostia, though small on the dry skull, are reduced in size in the living individual, so much so that they are minute. Hence, communication between the sinuses and the nasal fossa is easily impeded during respiratory congestion. Three of the four sinuses are bilateral. Although the sphenoidal sinus located in the midline is not bilateral, it is divided into two halves by an interposed plate of bone.

TABLE 14.1
Openings of the Paranasal Sinuses

Sinus	Opening	Location	Constancy
Maxillary	Maxillary ostium	Middle meatus via ethmoidal infundibulum	Constant
	Accessory maxillary ostium	Middle meatus	Inconstant
Frontal	Frontonasal duct	Frontal recess of middle meatus	Constant
	Frontal ostium	Middle meatus via the ethmoidal infundibulum	Inconstant
Ethmoidal Posterior air cells	Ostia of the posterior ethmoidal air cells	Superior meatus	Constant
Middle air cells	Ostia of the middle ethmoidal air cells	Middle meatus	Constant
Anterior air cells	Ostia of the anterior ethmoidal air cells	Middle meatus via ethmoidal infundibulum or via frontal recess	Constant Inconstant
Sphenoidal	Sphenoidal ostium	Sphenoethmoidal recess	Constant

Maxillary Sinus

The maxillary sinus, the largest paranasal sinus, is positioned lateral to the nasal cavity, inferior to the orbit, and often extends into the zygomatic process of the maxilla. The floor of the sinus is intimately related with the maxillary first and second molars, whose roots not only form considerable bulges but also may perforate the osseous floor of the sinus. Moreover, if the sinus is large, the third molar and second premolar may also be involved with its floor. The superomedial wall of the sinus consistently communicates with the ethmoidal infundibulum by way of the *maxillary ostium* and inconsistently communicates with the middle meatus via the accessory maxillary ostium.

Frontal Sinus

The frontal sinus pneumatizes the forehead and is incompletely subdivided into two or more compartments. The right and left sinuses are separated from each other by the frontal septum, which usually deviates to one side resulting in asymmetry of the two sinuses. The frontal sinus drains into the frontal recess of the middle meatus by way of the frontonasal duct or into the ethmoidal infundibulum via the same duct.

Ethmoidal Sinus

The ethmoidal sinus is composed of three sets of ethmoidal air cells, the anterior, middle, and posterior. These thin-walled, bony, honeycombed spaces collectively form the ethmoidal labyrinth located between the orbits and the nasal fossae. The posterior air cells drain into the superior meatus, the middle cells into the middle meatus just above the bulla ethmoidalis, and the anterior air cells into the ethmoidal infundibulum and thence into the middle meatus via the semilunar hiatus.

Sphenoidal Sinus

The sphenoidal sinus hollows out the body of the sphenoid bone and is separated into two asymmetrical halves by a plate of bone, the sphenoidal septum, that usually deviates to one side. The sphenoidal sinus drains into the sphenoethmoidal recess of the nasal fossa through the sphenoidal ostium.

Vascular and Nerve Supply of the Nasal Cavity and Paranasal Sinuses

Vascular Supply

The vascular supply of the nasal fossa is derived from several sources: branches of the facial, ophthalmic, and maxillary arteries. The vestibule receives septal branches from the facial artery. The ophthalmic artery supplies anterior and posterior ethmoidal branches to regions of the superior and middle conchae and meatuses, to the middle nasal septum, as well as to the frontal and ethmoidal sinuses.

The maxillary artery provides several branches to the nasal fossa. The greater palatine branches serve the anterior floor and posterior aspect of the nasal fossa. The sphenopalatine branch, entering via the sphenopalatine foramen, vascularizes portions of the nasal conchae and meatuses via its *posterior lateral nasal branches,* as well as the posterior segment of the median nasal septum by its *posterior septal branches.* Terminal branches of these vessels form a rich anastomotic plexus in the mucoperiosteum. The maxillary artery provides vascularization of the four paranasal sinuses (Table 14.2) via the *posterior lateral nasal branch* of the sphenopalatine artery. In addition, the anterior and posterior superior alveolar arteries serve the maxillary sinus, while the pharyngeal artery and the artery of the pterygoid canal supply the sphenoidal sinus.

The ophthalmic artery, via its *anterior* and *posterior ethmoidal branches,* assists in vascularizing the frontal, ethmoidal, and sphenoidal sinuses.

Venous drainage of the nose and paranasal sinuses is by way of the anterior and posterior ethmoidal veins into the ophthalmic vein, the sphenopalatine vein into the pterygoid plexus of veins, and the vein of the foramen cecum into the superior sagittal sinus. Since these venous elements usually do not possess valves, infection may be propagated throughout the entire system, affecting the dural venous sinuses—especially the cavernous sinus—and resulting in serious and, perhaps, life-threatening complications.

Nerve Supply

General sensory innervation to the respiratory mucosa is derived from the trigeminal nerve, in particular, from the ophthalmic and maxillary divisions. The olfactory epithelium receives its special visceral afferent fibers for smell from the olfactory nerves whose axons pass via perforations in the overlying cribriform plate of the ethmoid bone to the olfactory bulb. Secretomotor fibers derived from cranial nerve VII reach the mucoperiosteum via communications carried by branches of the maxillary division of the trigeminal nerve.

The paranasal sinuses also receive their sensory innervation via the ophthalmic and maxillary divisions of the trigeminal nerve (Table 14.2). The frontal sinus receives its sensory innervation via branches of the frontal and nasociliary nerves of the ophthalmic division of the trigeminal nerve.

TABLE 14.2
Vascular and Sensory Nerve Supply of the Paranasal Sinuses

Sinus	Arteries	Veins	Nerves
Maxillary	Maxillary Sphenopalatine Posterior lateral nasal Greater palatine Posterior superior alveolar Infraorbital Anterior superior alveolar	Sphenopalatine, greater palatine anterior, middle and posterior superior alveolar	Maxillary division Infraorbital Anterior superior alveolar Middle superior alveolar Posterior superior alveolar
Frontal	Ophthalmic Anterior ethmoidal Maxillary Sphenopalatine Posterior lateral nasal	Anastomosis of supraorbitals and superior ophthalmic	Ophthalmic division Frontal Nasociliary Anterior ethmoidal
Ethmoidal	Ophthalmic Anterior ethmoidal Posterior ethmoidal Maxillary Sphenopalatine Posterior lateral nasal	Anterior ethmoidal Posterior ethmoidal Sphenopalatine	Opthalmic division Nasociliary Anterior ethmoidal Posterior ethmoidal Maxillary division Orbital branch Posterior superior nasal
Sphenoidal	Ophthalmic Posterior ethmoidal Maxillary Artery of the pterygoid canal Pharyngeal branch Sphenopalatine Posterior lateral nasal	Posterior ethmoidal Sphenopalatine	Ophthalmic division Nasociliary Posterior ethmoidal Maxillary division Orbital branch

The ethmoidal sinuses are served by ethmoidal branches of the nasociliary nerve and by orbital and nasal branches of the maxillary division of the trigeminal nerve. The sphenoidal sinus is served by ethmoidal branches of the nasociliary nerve and orbital branches of the maxillary division. The maxillary sinus receives its innervation solely from the maxillary division, specifically, from the superior alveolar nerves.

CLINICAL CONSIDERATIONS

Nose and Nasal Passages

The nose usually is not affected by anomalous development, with the exception of incomplete fusion of the lateral nasal process with the maxillary process resulting in harelip and oblique facial clefts, as discussed in Chapter 5 on development of the head and neck. Occasionally, one or both nasal passages are blocked somewhere or are completely absent. This condition is known as *congenital atresia* of the nose. The occlusion may involve the anterior nares, the nasal fossae, and/or the choanae.

Frequently, a slight depression may be noted at the tip of the nose. This may be an indication of a very mild form of *bifid nose*, which may be severe enough to involve the entire bulb of the nose.

The nasal septum may be displaced to one side, so that one nasal fossa is larger than the other. In severe cases, the degree of *deviation of the nasal septum* is sufficiently great to cause atresia and/or reduced respiratory capability, infection, inflammation, and sinusitis, indicating the necessity for surgical treatment.

During fracture of the ethmoid bone, cerebrospinal fluid may leak into the nasal fossa and out through the external nares. This condition, *cerebrospinal rhinorrhea*, may lead to meningitis, with possibly fatal consequences.

Bleeding from the nose subsequent to injury is a common occurrence and is usually relatively easy to control. Normally, the source of blood flow is *Kiesselbach's area*, the anteroinferior region of the nasal septum, where the septal branch of the superior labial, anterior ethmoidal, nasopalatine, and greater palatine arteries anastomose. The bleeding is controlled by pressure or by packing the nose with cotton. Occasionally, bleeding is from higher up in the nose, where control may require more heroic action.

Paranasal Sinuses

Sinusitis, or inflammation of the mucosa of the paranasal sinuses, results in swelling of the mucoperiosteum, which blocks the ostia of the sinuses. This irritation causes fluid accumulation in the sinuses, resulting in increased pressure and displacement of the air normally located therein. This pressure causes "sinus headaches" of varied intensity, and if untreated, the infection may spread to the inner ear and the middle ear as well as to other areas.

Infection of the frontal sinus, if left untreated, may result in frontal bone osteomyelitis, since venous drainage of this sinus is intimately related to diploic veins and indirectly related with those of the dura and scalp.

The ethmoidal air cells are in close relationship with the orbit, with only a paper-thin lamina of bone separating these structures. Hence, in the case of severe infection, this bony separation may be perforated and the infection may involve the orbit, resulting in orbital cellulitis.

The maxillary sinus is quite prone to infection, since it is intimately associated with the first and second maxillary molars. Dental involvement may result from abscess, from carious lesions, or from tooth extractions with part of the floor of the maxillary sinus being removed in the process. A knowledge of the anatomy of the sinuses and roentgenographic analysis of the involved area should be a prerequisite to maxillary tooth extraction.

15

Submandibular Region and Floor of Mouth

The submandibular or suprahyoid region lies between the hyoid bone and the mandible. This region is located in the anterior triangle of the neck. It is more often studied with the head, since it is a transition zone between these two regions and because the structures contained therein function in association with the jaws and the floor of the mouth.

CONTENTS AND BOUNDARIES

Muscles contained within this region and/or forming its boundaries include the digastrics, stylohyoid, mylohyoid, and geniohyoid. Both intrinsic and extrinsic tongue musculatures—namely, the styloglossus, genioglossus, and hyoglossus—also occupy the region. Strictly described, the middle pharyngeal constrictor muscle also may be included, since it inserts upon the hyoid bone. The platysma, a muscle immediately deep to the skin, overlies this region.

Cutaneous sensation to the area is provided by branches of the cervical plexus. Branches of several cranial nerves, including the trigeminal, facial, and hypoglossal, provide sensory, special sensory, motor, and secretomotor innervation to the structures within this region.

The major vascular supply to the region is via branches of the lingual artery. Additional vascular supply is provided by branches of the facial and maxillary arteries. Venous drainage is accomplished by like-named veins and the anterior jugular vein.

Two of the three major salivary glands, the submandibular and sublingual, occupy the submandibular and sublingual regions, respectively. These two glands receive postganglionic parasympathetic innervation from the submandibular ganglion located near the submandibular gland.

The submandibular region is bounded superiorly by the inferior rim of the mandible and inferiorly by the anterior and posterior bellies of the digastric muscle, as these two muscles converge onto the hyoid bone to form the submandibular triangle. The mylohyoid muscle, spanning between each side of the mandible, is attached inferiorly to the anterior aspect of the hyoid bone. Its superior surface underlies the tongue, thus forming the floor of the mouth, while its inferior surface forms the floor of the submandibular triangle. Attached to much of the posterior aspect of the hyoid bone is the hyoglossus muscle ascending into the tongue. The interval between the two muscles permits the passage of neurovascular and lymphatic elements into and out of the floor of the oral cavity.

235

MUSCLES AND FASCIA

Muscles constituting the submandibular region and the floor of the oral cavity include the suprahyoid muscles of the anterior triangle of the neck and those attaching either to the mandible or hyoid bone forming the floor of the mouth and/or the tongue. Both intrinsic and extrinsic muscles of the tongue are generally described with this region, the exception being the palatoglossus muscle which originates from the palate and is thus more appropriately described with muscles of that region.

The suprahyoid structures are enclosed in the investing fascia of the neck. The fascia is attached to the hyoid bone and extends superiorly, attaching to the inferior border of the mandible. Enclosing the anterior belly of the digastric muscle, the fascia continues posteriorly and laterally to encase the submandibular gland. The deeper layers ensheath the muscles of the submandibular region, including those of the tongue. Fusing with the deep fascia of the posterior digastric, the investing fascia assists in forming the stylomandibular ligament. The fascial compartment reaches the floor of the mouth, the sublingual gland, and the tongue. Clefts between the fascial layers are continuous posteriorly, at the border of the mylohyoid muscle, into the lateral pharyngeal cleft and about the cleft around the submandibular gland.

Suprahyoid Muscles (Fig. 15.1)

Digastric

The digastric muscle consists of two portions: a *posterior belly*, which arises from the mastoid notch of the temporal bone, and an *anterior belly*, arising from the digastric fossa of the anterior lower border of the mandible. Both of these muscle bellies descend to the hyoid bone to be inserted by an intermediate tendon. A fibrous loop surrounds it, the body, and the greater cornu of the hyoid bone. At the loop, the tendon perforates the stylohyoid muscle at its attachment on the hyoid bone.

The combined function of the bellies is to elevate the hyoid bone and assist in opening the mandible when the hyoid bone is fixed by the infrahyoid muscles. Acting independently, the anterior belly draws the hyoid anteriorly, while the posterior belly draws it posteriorly. The digastric muscle is really two separate muscles, each derived from different branchial arches. The anterior belly originates from the mandibular arch (branchial arch I) and is innervated by a branch of the mylohyoid nerve from the mandibular division of the trigeminal nerve. The posterior belly develops in the hyoid arch (branchial arch II) and is innervated by a branch of the facial nerve which enters its deep surface at midbelly. The posterior belly of the digastric muscle is vascularized by the posterior auricular artery, with contributions from the suprahyoid branch of the lingual artery and muscular branches of the occipital artery. The anterior belly is vascularized by the submental branch of the facial artery.

Stylohyoid

The stylohyoid muscle arises from the posterior and lateral surfaces of the styloid process of the temporal bone. As this muscle descends to insert on the body of the hyoid bone, it is in close association with the posterior belly of the digastric muscle, which perforates it close to its insertion. The stylohyoid

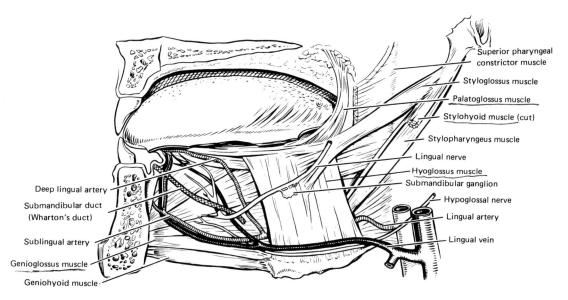

Figure 15.1. Suprahyoid region.

muscle functions to draw the hyoid bone superiorly and posteriorly, in addition to assisting in fixing it. Motor innervation to this muscle is provided by a branch of the facial nerve which enters its midbelly. Vascular supply is provided by posterior auricular and occipital branches of the external carotid artery. Additional vascular elements may reach the muscle via the suprahyoid branch of the lingual artery and from muscular branches of the facial artery.

Mylohyoid (Fig. 15.2)
The mylohyoid muscle forms the floor of the mouth as it unites in the midline with its counterpart from the opposite side of the mandible. This muscle arises from the entire length of the mylohyoid line of the mandible, from the symphysis menti to the region opposite the last molar tooth. Anteriorly, the fibers of each side insert into a median raphe, while the more posteriorly oriented fibers insert into the body of the hyoid bone.

The muscle assists in depressing the mandible when the hyoid bone is fixed. When the mandible is fixed, the muscle elevates the hyoid bone, and consequently the tongue, for swallowing.

The mylohyoid nerve from the inferior alveolar branch of the mandibular division of the trigeminal nerve innervates the muscle as the nerve approaches its inferolateral border. Vascular supply is provided by the anastomoses from the submental branch of the facial artery and the sublingual branch of the lingual artery.

Geniohyoid
Immediately superior to the mylohyoid is the geniohyoid muscle, originating from the inferior mental spine (genial tubercle) of the mandible before descending to the anterior surface of the body of the hyoid bone. At its insertion, the muscle is in contact with its counterpart from the opposite side of the mandible. This muscle functions to draw the hyoid bone anteriorly and, in so doing, draws the tongue as well.

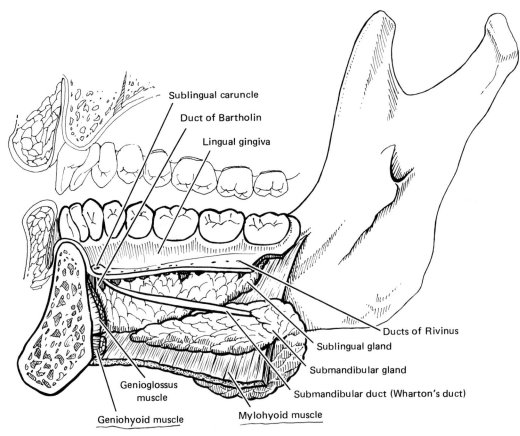

Figure 15.2. Submandibular and sublingual glands.

This muscle is innervated by fibers of the first cervical nerve, which are transported to it via the hypoglossal nerve. Vascularization is provided by the sublingual branch of the lingual artery.

Group Actions

The suprahyoid muscles, all of which attach to the hyoid bone and another structure superior to it, function as a group to assist in swallowing by lifting the hyoid bone, the floor of the mouth, and the tongue. As food passes down the esophagus, the stylohyoid and posterior digastric muscles retract the hyoid bone to prevent regurgitation. This muscle group may also assist in fixing the hyoid bone and in retracting the mandible when the hyoid bone is fixed by the infrahyoid muscles.

Tongue Muscles (Fig. 15.1)

The tongue muscles are composed of two groups: intrinsic and extrinsic. The *intrinsic muscles* of the tongue are confined within the structure itself and are described as longitudinal, transverse, and vertical muscles. The longitudinal group is subdivided into a superior and an inferior group. The intrinsic muscles function generally to alter the shape of the tongue as necessary in mastication, deglutition, and phonation. The varying shapes of the tongue can be predicted by relating the fiber orientations of the intrinsic muscles as named.

The *extrinsic muscles* of the tongue originate outside it. There are four such muscles: genioglossus, hyoglossus, styloglossus, and palatoglossus. The palatoglossus muscle, as was stated at the beginning of the chapter, is not discussed here, but rather it is described in Chapter 16, since it originates from the palatal region.

Genioglossus

The genioglossus muscle arises from the superior mental spine (genial tubercle) of the mandible directly above the geniohyoid muscle. From here, the muscle fans out to enter the entire length of the inferior surface of the tongue. The most anterior fibers curve upward to insert into the tip of the tongue. The posterior fibers pass to the base of the tongue, while some of the most inferior fibers are attached to the body of the hyoid bone. This muscle acts to protrude the tongue, while the most anterior fibers depress the tongue tip.

Hyoglossus

The hyoglossus muscle originates from the side of the body and greater cornu of the hyoid bone, passing vertically to enter the tongue, where the fibers intermingle with those of the styloglossus muscle. A separate slip of muscle, referred to by some as the *chondroglossus muscle* since it is separated from the hyoglossus by a small interval, is considered a part of the hyoglossus in this text. The hyoglossus functions as the major depressor of the tongue.

Styloglossus

The styloglossus muscle arises from the anterior surface of the styloid process of the temporal bone and the stylomandibular ligament. It then descends anteriorly and medially to enter the tongue from the lateral aspect, as it turns horizontally. Most fibers of the styloglossus continue on to the tip of the tongue. Some of the posterior fibers decussate with those of the hyoglossus muscle. This muscle functions to retract the tongue, while the more anterior fibers elevate the tip.

Innervation and Vascularization

All of the tongue musculature, with the exception of the palatoglossus, is innervated by the hypoglossal nerve. The palatoglossus muscle is innervated by the pharyngeal plexus. The vascular supply to the muscles of the tongue is provided primarily by the deep lingual artery, the terminal branch of the lingual artery. The exception, again, is the palatoglossus, which is served by the arteries of the palate.

Group Actions

Complex movements of the tongue are accomplished by intricate and coordinated contractions of both intrinsic and extrinsic muscles of the tongue. Generally, "movements" other than those that basically alter the shape of the tongue are the result of contractions of the extrinsic muscles, though one group seldom functions alone. The overlapping, intermingling, and decussating nature of the intrinsic and extrinsic muscle groups permit the fine coordinated effort so necessary in speech.

SALIVARY GLANDS (Fig. 15.2)

Two of the three major salivary glands are located within the submandibular/floor of the mouth region. These are the submandibular and sublingual glands. Most of the submandibular gland is located superficially in the submandibular triangle, with only a small portion extending into the floor of the mouth. The entire sublingual gland, however, is housed in the floor of the mouth.

Submandibular Gland

This salivary gland occupies much of the space within the submandibular triangle. Superficially, it is covered by skin, platysma, and the superficial layer of the deep cervical fascia. The superior extent of the gland is recessed under the cover of the mandible in the submandibular fossa. Inferiorly, the gland extends to the hyoid bone, overlapping the intermediate tendon of the digastric muscle. The gland extends anteriorly to the anterior belly of the digastric muscle and posteriorly as far as the stylomandibular ligament. The deep surface of the gland lies upon the hyoglossus, stylohyoid, styloglossus, and mylohyoid muscles. Usually, a finger-like projection extends into the sublingual space on the superior surface of the mylohyoid muscle. It is from this deep process that the *submandibular duct (Wharton's duct)* emerges to pass anteriorly between the mylohyoid, hyoglossus, and genioglossus muscle, then between the latter and the sublingual gland to open onto the *sublingual caruncula,* just lateral to the base of the lingual frenulum (Fig. 4.11).

The facial artery vascularizes the gland as the artery passes through the posterior portion on its way to the superficial face. The artery ascends across the lateral border of the mandible just anterior to the masseter muscle.

The sublingual branch of the lingual artery also provides additional vascular supply to the gland. Venous drainage follows the named arterial channels.

Sublingual Gland

The sublingual gland, smallest of the three major salivary glands, is housed in the floor of the mouth between the mucous membrane of the oral cavity and the mylohyoid muscle, inferiorly. This almond-shaped gland lies between the genioglossus muscle, medially, and the sublingual fossa of the mandible laterally. Posteriorly, it is in contact with the submandibular gland.

Ducts from the gland may open into the oral cavity as tiny excretory ducts (ducts of Rivinus) on the surface of the plica sublingualis located in the sublingual sulcus. Some ducts may unite to form the *sublingual duct (duct of Bartholin),* opening into the submandibular duct (Fig. 4.10).

The vascular supply to this gland is derived from two sources: the sublingual artery from the lingual artery and the submental artery, a branch of the facial artery.

Autonomic Innervation

Autonomic innervation to the submandibular and sublingual glands is provided by secretomotor fibers originating in the facial nerve and transmitted to the submandibular ganglion via the chorda tympani branch of the facial nerve and to the lingual nerve of the trigeminal nerve. Sympathetic innervation (vasomotor) is provided from the superior cervical ganglion via the carotid plexus and the facial artery. A more complete description of the autonomic system's relationships with these two glands is detailed in Chapter 18.

INNERVATION

Two cranial nerves may be observed coursing through the submandibular region. The trigeminal nerve is represented by two branches from the mandibular division. The other cranial nerve is the hypoglossal nerve serving the tongue musculature.

Trigeminal Nerve

The trigeminal nerve is represented by branches of the mandibular division in the vicinity of the submandibular region. Arising from the inferior alveolar nerve, just before that nerve enters the mandibular foramen, is the *mylohyoid nerve.* This nerve courses inferiorly in a groove on the deep surface of the mandibular ramus to reach the mylohyoid muscle, which it supplies with motor innervation. A small branch continues along the superficial surface of the mylohyoid muscle to supply motor innervation to the anterior belly of the digastric muscle.

The *lingual nerve* arises from the posterior division of the mandibular division of the trigeminal nerve within the infratemporal fossa. Here it is joined by the *chorda tympani,* a branch of the facial nerve, carrying special sensory fibers for taste and preganglionic parasympathetic fibers for the submandibular ganglion. The lingual nerve courses anteriorly between the mandible and medial pterygoid muscle, obliquely across the styloglossus muscle, and then into the submandibular region. It next passes between the submandibular gland and the hyoglossus muscle and over the submandibular duct on to the tip of the tongue, where it provides general sensation to the anterior two-thirds of the tongue, adjacent mucosa, and gingiva.

Special sensory fibers transmitted to the nerve from the chorda tympani are distributed to the taste buds on the anterior two-thirds of the tongue.

The *submandibular ganglion,* suspended from the lingual nerve by short filaments, lies upon the hyoglossus muscle in the vicinity of the posterior margin of the mylohyoid muscle. In this position, the parasympathetic ganglion is in close association with the submandibular gland (Fig. 15.1).

Preganglionic parasympathetic fibers from the chorda tympani leave the lingual nerve and enter the ganglion to synapse on postganglionic cell bodies. Some postganglionic fibers exit the ganglion to enter the submandibular gland, while some reenter the lingual nerve for distribution to the sublingual gland and minor salivary glands of the oral cavity, providing them with secretomotor innervation.

Hypoglossal Nerve (Fig. 15.1)

The hypoglossal nerve exits the cranial cavity through the hypoglossal canal to make its way to the tongue musculature. In its course, it passes anteriorly across the external carotid and lingual arteries, remaining above the hyoid bone and lying deep to the posterior digastric and stylohyoid muscles. It continues forward along the genioglossus muscle to the tip of the tongue, providing motor innervation to all of the muscles of the tongue, with the exception of the palatoglossus as described previously.

Near the posterior border of the hyoglossus muscle, branches communicated to the hypoglossal nerve from the first cervical nerve leave the hypoglossal nerve to pass to the thyrohyoid and geniohyoid muscles, providing them with motor innervation.

Nerves to the posterior one-third and root of the tongue are derived from branches of the glossopharyngeal and vagus nerves, respectively. Discussion of their contributions to innervation of the tongue is included later in Chapter 18.

VASCULAR SUPPLY

Vascular supply to the submandibular region and the floor of the mouth is provided mainly by the lingual and facial arteries. Other contributions of minor importance provide vascular supply to those structures originating outside the region or located on its periphery. This category includes the occipital and posterior auricular arteries, serving the posterior digastric and stylohyoid muscles, and the mylohyoid artery from the inferior alveolar branch of the mandibular portion of the maxillary artery, serving the mylohyoid muscle.

Lingual Artery

The lingual artery arises from the external carotid artery usually near the greater cornu of the hyoid bone. Sometimes, however, it arises in common with the facial artery. It passes deep to the posterior digastric, stylohyoid, and hyoglossus muscles to ascend to the tongue, turning anteriorly as it courses to its tip. During its passage, it gives off the following branches: suprahyoid, dorsal lingual, sublingual, and the deep lingual arteries.

The *suprahyoid artery* arises near the hyoid bone and, while staying above it, supplies most of the muscles attaching to the hyoid bone. The *dorsal lingual artery* arises deep to the hyoglossus muscle and ascends to the posterior dorsum of the tongue to supply the palatoglossal arch, mucous membrane of the tongue, palatine tonsil, and some of the soft palate, freely anastomosing with other vessels in the area.

The *sublingual artery* arises at the anterior margin of the hyoglossus muscle to course between the genioglossus and mylohyoid muscles on its way to the sublingual gland, which it supplies along with other nearby muscles in addition to the mucous membrane of the floor of the mouth and gingiva. This artery anastomoses with the submental branch of the facial artery by branches piercing the mylohyoid muscle.

The *deep lingual artery* is the terminal of the lingual artery lying immediately under the mucous membrane of the inferior surface of the tongue. It lies lateral to the genioglossus muscle and is accompanied by the lingual nerve. Anastomosis is accomplished with its counterpart of the opposite side at the tip of the tongue.

Facial Artery

The facial artery, as detailed in Chapter 7, arises from the external carotid artery just above the lingual artery. At first, it ascends deep to the posterior digastric and stylohyoid muscles, then enters the substance of the submandibular gland before crossing the lateral border of the mandible to enter the face. While in the neck four named branches arise. These are the ascending palatine, tonsillar, glandular, and submental arteries. These arteries are described in Chapters 7 and 16. Particularly important to this description are the glandular and submental branches. *Glandular branches* arise from the facial artery as it courses through the submandibular gland, which these branches supply. Postganglionic sympathetic fibers enter the gland via the facial artery as it courses through it.

The *submental artery* arises near the anterior border of the masseter muscle, after the facial artery has exited the submandibular gland but prior to its turning up onto the face. The submental artery courses upon the mylohyoid muscle, which it serves, in addition to providing branches to the anterior belly of the digastric muscle. A deep branch perforates the mylohyoid muscle to anastomose with the sublingual and mylohyoid arteries. At the symphysis menti, a branch turns upward onto the face to anastomose with the inferior labial artery.

Veins

The tongue and sublingual area are drained by several dorsal lingual veins and a large *deep lingual vein* visible on the underside of the tongue. These veins may empty directly into the internal jugular vein or they may drain into the *common facial vein,* as do the submental and sublingual veins.

LYMPHATICS

Several lymphatic channels drain the submandibular/sublingual area. The tongue is drained chiefly by vessels into the submandibular region, with nodes located along the posterior digastric and omohyoid muscles. One node of particular importance, the *principal node of the tongue,* lies in close association with the bifurcation of the common carotid artery.

Submandibular nodes located beneath the mandible in the submandibular triangle drain the area, including the nose, upper lip, lower lip, gingiva, and the tongue.

Efferents from the submental and submandibular nodes pass into the deep cervical nodes and eventually into the jugular trunk before emptying into the subclavian vein. The lymphatic system is detailed in Chapter 20.

CLINICAL CONSIDERATIONS

The sublingual artery, occasionally injured during dental procedures, may present problems to the surgeon attempting to ligate its source, since it may arise from the submental branch of the facial artery rather than from the lingual artery.

CHAPTER 16

Palate, Pharynx, and Larynx

PALATE

The palate forms the roof of the mouth and the floor of the nasal cavities. It consists of two regions, one containing a bony shelf, the immovable hard palate, and the other a muscular, movable soft palate.

Hard Palate (Figs. 6.9, 16.1)

The hard palate is a bony plate composed of the palatine process of the maxilla and the horizontal process of the palatine bone fused in the midline with their counterparts of the opposite side. Anteriorly and laterally, it is bounded by the alveolar arches, while posteriorly its boundary is demarcated by the beginning of the soft palate. The bone is covered by a specialized mucoperiosteum on both its oral and nasal surfaces. The posterior border of the hard palate possesses the palatine aponeurosis for attachment of the muscles of the soft palate. The oral aspect of the hard palate may be divided into several regions according to the composition of its soft tissues. Hence, the median raphe region, along the palatal midline, the anterior lateral adipose region, and the posterior lateral glandular region are recognized as regions of the hard palate (Fig. 4.12).

Soft Palate (Fig. 16.1)

The soft palate is a muscular structure, encased in a mucous membrane, suspended between the oral pharynx and the nasal pharynx. Its sides are attached to the lateral pharyngeal walls. The anterior portion of the soft palate, near its junction with the hard palate, is almost immobile, while its posteriormost extent, the uvula, is capable of great excursion.

Lateral to the uvula is the *palatoglossal fold (anterior fauces)*, extending into the side of the tongue, while posteriorly is the *palatopharyngeal fold (posterior fauces)* extending into the lateral pharyngeal wall. The palatine tonsils are located between the two fauces in the tonsillar sinus.

Muscles of the Soft Palate (Figs. 16.1, 16.2; Table 16.1)

The muscles of the soft palate are the levator veli palatini, tensor veli palatini, musculus uvulae, palatoglossus, and the palatopharyngeus.

245

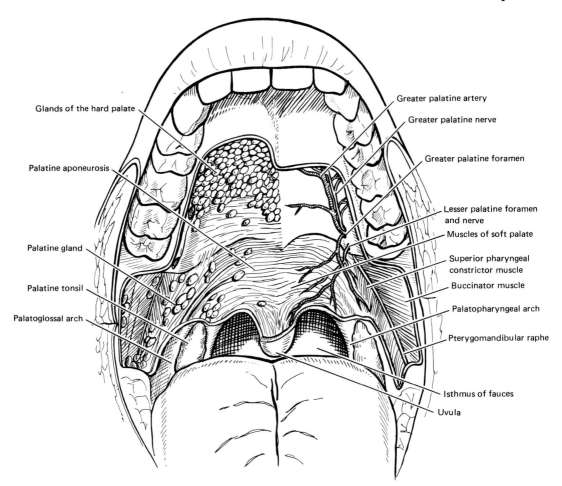

Figure 16.1. The palate.

Levator Veli Palatini.   The levator veli palatini is a thick, pencil-shaped muscle that is intimately associated with the lateral aspect of the choana. It has three regions of origin, one tendinous and two fleshy. The tendinous origin is the inferior aspect of the petrous portion of the temporal bone, on the proximal aspect of the apex just anteromedial to the entrance into the carotid canal. The fleshy origins are from the tympanic part of the temporal bone and from the cartilage of the auditory tube. The muscle fibers are directed medially, between the salpingopharyngeus and tensor veli palatini muscles to insert into the palatal aponeurosis, passing between the two layers of the palatopharyngeus muscle. As the levator inserts into the soft palate, its muscle fibers interdigitate with those of its counterpart from the other side. This muscle is innervated by branches of the pharyngeal plexus. The levator veli palatini, as its name implies, elevates the soft palate.

Tensor Veli Palatini.   The tensor veli palatini, a pyramid-shaped muscle, is situated anterior to the levator veli palatini and medial to the medial pterygoid muscle. It originates in the scaphoid fossa, on the spine of the sphenoid bone, and the cartilaginous auditory tube. The fibers collect into a tendinous cord

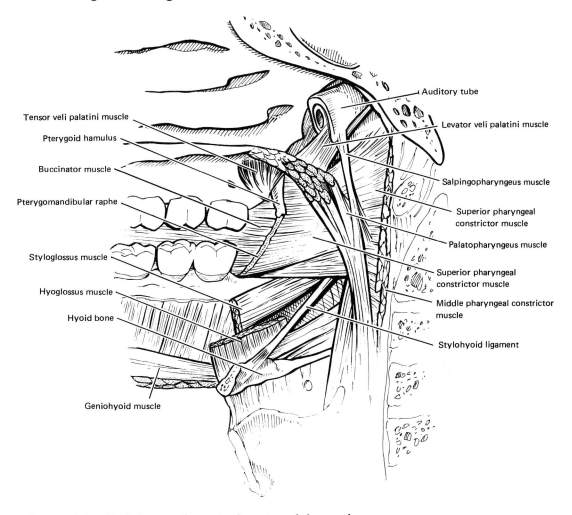

Figure 16.2. Medial view of a sagittal section of the oropharynx.

that wraps medially around the hamulus of the medial pterygoid plate to insert into the palatine aponeurosis. The tensor veli palatini is innervated by a branch of the nerve to the medial pterygoid, arising from the mandibular division of the trigeminal nerve. This muscle acts to flatten and tense the soft palate.

Musculus Uvulae. The musculus uvulae is a small, thin muscle lying between the two layers of the palatine aponeurosis. The muscle originates on the posterior nasal spine of the palatine bone and from the palatine aponeurosis to insert in common with its counterpart from the opposite side, forming the substance of the uvula. The musculus uvulae is innervated by branches of the pharyngeal plexus and acts to retract and elevate the uvula.

Palatoglossus. The palatoglossus muscle, a small longitudinally disposed muscle, is overlaid by a mucous membrane, thus forming the palatoglossal fold. It is a thin, cylindrical muscle originating in the fascia and musculature of

TABLE 16.1
Muscles of the Palate and Pharynx

Name	Origin	Insertion	Innervation	Action
Levator veli palatini	Petrous temporal, tympanic temporal, auditory tube	Palatal aponeurosis	Pharyngeal plexus	Elevates the soft palate; opens auditory tube. (?)
Tensor veli palatini	Scaphoid fossa, spine of sphenoid, auditory tube	Palatine aponeurosis	Mandibular division of the trigeminal	Tenses the soft palate. Opens auditory tube. (?)
Musculus uvulae	Posterior nasal spine, palatine aponeurosis	Uvula	Pharyngeal plexus	Elevates and retracts the uvula.
Palatoglossus	Fascia and muscles lateral aspect of soft palate	Side of the tongue	Pharyngeal plexus	Elevates root of tongue and constricts fauces.
Palatopharyngeus	Soft palate	Thyroid cartilage and muscular wall of pharynx	Pharyngeal plexus	Constricts pharyngeal isthmus and elevates larynx.
Stylopharyngeus	Styloid process	Muscular wall of the pharynx and thyroid cartilage	Glossopharyngeal	Elevates the larynx and pharynx.
Salpingopharyngeus	Auditory tube	Muscular wall of the pharynx	Pharyngeal plexus	Elevates pharynx; opens auditory tube. (?)
Superior pharyngeal constrictor	Medial pterygoid plate and hamulus; pterygomandibular raphe; mylohyoid line of mandible; alveolar process of mandible; root of tongue	Pharyngeal raphe	Pharyngeal plexus	Constricts the pharynx.
Middle pharyngeal constrictor	Lesser and greater cornua of hyoid bone; stylohyoid ligament	Pharyngeal raphe	Pharyngeal plexus	Constricts the pharynx.
Inferior pharyngeal constrictor	Cricoid cartilage; thyroid cartilage	Pharyngeal raphe	Pharyngeal plexus and external and recurrent laryngeal branches of vagus	Constricts the pharynx and acts as a pharyngoesophageal sphincter.

the lateral aspect of the soft palate. It inserts by interdigitating with the intrinsic muscles of the tongue in its lateral margin. Motor innervation to the muscle is derived from the pharyngeal plexus. The palatoglossus acts to elevate the posterior one-third of the tongue and, acting with its counterpart on the other side, constricts the fauces.

Palatopharyngeus. The palatopharyngeus muscle and its mucosal covering form the palatopharyngeal arch. It is a long, thin, cylindrical muscle arising by two fleshy slips from the side of the soft palate, with the levator veli palatini and the musculus uvulae being interposed between the two origins. The muscle inserts, along with fibers of the stylopharyngeus muscle, into the posterior aspect of the thyroid cartilage and also into the muscular coat of the pharynx. The palatopharyngeus receives its motor fibers from the pharyngeal plexus and functions to elevate the pharynx and to approximate the two palatopharyngeal arches.

Vascular and Nerve Supply (Fig. 16.1)

The vascular supply of the palate is derived chiefly from the greater and lesser palatine branches of the maxillary artery, the ascending palatine branch of the facial artery, and the ascending pharyngeal artery from the external carotid artery.

The greater and lesser palatine arteries descend in the pterygopalatine canal to enter the palate via the greater and lesser palatine foramina, respectively. The *greater palatine artery* passes anteriorly on the lateral aspect of the hard palate to supply the palatal mucosa, gingiva, and glands and then proceeds to anastomose with the nasopalatine artery in the incisive canal. The *lesser palatine artery* vacularizes the soft palate and tonsil and then anastomoses with the ascending palatine branch of the facial artery. The lesser palatine bifurcates and one branch travels along the surface of the levator veli palatini muscle to vascularize the soft palate. The other branch perforates the superior constrictor muscle to serve the auditory tube and the tonsil. The *ascending pharyngeal artery* from the external carotid artery travels along the lateral external surface of the superior constrictor muscle, reaches the levator veli palatini muscle, and gives off a palatine branch to serve the tonsil, auditory tube, and soft palate.

Venous drainage is by similarly named veins which are tributaries of the pterygoid and tonsillar plexus.

The sensory nerve supply of the palate is derived chiefly from the greater and lesser palatine branches of the maxillary division of the trigeminal nerve, which also carry sensory fibers from the facial nerve via the greater petrosal nerve. Additional sensory supply is derived from the nasopalatine nerve of the posterior superior nasal branch of the maxillary division of the trigeminal nerve and the tonsillar branches of the glossopharyngeal nerve.

Palatine Tonsil (Figs. 4.7, 16.1)

The palatine tonsil, located in the tonsillar sinus between the palatoglossal and palatopharyngeal arches, is an almond-shaped mass of lymphoid tissue covered by mucous membrane. The palatine tonsil is smaller than the tonsillar sinus and the small triangular recess above the tonsil is the supratonsillar fossa. However, it has been suggested that this is a misnomer, since tonsillar tissue surrounds this space and thus this recess is merely a large intratonsillar cleft.

The medial surface of the tonsil is visible when the tongue is depressed and presents tonsillar crypts which may invade nearly the entire depth of the tonsil. The lateral or deep surface is covered by a fibrous capsule, separating the tonsil from the pharyngeal musculature. The palatine tonsil forms a part of the *tonsillar circle (Waldeyer's ring)* which guards the oropharyngeal entrance (Figs. 4.7, 4.21).

The arterial supply of the palatine tonsil is derived from branches of four arteries. The facial artery via its tonsillar branch is the chief vascular supplier of the tonsil, but this artery also makes a minor contribution via its ascending palatine branch. Other minor vessels serving the palatine tonsil are the palatine branch of the ascending pharyngeal, the lesser palatine branch of the maxillary artery, and the tonsillar twig from the dorsal lingual branch of the lingual artery. Venous drainage is by way of the tonsillar plexus of veins on the deep aspect of the tonsil, a tributary of the pharyngeal venous plexus, and the facial vein. Sensory innervation to the palatine tonsil is from the glossopharyngeal nerve and palatine branches of the maxillary division of the trigeminal nerve. Contributions also come from the greater petrosal of the facial nerve via the trigeminal nerve.

PHARYNX (Figs. 4.20, 16.3, 16.4) ═══════════════════════════════════

The pharynx is a fibromuscular tube, 12–14 cm long, extending from the base of the skull to become continuous with the esophagus. It is broadest at its cranial extent and narrowest at its esophageal junction. Superiorly, it is attached to the basilar part of the occipital bone and the body of the sphenoid bone. Laterally, it is fixed to the medial pterygoid plate, pterygomandibular raphe, alveolar process of the mandible, lateral aspect of the tongue, hyoid bone, and the thyroid and cricoid cartilages. Posteriorly, the pharynx approximates the bodies of the first six cervical vertebrae, being separated from them by the prevertebral fascia. Anteriorly, the pharynx has no complete wall, instead it opens into the nasal, oral, and laryngeal cavities. Consequently, the pharynx is conveniently divided into nasal, oral, and laryngeal parts.

Nasal Pharynx

The nasal pharynx is the superiormost and broadest region of the pharynx. Its walls are rigid and present, on the two lateral aspects, several elevations. Anteriorly, it begins at the paired choanae; inferiorly, it is limited by the soft palate. During respiration, the soft palate is flaccid, and the nasal pharynx communicates with the oral pharynx through the *pharyngeal isthmus,* a space between the posterior wall of the pharynx and the free border of the soft palate. During deglutition, the soft palate is elevated and contacts the posterior wall of the pharynx blocking the communication between the nasal and oral cavities. The lateral wall of the nasal pharynx presents an opening, the *ostium of the auditory tube,* which is located inferoposterior to the inferior nasal concha. This ostium is located on the medial end of the cartilaginous auditory tube, which, protruding into the nasal pharynx, forms an elevation called the *torus tubarium.* Behind the torus is the *pharyngeal recess,* a mucosa-lined space extending to the base of the skull. Two folds extend from the torus, the smaller salpingopalatal fold covering the levator veli palatini muscle, extending from below the ostium of the internal auditory tube to the root of the soft palate,

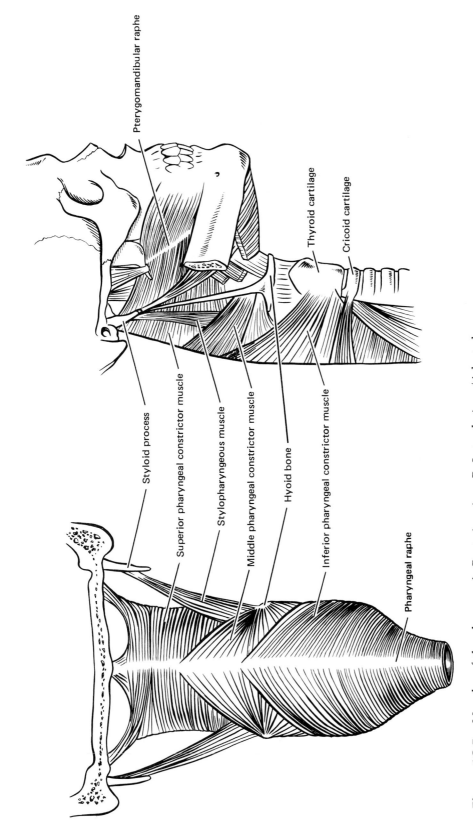

Figure 16.3. Muscles of the pharynx. **A.** Posterior view. **B.** Lateral view. (Adapted from W. H. Hollinshead, *Textbook of Anatomy*, 3rd ed., Hagerstown, Md., Harper & Row, 1974.)

Pterygomandibular raphe

Thyroid cartilage

Cricoid cartilage

Styloid process

Superior pharyngeal constrictor muscle

Stylopharyngeous muscle

Middle pharyngeal constrictor muscle

Hyoid bone

Inferior pharyngeal constrictor muscle

Pharyngeal raphe

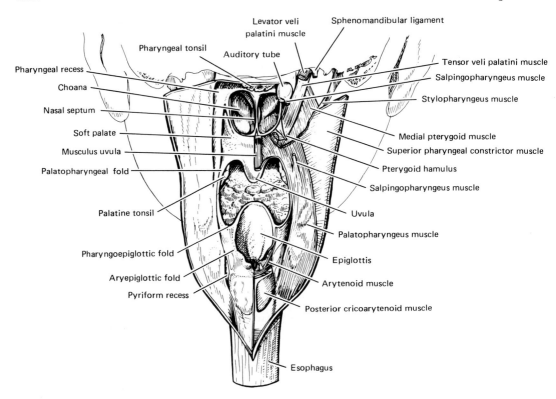

Figure 16.4. Posterior view of palate, pharynx, and larynx.

and the larger salpingopharyngeal fold, covering the salpingopharyngeus muscle. This latter fold extends from the posteroinferior aspect of the torus and passes inferiorly, becoming indistinguishable as the muscle merges with the muscles of the pharynx. The posterior wall of the nasopharynx contains a mass of lymphatic tissue, the *pharyngeal tonsil.*

Oral Pharynx

The oral pharynx is relatively uncomplicated, being that portion of the chamber which leads into the laryngeal pharynx. It extends from the soft palate to the cranial aspect of the epiglottis which is positioned at the level of the hyoid bone. Anteriorly, the oral pharynx begins at the oral cavity via the *oropharyngeal isthmus.* The lateral wall of the oral pharynx presents the palatine tonsil between the palatoglossal and palatopharyngeal arches (Figs. 4.7, 4.21, 16.1).

Laryngeal Pharynx

The laryngeal pharynx, the inferiormost region of the pharynx, extends from the epiglottis, at the level of the hyoid bone, to the esophagus, at the level of the inferior border of the cricoid cartilage. Anteriorly, it begins at the larynx, whose aperture appears to be guarded by the epiglottis, a movable flap-like structure. The *epiglottis* is connected to the midline and side of the pharyngeal root of the tongue by the *median* and *lateral glossoepiglottic folds,* respectively. The resultant fossa on either side of the median glossoepiglottic fold is known as the *epiglottic vallecula.* Inferior to the laryngeal opening, the anterior wall of the laryngeal pharynx consists of the posterior, mucosa-lined, aspect of the arytenoid and cricoid cartilages. The mucosal *aryepiglottic fold* connecting the epiglottis to the arytenoid cartilage constitutes the lateral boundary of the opening of the larynx. Lateral to this fold is a fossa, the *piriform recess,* whose lateral border is the thyroid cartilage with its thyrohyoid membrane. The internal laryngeal nerve and its branches pass just deep to the mucosal floor of this recess.

Pharyngeal Wall

The pharyngeal wall is composed of three layers: an innermost mucous layer, a middle fibrous and muscular layer, and an outer fibrous layer. The mucosa lining the pharynx is continuous with the mucosa of the chambers into which the pharynx opens. Hence, it is either a respiratory or an oral type of mucosa. Just deep to the mucosa is the *pharyngobasilar fascia,* a layer of fibrous connective tissue that is especially thick craniad but dwindles as it progresses caudally. The cranial portion of the pharyngobasilar fascia has no muscular covering. It is attached to the base of the skull at various points: at the basilar portion of the occipital bone, anterior to the pharyngeal tubercle, at the petrous temporal bone, and at the medial pterygoid plate. Further anteriorly, it is attached to structures in the neck, the thyroid cartilage, hyoid bone, stylohyoid ligament, and pterygomandibular raphe. A region of this fascia is attached posteriorly to a strong, longitudinally oriented, fibrous band of connective tissue, the *pharyngeal raphe,* which extends from the pharyngeal tubercle of the occipital bone to nearly the caudal border of the pharynx. The constrictors of the pharynx insert into the pharyngeal raphe. The muscular layer of the pharynx is positioned between the pharyngobasilar fascia and the thin outermost layer of the pharynx, the *buccopharyngeal fascia.* Cranially, in the region devoid of the superior constrictor, this fascia fuses with the pharyngobasilar fascia. Nerves and vessels traveling along the pharynx pass in the buccopharyngeal fascia.

Muscles of the Pharynx (Figs. 16.2, 16.3, 16.4; Table 16.1). The musculature of the pharynx is composed of the superior, middle, and inferior pharyngeal constrictors and the stylopharyngeus, salpingopharyngeus, and palatopharyngeus (the last muscle is discussed earlier in this chapter). The constrictors partly overlap each other and may be visualized as three sleeves telescoped inside one another.

SUPERIOR PHARYNGEAL CONSTRICTOR. The superior pharyngeal constrictor is a thin, quadrilateral-shaped muscle whose fibers originate from the pterygoid hamulus and an adjoining region of the medial pterygoid plate, the pterygomandibular raphe, the posterior quarter of the mylohyoid line, the alveolar process of the mandible, and the lateral aspect of the root of the tongue. The muscle fibers curve posteriorly to insert into the pharyngeal raphe. A thin slip of this muscle, couched on the internal surface of its cranial portion, passes lateral to the levator veli palatini muscle. It arises from the palatal aponeurosis and merges with the fibers of the main muscle mass of the superior constrictor. This muscle slip, the *palatopharyngeal sphincter,* produces a ridge, *Passa-*

vant's bar, on the posterior pharyngeal wall, which the elevated soft palate contacts during deglutition, effectively separating the nasal from the oral pharynx. The superior constrictor, innervated by branches from the pharyngeal plexus, acts to constrict the pharynx.

MIDDLE PHARYNGEAL CONSTRICTOR. The middle pharyngeal constrictor, a fan-shaped muscular sheet, originates on the lesser and greater cornua of the hyoid bone and the stylohyoid ligament. The cranial fibers pass superficial to the superior constrictor muscle, thus covering part of it, while the inferior fibers pass deep to the inferior constrictor muscle. The middle constrictor inserts into the median raphe. It is innervated by branches from the pharyngeal plexus and acts to constrict the pharynx.

INFERIOR PHARYNGEAL CONSTRICTOR. The inferior pharyngeal constrictor, the caudalmost of the three constrictors, envelops the lower part of the middle constrictor. It arises from the lateral aspect of the cricoid cartilage, from the region dorsal to the thyroid cartilage, and from the oblique line of the thyroid cartilage to insert into the pharyngeal raphe. The caudalmost fibers of the inferior constrictor are continuous with the cranialmost, circular inner muscle fibers of the esophagus. The inferior constrictor receives its motor supply from branches of the pharyngeal plexus and from the external and recurrent laryngeal branches of the vagus nerve. Functionally, the inferior constrictor may be considered to have two parts: the superior thyropharyngeal and the inferior cricopharyngeal. The former constricts the pharynx, while the latter acts as a pharyngo-esophageal sphincter, preventing reflux of esophageal contents into the pharynx.

STYLOPHARYNGEUS. The stylopharyngeus muscle, a long, thin cylinder-shaped muscle arises from the styloid process and passes inferomedially between the middle and superior pharyngeal constrictors to merge at its insertion with the fibers of those muscles. Additional fibers of the stylopharyngeus insert in common with the palatopharyngeus muscle on the dorsal aspect of the thyroid cartilage. The stylopharyngeus muscle receives its motor supply from the glossopharyngeal nerve. It acts to elevate the larynx and pharynx.

SALPINGOPHARYNGEUS. The salpingopharyngeus muscle is a thin, fusiform muscle arising from the inferior aspect of the cartilaginous auditory tube at its terminal end in the nasopharynx. The salpingopharyngeus passes inferiorly, deep to the pharyngeal mucosa, to insert into the muscular wall of the pharynx by interdigitating with the fibers of the palatopharyngeus muscle. The salpingopharyngeus is innervated by branches of the pharyngeal plexus. It functions in elevating the pharynx, and may assist in opening the auditory tube during deglutition.

Vascular and Nerve Supply

Arterial supply of the cranial portion of the pharynx is derived chiefly from the ascending pharyngeal branch of the external carotid artery, the pharyngeal branches of the maxillary artery, and the ascending palatine and tonsillar branches of the facial artery. The superior thyroid and, to a lesser extent, the inferior thyroid arteries supply the caudal portion of the pharynx. Venous drainage is via a plexus of veins, the *pharyngeal plexus*, located between the prevertebral fascia and the constrictor muscles. This plexus is drained by the pterygoid plexus of veins and the internal jugular and facial veins.

Nerve supply of the pharynx is via the *pharyngeal plexus of nerves*, derived from the cranial nerves IX, X, and XI. Motor fibers are delivered to this plexus by the vagus nerve, but are probably derived from the cranial nucleus of the accessory nerve. All muscles are innervated by this plexus, except for the tensor veli palatini which is innervated by the mandibular division of the trigeminal and the stylopharyngeus which is innervated by the glossopharyngeal nerve. Sensory innervation of the nasopharynx and part of the oropharynx is via branches of the maxillary division of the trigeminal, while the remainder of the pharynx is supplied by the glossopharyngeal and vagus nerves. Overlapping innervation in the region of the fauces is provided by the facial nerve via its greater petrosal branch, as indicated earlier.

ESOPHAGUS (Fig. 16.4)

The esophagus is a 25 cm-long muscular tube whose main function is to serve as a passageway for food from the pharynx to the stomach, where digestion will occur. Along its length, the esophagus resides in the neck, thorax, and abdomen. It is situated more or less anterior to the bodies of the vertebrae, until it pierces the diaphragm to enter the abdomen. The lumen of the esophagus is normally closed in its cervical and abdominal portions, while the thoracic portion is usually somewhat open and contains air.

The esophagus is in close association with various important structures along its descent through the neck and thorax, but only its cervical relations will be considered here. It begins at the level of the sixth cervical vertebra, as a continuation of the pharynx, near the inferior border of the cricoid cartilage, where the esophagus lies upon the prevertebral fascia over the longus colli muscle. The trachea lies directly anterior to the esophagus, thus creating a tracheoesophageal groove in which the recurrent laryngeal nerve makes its ascent. Lateral to the esophagus is the carotid sheath with its neurovascular contents. The thyroid gland, specifically its lateral lobes, are also in close association with the lateral aspect of the esophagus. Although the microscopic anatomy of the esophagus is not pertinent to the study of its gross morphology, mention should be made of the fact that the external muscular layers are composed of skeletal muscle in the cervical portion of the esophagus, smooth muscle in the lower thoracic and abdominal regions, and a combination of the two in the upper and middle thoracic regions.

Vascular supply of the cervical portion of the esophagus is via the inferior thyroid arteries and veins, while its nerve supply is derived from the recurrent laryngeal nerve and the cervical sympathetic trunk.

LARYNX (Figs. 16.3, 16.4, 16.5, 16.6)

The larynx, or voice box, is continuous with the laryngeal pharynx, cranially, and with the trachea, caudally. It is a passageway for inspired and expired air, a

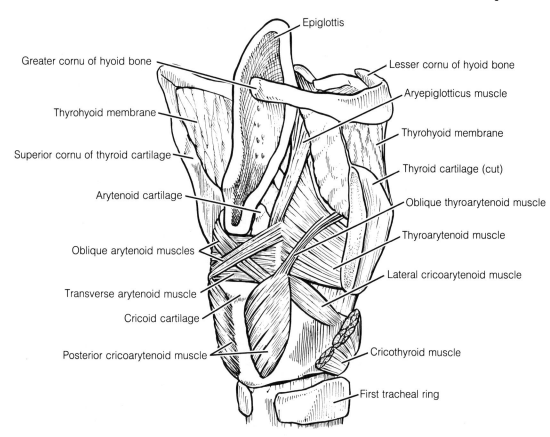

Epiglottis

Greater cornu of hyoid bone

Lesser cornu of hyoid bone

Aryepiglotticus muscle

Thyrohyoid membrane

Thyrohyoid membrane

Superior cornu of thyroid cartilage

Thyroid cartilage (cut)

Arytenoid cartilage

Oblique thyroarytenoid muscle

Thyroarytenoid muscle

Oblique arytenoid muscles

Lateral cricoarytenoid muscle

Transverse arytenoid muscle

Cricoid cartilage

Posterior cricoarytenoid muscle

Cricothyroid muscle

First tracheal ring

Figure 16.5. Posterolateral view of the laryngeal musculature.

sphincter preventing the entry of solids or liquids into the respiratory system caudal to itself, and an organ of phonation permitting the production and modulation of sound. It is composed of a series of cartilages, muscles, membranes, and ligaments which, acting in concert, accomplish these functions. It is interesting to note that the larynx of the male and female are the same size prior to puberty, while the adult male larynx is much larger than that of the adult female.

The larynx lies anteriorly in the midline of the neck and is covered by skin, infrahyoid muscles, and associated fascia. The great vessels of the neck pass posterolateral to it. It is lined by a mucous membrane, which is continuous with and similar to those of the pharynx and trachea. These membranes are modified in places to form two pairs of folds, the cranially-positioned ventricular and the caudally-placed vocal folds, the latter overlying the vocalis muscles and being responsible for the formation of sound. It is convenient to describe the *cavity of the larynx* as consisting of three compartments: the vestibule, ventricle, and the infraglottic cavity. The *vestibule* extends from the *superior laryngeal aperture* (aditus) to the *rima glottidis* (the space between the two vocal folds and the two arytenoid cartilages). The *ventricle* is a space lying directly between the ventricular and vocal cords, being lateral outpocketings of the vestibule. The *infraglottic cavity* is the space between the rima glottidis and the beginning of the tracheal cavity.

Cartilages

There are nine cartilages of the larynx: the unpaired thyroid, cricoid, and epiglottic and the paired arytenoid, cuneiform, and corniculate cartilages.

Thyroid Cartilage

The thyroid cartilage is composed of two quadrilateral plates, the right and left *laminae,* which fuse to form the *laryngeal prominence* (Adam's apple) of the neck. The angle of fusion is more acute in the male than in the female, accounting for the sexual dimorphism evidenced by this structure. Superiorly, this prominence ends in the *superior thyroid notch* and, inferiorly, in the inferior thyroid notch. The superior and inferior borders of each lamina end posteriorly in a *superior* and *inferior cornu,* respectively. The posterolateral surface of the cartilage bears the *oblique line,* extending from the superior to the inferior thyroid tubercles. The medial surface of the thyroid lamina is smooth and unremarkable.

Cricoid Cartilage

The cricoid cartilage is a ring-shaped structure whose width is greater posteriorly than anteriorly. It composes the antero- and lateroinferior walls as well as most of the posterior wall of the larynx. It consists of a quadrilateral, dorsal lamina and a ventral, narrow arch. At each junction of the lamina and the arch are the facets for articulation of the cricoid with the inferior cornua of the thyroid cartilage. The internal surface of the cricoid cartilage is smooth and

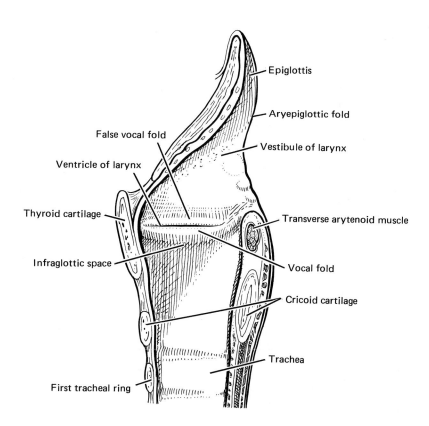

Figure 16.6.
Sagittal section of the larynx.

unremarkable. The superior margin of the lamina on either side of the midline bears two elliptical depressions for articulation with the arytenoid cartilages.

Epiglottic Cartilage

The epiglottic cartilage, an unpaired, leaf-like elastic cartilage, is attached by the thyroepiglottic ligament to the internal aspect of the laryngeal prominence, just inferior to the superior thyroid notch. This ligament attaches to the slender petiole, the narrow, inferior stalk-like extension of the epiglottic cartilage. The broad, leaf-shaped superior portion of the epiglottic cartilage extends craniad but in a posterior direction behind the tongue and hyoid bone, projecting above and anterior to the superior laryngeal aperture. Laterally, the aryepiglottic folds attach the epiglottis to the arytenoid cartilages.

The epiglottis is invested by a mucous membrane which is continuous with the mucosa of the root of the tongue and the lateral pharyngeal walls. The mucosa forms three folds between the tongue and the epiglottis, the single median glossoepiglottic fold and the two lateral glossoepiglottic folds. The depressions between these folds, on either side of the median glossoepiglottic fold, are known as the *epiglottic valleculae*.

Arytenoid Cartilage

The paired arytenoid cartilages are pyramid-shaped structures located on the superior border of the lamina of the cricoid cartilage. The arytenoid cartilage has a concave base which articulates with the arytenoid articular surface of the cricoid lamina, a dorsomedially-inclined apex to which the corniculate cartilage attaches, and three surfaces which provide attachments for muscles and ligaments.

The base has two free processes, the lateral angle, which is the *muscular process*, the point of insertion for the posterior and lateral cricoarytenoid muscles, and the anterior angle, or *vocal process*, to which the vocal cord attaches. The posterior surface serves for the attachments of the transverse arytenoid muscles. The ventrolateral surface presents a superiorly positioned triangular fovea containing mucous glands and providing attachment to the vestibular ligament. Positioned inferiorly is an oblong fovea which is the site of attachment for the vocalis and, frequently, the lateral cricoarytenoid muscles. The medial surface is smooth and is invested by a mucous membrane.

Corniculate and Cuneiform Cartilages

The corniculate and cuneiform cartilages are tiny pieces of elastic cartilage. The former articulates with the arytenoid apex, while the latter is attached to the aryepiglottic fold just anterior to the corniculate cartilage.

Membranes, Ligaments, and Muscles (Table 16.2)

Deep to the laryngeal mucosa is a thick intrinsic membrane of elastic lamina whose cranial portion is referred to as the *quadrangular membrane* and whose caudal portion is the *elastic cone*. The inferior free edge of the quadrangular membrane assists in the formation of the ventricular vocal cords. The elastic cone has a well-defined anterior portion, known as the *median cricothyroid ligament*, and two thickened lateral portions, the *vocal ligaments*, whose free edges assist in the formation of the vocal cords. Two extrinsic membranes of interest are the *thyrohyoid* and *cricothyroid membranes.* The former is a thick fibroelastic membrane between the body and greater cornua of the hyoid bone, superiorly, and the cranial aspect of the thyroid cartilage, inferiorly. The latter is a narrow band of fibroelastic tissue connecting the inferior rim of the cricoid cartilage with the superior rim of the first tracheal ring.

The muscles of the larynx may be classed in two groups, extrinsic and intrinsic. The extrinsic muscles have been described previously, therefore, only the main intrinsic muscles are treated in the following sections. The main intrinsic muscles are the cricothyroid, lateral cricoarytenoid, posterior cricoarytenoid, arytenoid, and thyroarytenoid muscles.

Cricothyroid Muscle

The cricothyroid muscle is situated on the ventrolateral aspect of the larynx, bridging the space between the cricoid and thyroid cartilages. It originates on the arch of the cricoid cartilage and fans out to insert onto the inferior margin of the lamina and the inferior cornu of the thyroid cartilage. The external branch of the superior laryngeal branch of the vagus nerve supplies the cricothyroid muscle. This muscle acts to raise the cricoid cartilage and draw the thyroid cartilage ventrally, thus placing tension on the vocal cords.

Lateral Cricoarytenoid Muscle

The lateral cricoarytenoid muscle is a small muscle originating on the arch of the cricoid cartilage to insert onto the muscular process of the arytenoid cartilage. This muscle is frequently fused with the thyroarytenoid muscle. Inferior laryngeal branches of the recurrent laryngeal nerve supply motor innervation

TABLE 16.2
Intrinsic Muscles of the Larynx

Name	Origin	Insertion	Innervation	Action
Cricothyroid	Arch of the cricoid cartilage	Lamina and inferior cornu of thyroid cartilage	External branch of superior laryngeal nerve	Tenses vocal cords.
Lateral cricoarytenoid	Arch of the cricoid cartilage	Muscular process of arytenoid cartilage	Inferior laryngeal nerve	Adducts vocal cords.
Posterior cricoarytenoid	Lamina of the cricoid cartilage	Muscular process of arytenoid cartilage	Inferior laryngeal nerve	Abducts vocal cords.
Arytenoid Transverse	Posterior surfaces of the two arytenoid cartilages		Inferior laryngeal nerve	Adducts vocal cords.
Oblique	Muscular process of one arytenoid cartilage	Apex of opposite arytenoid cartilage	Inferior laryngeal nerve	Adducts vocal cords.
Thyroarytenoid	Thyroid lamina and cricothyroid ligament	Lateral margin and base of the arytenoid cartilage	Inferior laryngeal nerve	Adducts vocal cords.
Vocalis	Thyroid lamina and cricothyroid ligament	Vocal ligament	Inferior laryngeal nerve	Modifies tension on vocal cord.

to this muscle. The lateral cricoarytenoid muscle acts to stretch the vocal cord by rotating the vocal process of the arytenoid cartilage in a medioinferior direction. This movement approximates the two vocal cords, narrowing the rima glottidis.

Posterior Cricoarytenoid Muscle
The posterior cricoarytenoid muscle arises from most of the inferomedial aspect of the cricoid lamina to insert on the muscular process of the arytenoid cartilage. It receives motor fibers from the inferior laryngeal branches of the recurrent laryngeal nerve and acts to tense the vocal cords and draw them away from each other.

Arytenoid Muscle
The arytenoid muscle, located on the dorsal aspect of the arytenoid cartilages, consists of transverse and oblique portions. The transverse portion *(transverse arytenoid)* is attached to the posterior surface of the lateral aspect of the two arytenoid cartilages. The oblique portion of the arytenoid muscle consists of two slender muscular filaments which cross over each other on the dorsal surface of the transverse arytenoid muscle. The oblique portion originates on the muscular process of one arytenoid cartilage to insert on the apex of the next. The muscle fibers frequently continue in the aryepiglottic region of the quadrangular membrane. This portion of the muscle is then called the *aryepiglotticus muscle.* The arytenoid muscle is innervated by the inferior laryngeal branch of the recurrent laryngeal nerve. This muscle draws the arytenoid cartilages toward each other, thus closing the rima glottidis.

Thyroarytenoid Muscle
The thyroarytenoid muscle is located on the lateral aspect of the larynx deep to the thyroid lamina. It originates on the medial aspect of the thyroid lamina and from the cricothyroid ligament to insert into the lateral margin and base of the arytenoid cartilage. A slip of this muscle, the *vocalis,* inserts into the vocal process of the arytenoid cartilage and is attached to the vocal ligament. The thyroarytenoid muscle is innervated by the inferior laryngeal branch of the recurrent laryngeal nerve. This muscle acts on the arytenoid cartilages to decrease the rima glottidis by bringing the vocal cords nearer to each other.

Movements of the Vocal Folds
The vocal folds may be adducted, that is moved towards each other, so that the intervening space, the rima glottidis, is almost obliterated. They may also be abducted, that is moved apart, so that the rima glottidis is opened. Air passing from the trachea through the rima vibrates the tensed vocal folds producing sounds.

The rima glottidis may be thought of as having two regions, an intermembraneous region, between the vocal folds, and an intercartilaginous region, between the arytenoid cartilages. During normal breathing, the intermembraneous portion is triangular, while the intercartilaginous portion is rectangular in outline. During forced breathing, the arytenoid cartilages are rotated laterally, so that the vocal folds are abducted greatly, describing a triangle whose apical angle is less acute than in normal respiration. The intercartilaginous portion of the rima also becomes triangular, thus the rima is shaped like a rhomboid.

During phonation, the rima is reduced to a thin slit in both its inter-membraneous and intercartilaginous portions, and the vocal folds are tensed by the cranial tilting of the cricoid cartilage by the cricothyroid muscle. The pitch of the sound is directly dependent upon the degree of tilting. During very soft speech, the intercartilaginous portion of the rima opens, while the inter-membraneous portion is almost obliterated.

Vascular and Nerve Supply

The arterial supply of the larynx is derived mainly from the superior thyroid artery and the inferior thyroid branch of the thyrocervical trunk. These vessels provide superior and inferior laryngeal branches (respectively) which vascular-ize the larynx. The cricothyroid branch of the superior thyroid artery also serves the larynx. Venous drainage is accomplished by the superior and inferior laryngeal veins, tributaries of the superior and inferior thyroid veins, respec-tively.

Sensory innervation of the larynx, above the vocal cords, is via the internal laryngeal branch of the superior laryngeal nerve of the vagus. The internal laryngeal nerve accompanies the superior laryngeal branch of the superior thy-roid artery, pierces the thyrohyoid membrane, and distributes deep to the mu-cosa of the epiglottis, aryepiglottic fold, and larynx. Taste buds of this region are also supplied by the internal laryngeal nerve. Sensory innervation below the vocal cords is via sensory fibers of the recurrent laryngeal branches of the vagus nerve. Motor innervation of the larynx has been detailed earlier, but in summary, all intrinsic muscles of the larynx, with the exception of the crico-thyroid, are innervated by the recurrent laryngeal branch of the vagus nerve. The cricothyroid muscle is served by the external laryngeal branch of the vagus nerve.

TRACHEA (Figs. 7.11, 16.3, 16.5)

The trachea begins at the inferior border of the larynx to which it is attached by the cricotracheal ligament. The trachea enters the thoracic cavity, where it bifurcates forming the right and left bronchi. The cervical portion of the tra-chea is superficial, being only partially covered by the infrahyoid muscles. Its superior portion may be palpated between the sternal heads of the sterno-cleidomastoid muscles, as well as in the jugular notch. It is a membraneous structure, whose lumen is maintained by incomplete cartilaginous rings dis-tributed more or less evenly along the length of the tube. The complete portion of the ring is placed anteriorly, while the posteriorly placed interval contains smooth muscle fibers which are able to regulate the size of the lumen to a limited extent.

DEGLUTITION

Deglutition, or the act of swallowing, is a complex neuromuscular phenome-non which is by no means understood completely. For this reason, the anat-omy of deglutition is an area rife with disagreement. The present discussion focuses on generally accepted aspects of deglutition.

Although the act of swallowing, once initiated, is a continuous process, it is divided into three phases here for the sake of convenience: voluntary, involuntary, and final stages. The voluntary, or first stage, involves the formation of the bolus of food by the actions of the tongue against the hard palate and by the assistance of the soft palate as it approximates the back of the tongue. Once the bolus is ready, the suprahyoid muscles elevate and fix the hyoid bone and the tongue forces the bolus through the oropharyngeal isthmus.

Once the bolus enters the oral pharynx, the involuntary or second stage of deglutition is initiated. The levator veli palatini and tensor veli palatini muscles elevate and tense the soft palate, which comes into contact with the bar of Passavant, thus isolating the nasopharynx from the oral pharynx. The actions of the tensor veli palatini and salpingopharyngeus muscles also open the auditory tube. The paired palatoglossus muscles also contract, bringing the palatoglossal folds in close proximity to the back of the tongue. Thus, the bolus cannot pass laterally, superiorly, or ventrally, only inferiorly. Simultaneously, the stylopharyngeus, palatopharyngeus, salpingopharyngeus, and thyrohyoid muscles elevate the larynx and pharynx in a dorsal direction, approximating the laryngeal part of the pharynx to the descending bolus and pulling the laryngeal inlet out of the way. In order to protect the larynx, the aryepiglottic, thyroarytenoid, and oblique arytenoid muscles contract to bring the aryepiglottic folds medially, creating a chute leading to the piriform recess. The bolus of food, sliding along the sides of the epiglottis, descends via this chute to the piriform recess, where the action of the inferior constrictor muscle initiates the final stage of deglutition by forcing the bolus into the esophagus whose cranial portion is completely relaxed. The esophagus, via its musculature, then performs peristaltic actions to transmit the bolus of food into the stomach.

CLINICAL CONSIDERATIONS ══════════════════════════════════

Congenital

Congenital defects of the palate, such as the various degrees of cleft palate, are discussed in Chapter 5.

A somewhat common type of developmental defect is the tracheoesophageal fistula, which usually occurs just cranial to or at the bifurcation of the trachea. This anomaly is less common in females than in males. The fistula provides esophageal (and occasionally gastric) contents with free access to the respiratory system.

Palate

Osseous protrusions, palatal tori, may be observed on the hard palate. These tori, usually bilateral, are asymptomatic, though they interfere with fitting of maxillary dentures. They may need to be excised surgically prior to the making of impressions.

The soft palate is a movable structure and must be avoided by the posterior aspect of a maxillary denture, since its muscular action will break the palatal seal and dislodge the prosthesis.

The posterior aspect of the soft palate is sensitive to touch and may induce vomiting upon tactile stimulation.

Pharynx

The palatine tonsils of a child are much larger than those of an adult. They are commonly prone to infection, since they tend to accumulate debris in the tonsillar crypts. Frequent tonsillitis may indicate the need for tonsillectomy, a relatively minor surgical procedure. However, the proximity of the tonsils to the common carotid artery and the rich vascular supply of the tonsils necessitate extreme care in the procedure.

Adenoids is the term that commonly refers to the pathologic state when the pharyngeal tonsil becomes hypertrophied due to infection. Excessive hypertrophy partially (or completely) blocks the posterior choanae, necessitating mouth breathing, and causing nasal speech and loud snoring during sleep. Persistent inflammation and infection of the pharyngeal tonsil may lead to spreading of the infection into the internal auditory tube and eventually into the mastoid air cells. Although in the past this was a relatively common disease (treated with mastoidectomy), the advent of antibiotics had done much to control and subdue it.

The laryngopharynx, specifically the piriform recess, is a common site for lodging of sharp objects, such as chicken and fish bones. The presence of foreign material in this region causes gagging, and the person is unable to remove the irritant. Care must be exercised in working in the piriform recess, for deep to the mucous membrane is the internal laryngeal nerve, which may be damaged during probing procedures.

Larynx

The intrinsic laryngeal musculature is served by two nerves, the inferior laryngeal branch of the recurrent laryngeal nerve and the external branch of the superior laryngeal nerve, both branches of the vagus nerve. Since these two nerves are prone to damage, it is essential that they be protected from injury during surgical procedures. The external laryngeal nerve, passing deep to the superior thyroid artery, supplies only a single muscle, the cricothyroid. Its section does not cause excessive damage to phonation. It will, however, affect the ability to tense the vocal cords and thus to produce high-pitched sounds. In addition, damage to it causes some hoarseness and easy tiring of the voice. On the other hand, damage to the recurrent laryngeal or the inferior laryngeal nerves will result in serious complications, whose severity depends on the degree of damage and whether or not the injury is bilateral. The involvement may range from slight hoarseness to complete inability to vocalize and breathe, necessitating the performance of a tracheotomy.

Tracheotomy is a surgical procedure performed to provide an airway passage to relieve dyspnea. This procedure is now generally employed only for long-term maintenance of airway passage. Though the procedure may be performed any place along the trachea between the cricoid cartilage and the jugular notch, several complications may result due to the possibility of severing major venous channels and the isthmus of the thyroid gland overlying the trachea. A much safer emergency procedure for opening the airway is *cricothyrotomy*, where opening the passageway is accomplished by incising the cricothyroid membrane between the thyroid and cricoid cartilages. This procedure is easily performed with but few possible complications.

CHAPTER 17

Brain and Spinal Cord

The brain and spinal cord together compose the receiving, integrating, analyzing, and responding portion of the body, called the Central Nervous System (CNS). These are delicate, almost gelatinous-like structures that consist of cells with very little intercellular connective tissue material. Since the CNS is so fragile and so important for the life and proper functioning of the individual, the brain and spinal cord are housed in bony compartments which protect them from injury. In order to provide further protection, the brain and spinal cord are surrounded by meningeal membranes and are bathed in cerebrospinal fluid. This chapter does not provide a thorough account of the central nervous system; that is to be found in textbooks of neuroanatomy. Rather, a general accounting is included here to provide students with some terminology and a descriptive introduction to the morphology of the meninges, brain, and spinal cord.

MENINGES (Figs. 9.1, 9.2)

The brain and spinal cord are invested by three layers of membranes which, in addition to providing support and protection, act as a covering for blood vessels that supply the CNS. These three layers include the externalmost dura mater, the middle arachnoid, and the innermost pia mater.

The *dura mater*, the outer, coarse, fibrous covering of the brain, also covers the spinal cord, and the two are continuous with each other through the foramen magnum. The dura of the brain is described in Chapter 9; that of the spinal cord is similar in concept, but it forms no reflections as does the cranial dura. Instead, the spinal dura is a cylindrical sheath which surrounds the spinal cord as well as the spinal nerve roots that pass through the intervertebral foramina. The external aspect of the spinal dura is not attached to bone, but rather a fatty connective tissue layer, the *epidural fat*, separates it from the periosteum and provides further cushioning of the spinal canal. The epidural fat contains the internal vertebral venous plexus, which empties into the venous sinuses of the cranial dura. The internal aspect of the cranial and spinal dura mater is lined by a simple squamous type of epithelium, which separates the dura from the arachnoid. A potential space, the *subdural space*, is interposed between the epithelia lining the dura and the arachnoid.

265

The *arachnoid*, a thin avascular layer, is covered by a simple squamous epithelium and extends thin web-like processes into the *subarachnoid space*, a fluid-filled region between the arachnoid and pia mater. The arachnoid and dura, although separated from each other by the potential subdural space, follow each others' contours. These membranes display connections at the spinal and cranial nerves, at the infundibulum of the hypophysis, in regions where vessels penetrate the dura to and from the subarachnoid space, as well as at the points where the *denticulate ligaments* of the pia attach and fix the pia to the dura. The subarachnoid space contains blood vessels and cerebrospinal fluid. This fluid exits the subarachnoid space via the specialized *arachnoid granulations*, which, piercing the meningeal dura in the parietal region, deliver the cerebrospinal fluid into the *lacunae lateralis*, located in the fovea granularis of the parietal bone. These lacunae are drained by short vessels which empty into the superior sagittal sinus. The subarachnoid space becomes dilated in certain regions, forming cisterns, which are detailed later in this chapter.

The *pia mater* is a delicate membrane that closely follows the contours of the brain and spinal cord, and the nerves emanating from them. Blood vessels passing through the subarachnoid space branch extensively on the superficial surface of the pia, which they pierce to enter the substance of the brain. Here, glial cells (supporting cells of the CNS), form a protective coating around the vessels to establish an effective *blood-brain barrier*, controlling the entry of materials into the intercellular spaces of the brain and spinal cord.

The central nervous system is a hollow structure lined by a special type of epithelium, known as *ependyma*. This epithelium, which is modified in certain areas of the brain, surrounds vascular intrusions of pial elements to form the *choroid plexus*, which functions in the elaboration of cerebrospinal fluid.

BRAIN

The brain is an immensely complex structure whose organizational hierarchy is not completely understood. This section of the chapter does not attempt to discuss the functional aspects of neuroanatomy; instead, only the gross morphology of the brain is described.

Divisions

The brain, during embryogenesis, is noted to be clearly divided into five continuous parts: the telencephalon, diencephalon, mesencephalon, metencephalon, and myelencephalon, arranged in an anteroposterior (rostro-caudal) direction. Regions of the developing brain become greatly enlarged and some of these portions overgrow others so that the brain begins to fold upon itself, so much so that parts of the brain become submerged and surrounded by more rapidly growing elements. Hence, only three regions are evident upon a cursory examination of the whole adult brain: the cerebral hemispheres, cerebellum, and brainstem.

Cerebral Hemispheres (Figs. 17.1, 17.2, 17.3)
The largest portion of the brain is composed of the two cerebral hemispheres. The two hemispheres, derived from the telencephalon, are partly separated

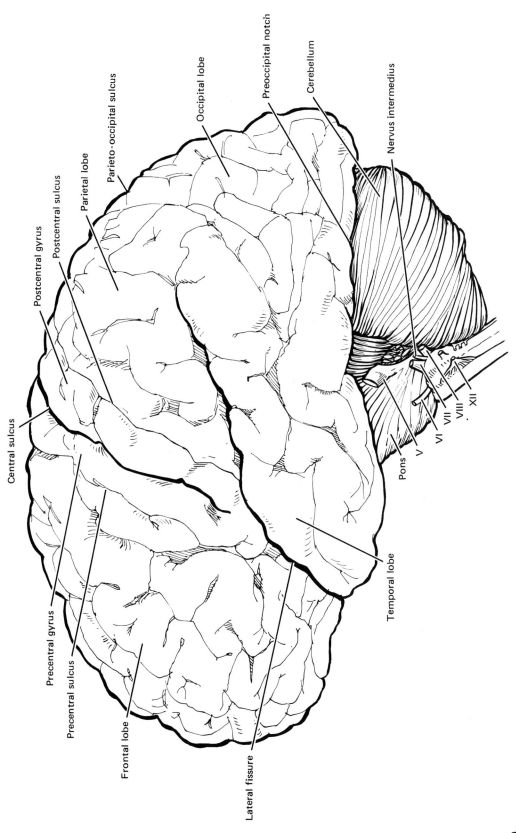

Central sulcus

Postcentral gyrus

Postcentral sulcus

Parietal lobe

Parieto-occipital sulcus

Occipital lobe

Preoccipital notch

Cerebellum

Nervus intermedius

Precentral gyrus

Precentral sulcus

Frontal lobe

Lateral fissure

Temporal lobe

Pons

V

VI

VII

VIII

XII

Figure 17.1. Lateral view of the whole brain.

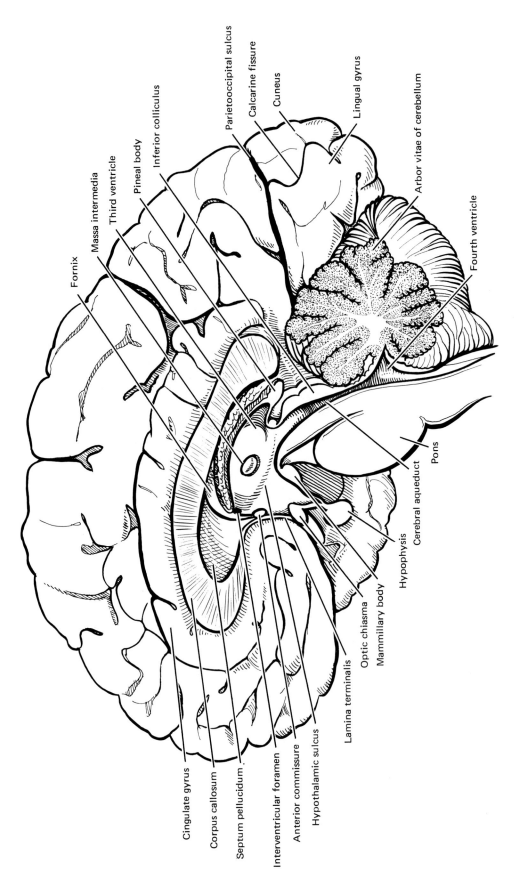

Figure 17.2. Midsagittal section of the whole brain.

Cingulate gyrus

Corpus callosum

Septum pellucidum

Interventricular foramen

Anterior commissure

Hypothalamic sulcus

Lamina terminalis

Optic chiasma

Mammillary body

Hypophysis

Cerebral aqueduct

Pons

Fourth ventricle

Arbor vitae of cerebellum

Lingual gyrus

Cuneus

Calcarine fissure

Parietooccipital sulcus

Inferior colliculus

Pineal body

Third ventricle

Massa intermedia

Fornix

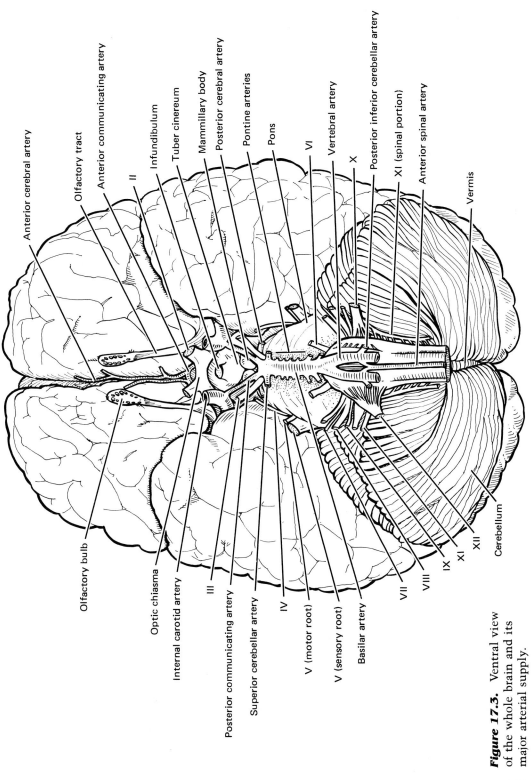

Anterior cerebral artery

Olfactory tract

Anterior communicating artery

II

Infundibulum

Tuber cinereum

Mammillary body

Posterior cerebral artery

Pontine arteries

Pons

VI

Vertebral artery

X

Posterior inferior cerebellar artery

XI (spinal portion)

Anterior spinal artery

Vermis

Olfactory bulb

Optic chiasma

Internal carotid artery

III

Posterior communicating artery

Superior cerebellar artery

IV

V (motor root)

V (sensory root)

Basilar artery

VII

VIII

IX

XI

XII

Cerebellum

Figure 17.3. Ventral view of the whole brain and its major arterial supply.

269

from each other by the deep *longitudinal fissure,* a space occupied by the falx cerebri. The surface of the brain is intimately invested by the almost invisible pia mater, which follows the convoluted elevations and depressions of the surface. Each elevation or *gyrus,* is bounded by the depressions, or *sulci.* The locations of these sulci and gyri are more or less constant. The cerebral hemispheres completely fill the supratentorial space of the skull and may be subdivided into regions reflecting their anatomical position. Hence, there are frontal, parietal, temporal, occipital, and insular lobes. The surface of each cerebral hemisphere is the cortex, consisting of *gray matter.* Deep to the cortex is *white matter,* consisting of fiber tracts passing to and from the cortex and other parts of the brain. Deep within this fibrous region of the cerebrum reside *subcortical nuclei,* groups of cell bodies which constitute the *basal ganglia* associated with somatic motor functions.

The lateral convex surface of the cerebral hemisphere resembles a boxing glove, of which the thumb, pointing inferiorly, is the temporal lobe. A deep fissure, the *lateral sulcus,* separates the temporal from the frontal and parietal lobes. Deep to the temporal lobe, forming the floor of the lateral fissure, is the insula, a cortical lobe also covered by the frontal and parietal lobes. The occipital lobe, a relatively small, triangular portion of the cerebrum lies caudal to the parietal lobe, forming the posterior terminus of the cerebrum. The *central sulcus,* running obliquely from just behind the center of the hemisphere to, but not into, the lateral fissure, separates the frontal and parietal lobes. The gyri, anterior and posterior to the central sulcus, are known as the *precentral gyrus* and the *postcentral gyrus,* respectively. The former is a motor area, while the latter is a sensory area of the cortex. The sulcus caudal to the postcentral gyrus is the *postcentral sulcus* and the one anterior to the precentral gyrus is the *precentral sulcus.*

The largest, or *frontal lobe,* of the cerebral hemisphere is bounded anteriorly by the anterior pole, posteriorly by the central sulcus, and inferiorly by the lateral sulcus. The precentral sulcus and precentral gyrus complete the frontal lobe. The region of the frontal lobe which covers the insula is known as the *frontal operculum.* The operculum and part of the inferior frontal gyrus function in speech. The *parietal lobe* is incompletely defined morphologically. Its anterior boundary is the central sulcus, while posteriorly the lobe is separated from the occipital lobe by an imaginary line extending from the *parieto-occipital sulcus* to the *preoccipital notch.* The region of the parietal lobe covering the insula is the *parietal operculum.* The *temporal lobe* has well-defined superior and inferior boundaries, the lateral sulcus and the inferior extent of the convexity of the cerebrum, while its posterior boundary is the imaginary line between the parieto-occipital sulcus and the preoccipital notch. Several short gyri may be observed on the inner aspect of the temporal lobe forming the inferior border of the lateral sulcus. These transverse gyri represent the primary auditory cortex.

The *occipital lobe* is the posteriormost aspect of the cerebral hemisphere and is separated from the parietal and temporal lobes by the imaginary line connecting the parieto-occipital sulcus and the preoccipital notch. The occipital lobe functions as the visual cortex.

The *insula* is the region of the cerebral hemispheres that is hidden from view by the parietal, frontal, and especially the temporal opercula. It forms the floor of the lateral sulcus and is reported to function in taste.

The two cerebral hemispheres are structurally and functionally connected to each other by commissures, the larger of which is the *corpus callosum,* a midline structure forming the floor of the longitudinal fissure. The other commissure is the much smaller *anterior commissure.* The *fornix* also contains some commissural fibers, though these are not well developed in the human brain. The corpus callosum is best appreciated in the midsagittal view, where it is noted as a white, dense, salient feature of the brain. Fortuitous hemisection of the brain displays the *septum pellucidum* (stretched between the inferior aspect of the corpus callosum and the fornix), which intervenes between the two *lateral ventricles* of the cerebral hemisphere. The two lateral ventricles communicate with each other and the third ventricle via the *interventricular foramen,* which is located just inferior to the anterior portion of the fornix. The medial aspect of the hemisected brain displays the *cingulate gyrus,* located superior to the corpus callosum. The well-defined parieto-occipital sulcus, delineating the anterior border of the occipital lobe, is also evident. The occipital lobe is subdivided into a superior *cuneus* and an inferior *lingula* by the *calcarine sulcus.*

When the cerebral hemisphere is viewed from the inferior perspective, the occipital and part of the temporal lobes are hidden by the cerebellum and the brainstem. The anteroinferior aspect presents the midline longitudinal cerebral fissure, lateral to which is the thin *gyrus rectus* and the *olfactory sulcus* with the attendant *olfactory bulb* and *tract.* Olfactory nerves synapse in the inferior aspect of the bulb after passing through the cribriform plate of the ethmoid bone.

Cerebellum

The cerebellum is a large structure displaying thin, leaf-like plates, the cerebellar folia, giving the cerebellum its distinctive appearance. The cerebellum lies deep to the tentorium cerebelli and is composed of two *cerebellar hemispheres* and the intervening *vermis.* This portion of the brain is derived from the metencephalon. The cerebellum consists of a thin gray matter mantle, known as the *cerebellar cortex,* overlying the centrally located white matter containing several nuclei. Functionally, the cerebellum may be divided into three areas. The *neocerebellum* is responsible for precise coordination of muscle action, especially that related to movements of the hand. The *paleocerebellum* functions in maintaining proper posture in response to gravity. The *archicerebellum* is responsible for proprioception, especially that involved with spatial orientation.

Brainstem (Figs. 17.2, 17.4, 17.5)

The brainstem, the oldest part of the central nervous system, is obscured by the large cerebral and cerebellar hemispheres to such an extent that only its ventral and lateral aspects are visible in the whole brain. Removal of the cerebrum and cerebellum exposes the entire brainstem, which extends from the diencephalon rostrally to the myelencephalon (medulla oblongata) caudally. All cranial nerves arise from the ventral aspect of the brainstem, except for the trochlear nerve which originates from its dorsal surface.

Diencephalon. The diencephalon is the rostralmost portion of the brainstem. It is composed of four regions, the epithalamus, thalamus, hypothalamus, and

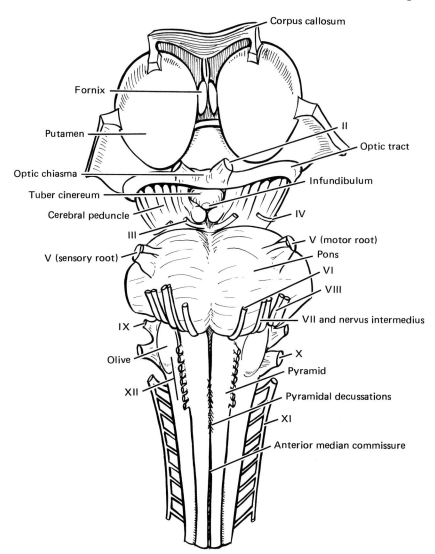

Figure 17.4. Ventral view of the brainstem.

subthalamus. The diencephalon surrounds an ependyma-lined space, the third ventricle, which communicates with the lateral ventricles of the cerebrum via the *interventricular foramen* and with the fourth ventricle through the *cerebral aqueduct.*

The *epithalamus* is the dorsal surface of the diencephalon and is composed of the *pineal body* (whose function in humans is relatively unknown, though it appears to be an endocrine gland), the *stria medullaris,* and the *habenular trigone,* whose nuclei and interhabenular connections are associated with the olfactory system.

The *thalamus* is the largest portion of the diencephalon and is separated into right and left halves by the third ventricle. The two thalami are interconnected by a bridge of gray matter, the *massa intermedia* (or interthalamic adhesion). All sensory stimuli, with the exception of olfaction, enter the thala-

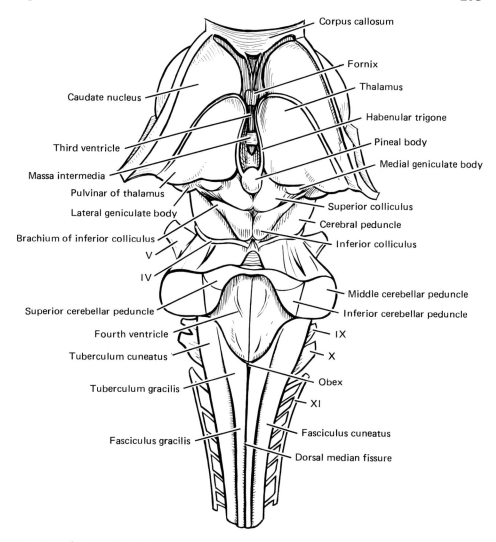

Figure 17.5. Dorsal view of the brainstem.

mus and are redistributed to the sensory cortex for finer perception via the thalamocortical radiations. The thalamus contains many nuclei, some of which create prominent bulges on the surface of the diencephalon. The *pulvinar* is one such large caudal region of the thalamus, located just above the midbrain. Two other nuclei, the *medial* and *lateral geniculate bodies*, associated with hearing and sight, respectively, are located in the vicinity of the pulvinar.

The *hypothalamus* is separated from the thalamus by a groove, the hypothalamic sulcus, located on either wall of the third ventricle. This small region of the diencephalon is associated with endocrine function, sleep, emotion, and regulation of temperature. Structures of the hypothalamus evident on the ventral surface of the brainstem are the *hypophysis* (pituitary gland), the small, elevated *tuber cinereum* with the attendant *infundibulum* of the hypophysis, and the two *mammillary bodies,* located caudal to the tuber cinereum.

The *subthalamus* contains one major nucleus, the subthalamic nucleus, and a few small bundles of fiber tracts. This subdivision of the diencephalon is associated with somatic efferent functions.

Mesencephalon. The mesencephalon (midbrain) is a short segment surrounding the cerebral aqueduct, situated between the diencephalon and the pons. The dorsal aspect, or *tectum*, contains four marked elevations: the *corpora quadrigemina*, consisting of the two rostrally-placed *superior colliculi* functionally related to the visual system, and the caudally-placed *inferior colliculi*, associated with hearing. The lateral geniculate body is connected to the superior colliculus via fiber bundles, the *brachium of the superior colliculus*, while the *brachium of the inferior colliculus* connects the inferior colliculus to the medial geniculate body. Just inferior to this colliculus, the slender trochlear nerve (cranial nerve IV) emerges from the mesencephalon. This is the only cranial nerve to leave the dorsal aspect of the brainstem. The two *cerebral peduncles*, fiber tracts connecting the cerebrum to the brainstem, are located ventrally, below the cerebral aqueduct in a region known as the tegmentum. The *interpeduncular fossa*, between the two peduncles, displays the oculomotor nerve (cranial nerve III) leaving the brainstem.

Metencephalon. The metencephalon is hidden from view by the cerebellum, but its ventral surface is clearly visible as the bulging *pons.* It is separated from the mesencephalon by the superior pontine sulcus and from the myelencephalon by the inferior pontine sulcus. The dorsal aspect of the pons, which forms the floor of the fourth ventricle, is known as the *tegmentum.* The tegmentum contains the nuclei of cranial nerves V, VI, VII, and VIII. As the facial nerve passes over the nucleus of VI, it forms a bulge on the floor of the fourth ventricle, the *facial colliculus.* The *superior* and *middle cerebellar peduncles* connect the cerebellum to the brainstem, and cranial nerve V pierces the rostal part of the middle cerebellar peduncle. The other three cranial nerves associated with the metencephalon leave this structure at the inferior pontine sulcus.

Myelencephalon. The myelencephalon *(medulla oblongata)* is the caudalmost portion of the brainstem. It extends from the inferior pontine sulcus to the spinal cord, demarcated approximately by the foramen magnum. The V-shaped lateral walls close over the fourth ventricle at the apex, the *obex.*

Bilateral, cylindrical structures, the *pyramids,* are evident on the ventral surface of the medulla. *Pyramidal decussations,* or crossings of fibers, appear across the anterior midline fissure from one pyramid to the other. Lateral to each pyramid is an olive pit-shaped bulge, the *olive.* Filaments of cranial nerve XII are lodged in the groove *(anterior lateral sulcus)* between the pyramid and the olive. Cranial nerves IX, X, and XI are located in the groove dorsal to the olive. Fiber connections between the medulla and the cerebellum are via the *inferior cerebellar peduncle.* Located in the midline of the dorsal surface of the medulla is the *posterior median fissure,* lateral to which is the *tuberculum gracilis,* a swelling demarcating the underlying *nucleus gracilis,* upon which many lower sensory neurons synapse. Lateral to the tuberculum gracilis is a similar swelling, the *tuberculum cuneatus* with the underlying *nucleus cuneatus,* where many sensory neurons from the upper part of the body synapse. The most lateral swelling is the *tuberculum cinereum,* representing the descending tract of the trigeminal nerve.

Cerebrospinal Fluid and Ventricles

Cerebrospinal Fluid

The central nervous system develops from a hollow cylindrical tube and retains this space in the adult as the ventricles of the brain and the central canal of the spinal cord. The ventricles and the central canal form a continuous channel filled with cerebrospinal fluid, a clear, colorless, acellular liquid produced by specialized structures, the *choroid plexus,* located mostly in the ventricles. The cerebrospinal fluid is elaborated continuously, bathing the CNS. Some of the fluid enters the subarachnoid space via specialized foramina of the myelencephalon, the paired lateral *foramina of Luschka* and the single, medial *foramen of Magendie.* This fluid circulates in the subarachnoid space eventually to be resorbed into the superior sagittal sinus by *arachnoid granulations,* structures composed of pia and arachnoid cells. The subarachnoid space closely follows the contours of the brain, except in certain regions where the arachnoid diverges, forming larger spaces known as *cisterns.* The three foramina of the myelencephalon empty into the *cisterna magna (cisterna cerebellomedullaris),* the largest of the cisterns, located between the cerebellum and the medulla oblongata. Two other large cisterns in the head are worthy of mention, the *cisterna superior,* between the cerebellum and the midbrain, and the *cisterna interpeduncularis,* located between the two cerebral peduncles. Hence the central nervous system is completely surrounded by cerebrospinal fluid, which may act as a hydrodynamic protective cushion, absorbing sudden traumas in addition to providing its possible nutrient functions.

Ventricles

The ventricles of the brain are ependyma-lined spaces containing cerebrospinal fluid. There are four: the paired *lateral ventricles* of the cerebral hemispheres and the *third* and *fourth ventricles.*

The paired lateral ventricles, the largest of the four, hollow out the cerebral hemispheres. These two ventricles are separated from each other by the intervening *septum pellucidum,* although a connection, the *interventricular foramen,* permits communication between the lateral ventricles and the third ventricle. Each lateral ventricle has a body, and anterior, posterior, and inferior horns.

The third ventricle is surrounded by the right and left halves of the thalamus and is interrupted by a mass of gray matter, the massa intermedia, which crosses this ventricle. The third ventricle communicates with the fourth ventricle by the *cerebral aqueduct.*

The fourth ventricle is located in the hindbrain and also communicates with the central canal of the medulla. Cerebrospinal fluid leaves the fourth ventricle to enter the subarachnoid space by way of the paired lateral foramina of Luschka and the median foramen of Magendie.

Blood Supply

Arterial Supply (Fig. 17.3)

Arterial supply to the brain is derived from the two vertebral and two internal carotid arteries. The vertebral arteries enter the cranial cavity through the foramen magnum and, just prior to reaching the pons, fuse to form the single basilar artery. The two internal carotid arteries gain the cranial cavity via the carotid canals, pass through the cavernous sinus, and give branches to the brain.

Vertebral Artery. The vertebral artery, a branch of the first part of the subclavian artery, supplies three named branches to the central nervous system. These are the single anterior spinal artery and the posterior spinal artery, serving the medulla and the spinal cord, and the *posterior inferior cerebellar artery,* vascularizing the inferior aspect of the caudal portion of the cerebellum.

The vertebral arteries of the two sides join to form the single *basilar artery,* which travels along the ventral aspect of the pons in the basilar groove. Branches of the basilar artery are the anterior inferior cerebellar, labyrinthine, pontine, superior cerebellar, and the posterior cerebral arteries.

The *anterior inferior cerebellar artery,* the caudalmost branch of the basilar artery, supplies the inferior aspect of the anterior portion of the cerebellum. The small *labyrinthine artery* serves the cochlea and vestibular apparatus. Several small *pontine arteries* vascularize the pons, while the *superior cerebellar artery* passes between the cerebral hemispheres and the cerebellum to serve the superior aspect of the latter structure. The basilar artery bifurcates to give rise to the two *posterior cerebral arteries,* which serve the inferomedial aspect of the temporal and occipital lobes of the cerebrum. The posterior cerebral artery possesses an arterial connection to the internal carotid artery, the *posterior communicating artery,* thus forming the posterior arch of the *cerebral arterial circle of Willis.*

Internal Carotid Artery. Branches of the internal carotid artery are the anterior choroidal, middle cerebral, anterior cerebral, and ophthalmic arteries.

The *anterior choroidal artery* supplies the choroid plexus as well as portions of the cerebral hemispheres. The *middle cerebral artery* courses laterally to pass between the temporal and parietal lobes. It supplies the lateral surfaces of most of the frontal, parietal, and temporal lobes. The *anterior cerebral artery* passes anteriorly, on the inferomedial aspect of the gyrus rectus, to vascularize the medial and superior aspects of the frontal and parietal lobes. The two anterior cerebral arteries are interconnected by the short *anterior communicating artery,* thus completing the cerebral arterial circle. This arterial circle, circumscribing the mammillary bodies, the hypophysis, and the optic tracts, is composed of the two posterior cerebral, two posterior communicating, two internal carotid, two anterior cerebral, and the single anterior communicating arteries. The *ophthalmic artery* is not associated with the vascularization of the brain. It passes through the optic foramen to enter and supply the orbit and its contents.

Venous Drainage

Venous drainage of the brain arises from the pial venous plexus derived from the confluence of minute venous vessels. The cerebral veins are divisible into external and internal groups. The external veins drain into the regional venous sinuses. Venous drainage of the deeper regions of the brain eventually empty into the straight sinus via the *great cerebral vein.* Cerebellar veins also are of two groups, *superior* and *inferior cerebellar veins.* These drain into the straight sinus or other regional sinuses.

SPINAL CORD (Figs. 3.9, 3.11)

The spinal cord is an anteroposteriorly flattened cylindrical continuation of the medulla, extending from the cranial border of the first cervical vertebra to the first or second lumbar vertebra. Thus, the spinal cord of the adult does not fill the whole vertebral canal, but ends in a conical structure, the *conus medullaris*. The pial covering continues as a thread-like filament, the *filum terminale*, anchoring the conus medullaris to the coccyx. The spinal cord is fixed also to the lateral wall of the dural covering by toothlike extensions of pia, the *denticulate ligaments*, located equidistant between the ventral and dorsal roots of each spinal nerve. Although the spinal cord extends only to L1 or L2 vertebral levels, the dural covering continues to line the entire extent of the vertebral canal, creating a large, fluid-filled subarachnoid space, the *lumbar cistern*, utilized for spinal fluid taps and lumbar punctures. The lumbar cistern contains, in addition to the filum terminale and cerebrospinal fluid, the *cauda equinae*, root filaments of lumbar and sacral spinal nerves which must pass from the spinal cord to the intervertebral foramina of their destination.

The spinal cord, in cross section, displays the peripheral white matter with the central gray matter arranged in a characteristic H-shaped configuration (Fig. 3.11). The horizontal crossbar of the *H* is represented by the *dorsal* and *ventral gray commissures*, posterior and anterior to the ependyma-lined central canal, respectively. The legs of the *H* are represented by the ventral and dorsal horns. The *ventral horns* house the motor neurons, whose axons leave the spinal cord as ventral rootlets. Sensory fibers enter the spinal cord as dorsal rootlets via the *dorsal horns*. Internuncial cell bodies occupy the *dorsal gray column*, while, at thoracic levels (T1 to L2), the *intermediolateral cell column* houses all presynaptic sympathetic cell bodies.

The right and left sides of the spinal cord are partly separated from each other by the *dorsal median septum* and the somewhat wider *ventral median fissure*, neither of which penetrates the gray matter. Each half of the spinal cord is an apparent mirror image of the other and the white matter of each half contains groups of nerve fiber tracts (or fasciculi) ascending or descending in the cord.

CHAPTER 18

Cranial Nerves

There are twelve pairs of cranial nerves that originate in the brain, leave its surface, and pass through certain foramina of the skull to be distributed in and about the head and neck. One cranial nerve, the vagus, continues on into the thorax and abdomen to innervate some of the viscera. The cranial nerves are named and numbered sequentially with Roman numerals, progressing rostrally to caudally. The names correspond with the numbers as follows:

I Olfactory	VII Facial
II Optic	VIII Acoustic
III Oculomotor	IX Glossopharyngeal
IV Trochlear	X Vagus
V Trigeminal	XI Accessory
VI Abducent	XII Hypoglossal

Two figures appearing earlier in the book may be reviewed to observe the relative positions of the cranial nerves emerging from the brain (Fig. 17.3) and their relative positions in the floor of the cranial vault (Fig. 9.2).

As explained earlier, peripheral nerves consist of several nerve fiber types specific for their function. Typically, each peripheral nerve contains somatic and visceral components, each with afferent and efferent fibers. The peripheral nerves emanating from the brain (cranial nerves) are more complex in that these nerves serve special sensory functions—such as hearing, seeing, smelling, and tasting—in addition to supplying special muscles of branchiomeric origin. The cranial nerves, then, carry certain components in addition to the general somatic and general visceral components carried by spinal nerves. These other components carried by the cranial nerves are designated as special somatic afferent, special visceral afferent, and special visceral efferent:

General somatic afferent—General sensation in function. For example, the trigeminal nerve serves much of the skin and the mucous membranes of the face, while the facial and vagus nerves serve the area of the ear.

General somatic efferent—General motor in function to skeletal muscles. This grouping is carried by the oculomotor, trochlear, abducent, and hypoglossal nerves innervating musculature derived from somites.

General visceral afferent—General sensation from the viscera included in the facial, glossopharyngeal, and vagus nerves.

General visceral efferent—Visceral motor (parasympathetic) to the viscera. Only four cranial nerves transmit parasympathetic fibers: the oculomotor, facial, glossopharyngeal, and vagus nerves.

Special somatic afferent—Special sensory in function from the eye and ear. The cranial nerves carrying this component are the optic and acoustic nerves.

Special visceral afferent—Special sensory in function from the viscera. These fibers are associated with the special senses of smell, carried in the olfactory nerve and that of taste, transmitted in the facial, glossopharyngeal, and vagus nerves.

Special visceral efferent—Special motor to the branchiomeric musculatures. This component is carried to the muscles derived from the branchial arches and is transmitted by the nerves of those arches: the trigeminal, facial, glossopharyngeal, accessory (contributions to the pharyngeal plexus), and vagus nerves.

As with the typical spinal nerve, cell bodies of afferent nerve fibers within the cranial nerves are located in sensory ganglia outside the central nervous system, that is, outside the brain. Central processes of these fibers pass via the cranial nerves into the brain to terminate on neurons that relay impulses for processing, sorting out, and coordinating the information prior to initiation of a motor response that may or may not be at a conscious level. All of the interconnections and workings of the brain are extremely complicated and beyond the scope of this text. Those desiring more information on this subject are referred to standard textbooks of neuroanatomy.

CRANIAL NERVES

Each of the twelve cranial nerves is described in the following sections, including information on the location of the cell bodies, the components carried, connections with other nerves, and finally the distribution and function. A summary of this information is presented in tabular form in Table 18.1.

I Olfactory Nerve (Fig. 18.1)

Cell bodies of the olfactory nerve, the nerve of smell, are found in the olfactory mucosa situated over the superior nasal concha. Axons of the olfactory nerve pass through the cribriform plate of the ethmoid bone to terminate in the *olfactory bulb,* which is connected to the brain by the *olfactory tract,* technically a part of the brain.

II Optic Nerve (Fig. 18.2)

The cell bodies of the optic nerve, the nerve of sight, are located in the ganglionic layer of cells composing the retina. Axons of these cells are gathered into bundles that leave the bulb of the eye as the optic nerve, passing posteriorly through the orbit to exit through the optic foramen. Here the axons join the optic nerve of the opposite side, forming the *optic chiasma.* Optic tracts continue from the chiasma to enter the base of the brain near the cerebral peduncle.

TABLE 18.1
Cranial Nerves

Nerve	Components	Cell bodies	Peripheral distribution	Function
I Olfactory	SVA	Olfactory epithelial cells	Olfactory nerves	Smell
II Optic	SSA	Ganglion cells of retina	Rods and cones	Vision
III Oculomotor	GSE	Nucleus III	Levator palpebrae; recti: superior, medial, inferior; and inferior oblique	Eye movement
	GVE	Edinger-Westphal nucleus	Ciliary ganglion— Ciliary body— Sphincter pupillae	Contraction of pupil and accomodation
	GP	Mesencephalic nucleus V	Ocular muscles	Kinesthetic sense
IV Trochlear	GSE	Nucleus IV	Superior oblique	Ocular movement
	GP	Mesencephalic nucleus V	Superior oblique	Kinesthetic sense
V Trigeminal	GSA	Trigeminal ganglion	Ophthalmic, maxillary, and mandibular divisions to mucous membranes and skin of face and head	General sensation
	SVE	Motor nucleus V	Temporalis, masseter, pterygoids, anterior belly of digastric, mylohyoid, tensors palatini and tympani	Mastication
	GP	Mesencephalic nucleus V	Muscles of mastication	Kinesthetic sense
VI Abducent	GSE	Nucleus VI	Lateral rectus	Eye movement
	GP	Mesencephalic nucleus V	Lateral rectus	Kinesthetic sense
VII Facial	SVE	Motor nucleus VII	Muscles of facial expression, stapedius, stylohyoid, post. belly of digastric	Facial expression
	GVE	Salivatory nucleus	Greater petrosal— pterygopalatine ganglion—nasal mucosa, lacrimal gland; chorda tympani—lingual nerve, submandibular ganglion— submandibular, sublingual glands	Secretomotor
	SVA	Geniculate ganglion	Chorda tympani— lingual nerve-taste buds anterior two-thirds tongue	Taste
	GVA	Geniculate ganglion	Greater petrosal, chorda tympani	Visceral sensation

TABLE 18.1 (CONTINUED)

Nerve	Components	Cell bodies	Peripheral distribution	Function
	GSA	Geniculate ganglion	Auricular branch—ear and mastoid	Cutaneous sensation
VIII Acoustic	SSA	Spiral ganglion	Organ of Corti	Hearing
	SP	Vestibular ganglion	Vestibular mechanism	Balance
IX Glossopharyngeal	SVA	Inferior ganglion IX	Lingual br.—taste buds posterior one-third tongue, circumvallate papillae	Taste
	GVA	Inferior ganglion IX	Tympanic nerve—middle ear, pharynx, tongue, carotid sinus	Visceral sensation
	GVE	Salivatory nucleus	Tympanic—lesser petrosal—otic ganglion, auriculotemporal to parotid gland	Secretomotor
	SVE	Nucleus ambiguus	Stylopharyngeus	Swallowing
X Vagus	GVE	Dorsal motor nucleus X	Cardiac nerves and plexus, ganglia on heart; pulmonary plexus, ganglia respiratory tract; esophageal, gastric, celiac plexus; myenteric and submucous plexus—to transverse colon	Smooth muscle and glands
	SVE	Nucleus ambiguus	Pharyngeal br., superior, inferior laryngeal nerves	Swallowing, speaking
	GVA	Inferior ganglion X	All fibers in all branches	Visceral sensation
	SVA	Inferior ganglion X	Br. to epiglottis, base of tongue, taste buds	Taste
	GSA	Superior ganglion X	Auricular br.—ear, meatus	Cutaneous sensation
XI Accessory	SVE	Nucleus ambiguus	Communication to vagus—muscles of pharynx and larynx	Swallowing, speaking
	SVE (Assuming branchiomeric origin)	Upper spinal cord—lat. column	Spinal portion—sternocleidomastoid, trapezius	Movement, head and shoulder
XII Hypoglossal	GSE	Nucleus XII	Brs. intrinsic, extrinsic muscles of tongue	Tongue movement

Components Code: GSA, General Somatic Afferent; GVA, General Visceral Afferent; SVA, Special Visceral Afferent; SSA, Special Somatic Afferent; GP, General Proprioception; SP, Special Proprioception; GSE, General Somatic Efferent; GVE, General Visceral Efferent; SVE, Special Visceral Efferent

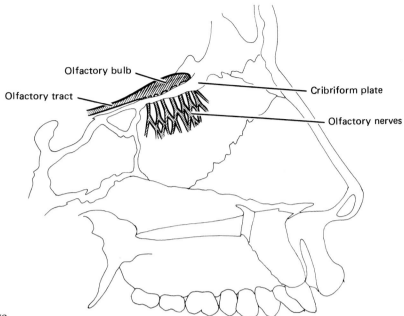

Figure 18.1.
I. Olfactory nerve.

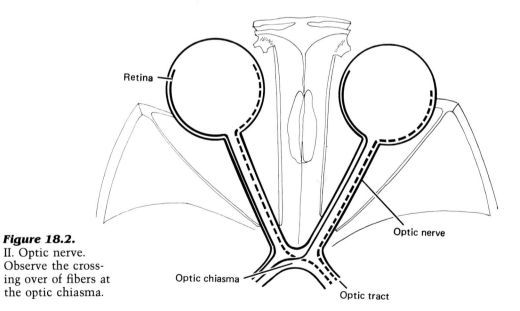

Figure 18.2.
II. Optic nerve. Observe the crossing over of fibers at the optic chiasma.

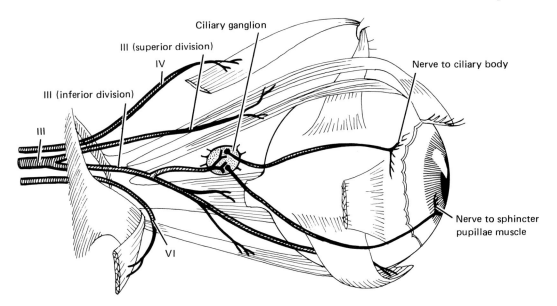

Figure 18.3. III. Oculomotor nerve. IV. Trochlear nerve. VI. Abducent nerve. Observe that the trochlear and abducent nerves innervate but one muscle each. Note the ciliary ganglion and the distribution of the postganglionic parasympathetic fibers from it.

III Oculomotor Nerve (Fig. 18.3)

The oculomotor nerve serves most of the extrinsic muscles of the eye, excluding the superior oblique and the lateral rectus muscles, with general somatic efferent innervation. A specialized group of motor cells in the oculomotor nucleus within the brain is termed the *Edinger–Westphal nucleus.* These are preganglionic parasympathetic cells, whose fibers are destined for the ciliary ganglion within the orbit. Postganglionic fibers from the ganglion pass to the orb via short ciliary nerves and on to the ciliary body and sphincter pupillae muscles of the eye.

The oculomotor nerve exits the brain near the medial side of the cerebral peduncle, passes through the free and attached borders of the tentorium cerebelli, then passes through the lateral wall of the cavernous sinus to enter the superior orbital fissure for distribution. While in the cavernous sinus, contributions from the carotid plexus are communicated to the oculomotor nerve. These communications are the postganglionic sympathetic fibers from the superior cervical ganglion destined for the dilatator pupillae muscle.

Once in the orbit, the nerve divides into superior and inferior divisions, facilitating innervation of the extra-ocular muscles. The ciliary ganglion is suspended from the inferior division by the parasympathetic motor root of the ganglion. Additional communications to the ganglion are from the nasociliary nerve, a branch of the ophthalmic division of the trigeminal nerve. These communications are purely sensory, passing through the ganglion without synapsing. They reach the orb by way of the short ciliary nerves. Postganglionic sympathetic fibers may also communicate with the ganglion in a fashion similar to that of the nasociliary nerve. These sympathetic fibers are destined for the dilatator pupillae muscle. The functions of these intrinsic muscles are detailed in Chapter 10.

Proprioceptive fibers in the extra-ocular muscles are carried in the oculo-motor nerve, then transmitted to the ophthalmic division of the trigeminal nerve to join it in the orbit or via communications while it passes through the walls of the cavernous sinus. Terminations of these fibers are described in the section on the trigeminal nerve.

IV Trochlear Nerve (Fig. 18.3)

The trochlear nerve, the smallest of the cranial nerves, supplies the superior oblique muscle of the eye with motor innervation. This nerve is the only cranial nerve originating on the dorsal surface of the brainstem. From there, it passes around the midbrain to pierce the tentorial dura, thus entering the cavernous sinus. While coursing through the cavernous sinus, the trochlear nerve communicates with the carotid plexus and the ophthalmic division of the trigeminal nerve. Proprioceptive fibers from the superior oblique muscle are thought to communicate to the ophthalmic nerve at that point. Upon entering the orbit through the superior orbital fissure, the nerve terminates in the superior oblique muscle, which it provides with motor innervation.

V Trigeminal Nerve (Figs. 18.4, 18.5, 18.6, 18.7)

The largest of the cranial nerves, the trigeminal nerve, serves much of the face, the teeth and supporting structures, and the mucous membranes of the head with cutaneous sensation and also provides motor innervation to the muscles of mastication. The nerve has two roots emanating from the pons. The larger, sensory root, which lies lateral to the motor root, contains the central processes of the neurons whose cell bodies are found in the *trigeminal (semilunar) ganglion*, the sensory ganglion of the trigeminal nerve. This ganglion is located under the cover of the dura in a pocket (Meckel's cave) on the trigeminal impression located near the apex of the petrous portion of the temporal bone. Peripheral processes of the sensory neurons located in the flat, semilunar-shaped ganglion are gathered in three separate bundles. These bundles leave the ganglion as the ophthalmic, maxillary, and mandibular divisions. The motor root, passing along with the sensory root, but medial to it, courses beneath the trigeminal ganglion to exit the cranial vault through the foramen ovale along with the mandibular division of the nerve. The ophthalmic and maxillary divisions remain purely sensory. The mandibular division is joined by the motor root outside the skull; thus, this division becomes mixed in function.

Four parasympathetic ganglia of the head are in close association with the trigeminal nerve, although, functionally, these ganglia are not part of the trigeminal nerve. Postganglionic parasympathetic fibers arising in these ganglia are transmitted to the structures they serve by joining branches of the trigeminial nerve for distribution. The parasympathetic ganglia, the preganglionic motor root, and the associated divisions of the trigeminal nerve are listed in Table 18.2.

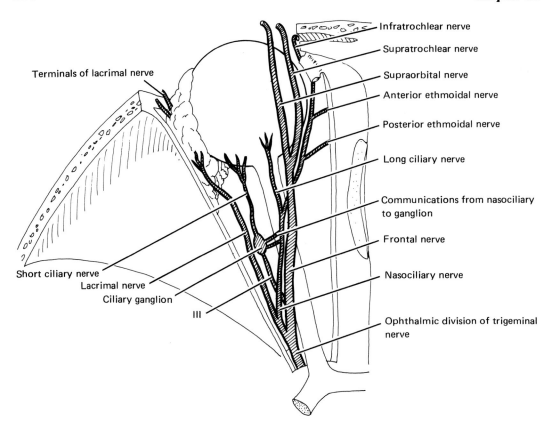

Figure 18.4. V. Trigeminal nerve, ophthalmic division. Note the communications to the ciliary ganglion from the nasociliary nerve.

Ophthalmic Nerve V₁ (Fig. 18.4)

The ophthalmic nerve, providing the bulb and conjunctiva of the eye, lacrimal gland, skin over the forehead, eyes and nose, and the mucous membranes of the paranasal sinuses with sensory innervation, leaves the superior aspect of the trigeminal ganglion, then lies in the lateral wall of the cavernous sinus as it

TABLE 18.2
Parasympathetic Ganglia of the Head

Ganglion	Preganglionic motor nerve origin	Trigeminal association
Ciliary	Oculomotor (III) Inferior division of nerve	Ophthalmic division Nasociliary nerve
Pterygopalatine	Facial (VII) Greater petrosal nerve	Maxillary division Trunk of nerve
Submandibular	Facial (VII) Chorda tympani nerve	Mandibular division Lingual nerve
Otic	Glossopharyngeal (IX) Lesser petrosal nerve	Mandibular division Medial pterygoid nerve

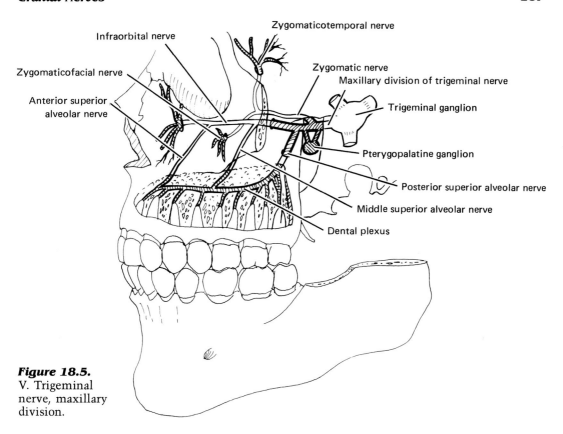

Figure 18.5.
V. Trigeminal
nerve, maxillary
division.

courses to the orbit. Along the way, tentorial branches are supplied to the tentorium. Just prior to entering the orbit through the superior orbital fissure, the nerve divides into three separate nerves: the lacrimal, frontal, and naso-ciliary nerves. In its course, the ophthalmic nerve communicates with the carotid plexus in the cavernous sinus and with other cranial nerves represented in the orbit. Discussion of these communications is not warranted here, how-ever.

Lacrimal Nerve. The lacrimal nerve, smallest of the ophthalmic division, runs along the lateral rectus muscle distributing to the lacrimal gland and adjacent conjunctiva. It then exits the orbit to be distributed to the skin of the lateral aspect of the upper eyelid. While in the orbit, it communicates with the zygomaticotemporal branch of the zygomatic nerve of the maxillary division of the trigeminal nerve, which is carrying postganglionic parasympathetic fi-bers communicated to it from the pterygopalatine ganglion. These parasympa-thetic fibers are thus transmitted to the lacrimal gland, providing it with secretomotor innervation.

Frontal Nerve. The frontal nerve, the largest of the branches, divides shortly after entering the superior aspect of the orbit into a supratrochlear and the larger supraorbital nerve, the former passing medial to the latter as the nerves course anteriorly above the levator palpebrae superioris muscle. The *supra-*

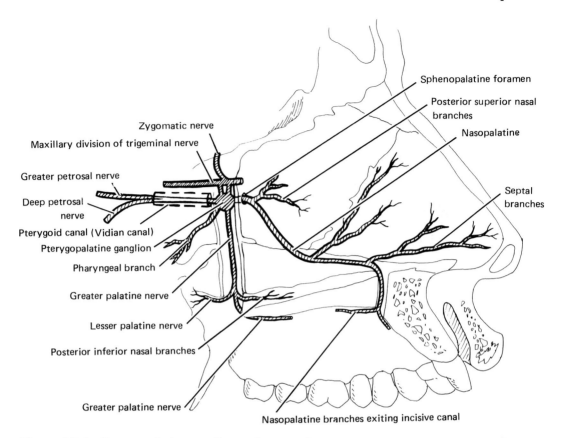

Figure 18.6. Pterygopalatine ganglion and connections.

trochlear nerve bends to pass superior to the pulley of the superior oblique muscle. Here it provides sensory innervation to the conjunctiva and skin of the medial aspect of the eye before leaving the orbit to turn upward to supply the skin over the forehead. The *supraorbital nerve* continues forward to exit the orbit at the supraorbital notch. While passing the notch, it sends a filament into the frontal sinus. The nerve supplies sensory innervation to the upper lid, forehead, and scalp as far posteriorly as the lambdoidal suture.

Nasociliary Nerve. The nasociliary nerve enters the orbit between the lateral rectus muscle and the oculomotor nerve. It then passes obliquely over the optic nerve to the medial wall of the orbit, where it enters the anterior ethmoidal foramen. Just prior to entering the foramen, the nasociliary nerve gives off an *infratrochlear branch,* which courses anteriorly along the medial wall to exit the orbit at its medial margin. Along the way, the branch provides sensory innervation to the conjunctiva, eyelid, lacrimal sac, caruncula, and side of the nose. *Anterior* and *posterior ethmoidal branches* enter the respective foramina to supply the ethmoidal, sphenoidal, and frontal sinuses. The *anterior ethmoidal nerve* continues through the ethmoid bone to enter the nasal cavity. *Internal nasal branches* innervate the mucous membranes. The nerve continues on to exit the nasal cavity at the inferior border of the nasal bone as the *external nasal branch,* providing general sensation to the ala and globe of the nose.

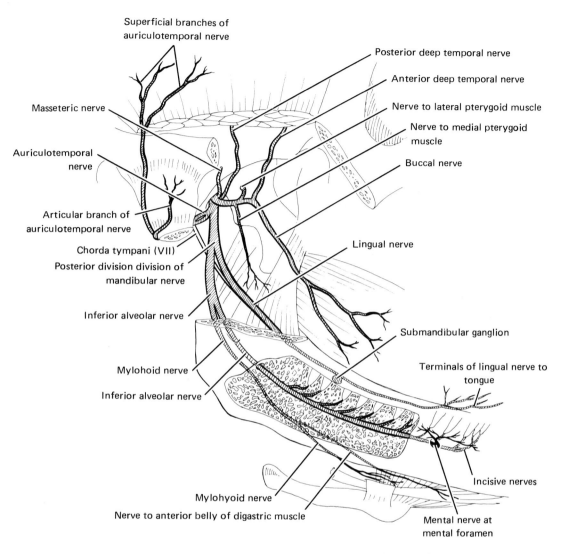

Superficial branches of
auriculotemporal nerve

Posterior deep temporal nerve

Anterior deep temporal nerve

Nerve to lateral pterygoid muscle

Masseteric nerve

Nerve to medial pterygoid
muscle

Buccal nerve

Auriculotemporal
nerve

Articular branch of
auriculotemporal nerve

Chorda tympani (VII)

Posterior division division of
mandibular nerve

Lingual nerve

Inferior alveolar nerve

Submandibular ganglion

Terminals of lingual nerve to
tongue

Mylohoid nerve

Inferior alveolar nerve

Incisive nerves

Mylohyoid nerve

Nerve to anterior belly of digastric muscle

Mental nerve at
mental foramen

Figure 18.7. V. Trigeminal nerve, mandibular division. Observe the chorda tympani from the facial nerve joining the lingual nerve.

While in the orbit, the nasociliary nerve sends *long ciliary nerves* to the orb as the nerve crosses the optic nerve. Other short filaments pass to the ciliary ganglion, establishing a close association with this parasympathetic ganglion. The long ciliary nerves and those filaments which pass to the ganglion and on to the orb as part of the short ciliary nerves are purely sensory and are destined for the iris and cornea. Postganglionic sympathetic fibers communicate to the ophthalmic nerve from the carotid plexus while passing through the cavernous sinus; they may accompany the long ciliary nerves or the short filaments to the ganglion and on to the orb via the short ciliary nerves. These fibers are destined for the dilatator pupillae muscle within the iris.

Maxillary Nerve V₂ (Figs. 18.5, 18.6)
The maxillary nerve, the second division of the trigeminal nerve, is purely sensory and serves the skin of the side of the nose, cheek, eyelids, midface, the

nasopharynx, tonsil, palate, maxillary sinus, gingiva, teeth, and associated structures of the upper jaw. The nerve exits the cranial vault via the foramen rotundum after passing through the posterior portion of the cavernous sinus. From the foramen rotundum, the nerve courses through the pterygopalatine fossa to enter the floor of the orbit at the inferior orbital fissure. Here, the nerve becomes the infraorbital nerve, enters the infraorbital canal, and then exits upon the face through the infraorbital foramen.

The maxillary nerve provides several branches in the cranial vault, pterygopalatine fossa, and orbit, as well as on the face. While in the cranial vault, the *middle meningeal nerve* supplies the dura. Several branches also arise from the nerve as it traverses the pterygopalatine fossa.

Zygomatic Nerve. The zygomatic nerve passes into the orbit and divides into the *zygomaticofacial* and *zygomaticotemporal nerves*. Both of these nerves enter the zygomatic bone and exit it through like-named foramina on its surface. The zygomaticofacial nerve exits upon the face, providing sensation for the cheek. The zygomaticotemporal nerve exits in the temporal fossa to distribute to the skin of the side of the forehead. Prior to leaving the orbit, this nerve supplies a communication to the lacrimal nerve. The communication is a postganglionic parasympathetic fiber passed to the zygomatic nerve from the pterygopalatine ganglion, which lies in close association with the maxillary nerve within the pterygopalatine fossa and is connected to it via two *pterygopalatine nerves.*

Pterygopalatine Nerves. The pterygopalatine nerves are a part of the maxillary nerve rather than part of the ganglion, though they serve as functional communications permitting the passage of postganglionic parasympathetic fibers from the ganglion to the nerve trunk for distribution to the lacrimal gland. Other postganglionic parasympathetic fibers are communicated from the ganglion to the branches of the maxillary nerve destined for glands in the palate and nasal cavity, where these fibers serve secretomotor function.

There are several branches of the maxillary nerve which appear to originate from the ganglion but actually are further branchings of the two pterygopalatine nerves. These branchings emerge after the pterygopalatine nerves have passed through the ganglion. They are the orbital, palatine, posterior superior nasal, and pharyngeal branches.

Orbital Branches. The orbital branches enter the orbit to supply the periorbita and the posterior ethmoidal and sphenoidal sinuses.

Greater Palatine Nerve. The greater palatine nerve descends from the ganglion to enter and descend in the pterygopalatine canal, finally to emerge upon the palate through the greater palatine foramen. The nerve serves the adjacent soft palate, hard palate, gingiva, and mucous membranes of this region as far anteriorly as the incisive teeth, where it communicates with the nasopalatine nerve. In its descent in the canal, *posterior inferior nasal branches* are given off, innervating the inferior concha and the middle and inferior meatuses. The greater palatine nerve splits while in the canal to form a *lesser palatine nerve,* which exits upon the palate through a like-named foramen serving the soft palate, tonsil, and uvula. Many of the afferents to this region are from the facial nerve communicated to the lesser palatine nerve through the pterygopalatine ganglion by way of the greater petrosal nerve and nerve of the pterygoid canal. These nerves are described with the facial nerve.

Posterior Superior Nasal Branches. Posterior superior nasal branches enter the nasal cavity from the sphenopalatine foramen to supply the mucous membrane over the middle and superior conchae, the septum, and the ethmoidal sinus. One of these branches, called the *nasopalatine nerve,* is larger than the others and continues anteriorly between the septum and the mucous membrane to reach the incisive canal, through which it passes to communicate with its counterpart from the opposite side. It serves the anterior palate as far posteriorly as the cuspid teeth, where it overlaps the distribution of the greater palatine nerve.

Pharyngeal Branch. A pharyngeal branch leaves the posterior aspect of the ganglion to enter the pharyngeal canal. It serves the mucous membrane and the nasopharynx as far as the auditory tube.

Posterior Superior Alveolar Nerve(s). Arising from the main trunk of the maxillary nerve, while still in the pterygopalatine fossa, is the posterior superior alveolar nerve(s). This nerve passes down over the tuberosity of the maxilla providing branches to the mucous membrane of the cheek and the adjacent gingiva. The posterior superior alveolar nerve then enters the same-named foramen to supply the maxillary sinus and the molar teeth, with the exception of the mesial buccal root of the first molar. Sensory innervation to this root is provided by the middle superior alveolar nerve to be described in the next section.

Infraorbital Nerve. Upon entering the floor of the orbit, the infraorbital nerve sends a *middle superior alveolar nerve* over the lateral wall of the maxillary sinus, which it innervates. This nerve then enters the mesial buccal root of the first molar and all of the roots of the premolar teeth. Continuing anteriorly, the infraorbital nerve provides an anterior superior alveolar nerve just prior to its exit from the infraorbital foramen. The *anterior superior alveolar nerve* supplies the anterior maxillary sinus and the anterior teeth. Also, small twigs of this nerve enter the nasal cavity to supply its floor, the inferior meatus, and adjacent mucous membrane. The posterior, middle, and anterior superior alveolar nerves intermingle, forming a dental plexus prior to innervating the upper teeth.

As the infraorbital nerve exits the same-named foramen, it provides three major groups: one ascending to the lower lid, the *inferior palpebral branches,* another to the side of the nose, the *external nasal branches,* and finally the descending group to the upper lip region, the *superior labial branches.*

Mandibular Nerve V₃ (Fig. 18.7)

The mandibular nerve, the largest division of the trigeminal nerve, is the only division containing a motor component in addition to the sensory component. The sensory fibers serve the skin about the lower face, cheek and lower lip, the ear, external acoustic meatus, temporomandibular joint, and the skin about the temporal region. This sensory component also supplies the mucous membranes of the cheek, tongue, the mandibular teeth, and supporting tissues and gingiva, mastoid air cells, the mandible, and portions of the dura. The motor component supplies all of the musculature developed within the first branchial arch: the muscles of mastication, including the temporalis, masseter, internal and external pterygoid muscles, as well as the tensors tympani and veli palatini, and the anterior belly of the digastric and the mylohyoid muscles.

As described earlier, the motor and sensory roots do not unite before exiting the skull. Both roots pass through the foramen ovale and unite just outside the skull forming the mandibular trunk, a mixed nerve that soon divides into a smaller, primarily motor anterior division, and a larger posterior division that is mostly sensory in function. Lying just outside the foramen ovale, immediately behind the mandibular nerve trunk, is the otic ganglion. Though this parasympathetic ganglion is in close association with the mandibular nerve via the nerve to the medial pterygoid muscle, preganglionic fibers synapsing within the ganglion are from the lesser petrosal nerve, a branch of the glossopharyngeal nerve. Postganglionic fibers from the ganglion utilize the auriculotemporal nerve for distribution to the parotid gland.

The mandibular nerve possesses several branches, some from the nerve trunk, others from the anterior division, and still others from the posterior division; and they are described in that order in the following sections.

Branches From the Main Mandibular Trunk. Two nerves branch from the main trunk of the nerve: the recurrent meningeal nerve and the nerve to the medial pterygoid muscle.

RECURRENT MENINGEAL NERVE. The recurrent meningeal nerve leaves the nerve trunk and ascends back into the skull through the foramen spinosum in company with the middle meningeal artery. This nerve supplies the dura, while some fibers supply the mastoid air cells.

MEDIAL PTERYGOID NERVE. The medial pterygoid nerve arises from the posterior aspect of the nerve trunk, penetrates the otic ganglion, then enters the deep surface of the medial pterygoid muscle supplying it with motor innervation. Two small branches are given off: the *nerve to the tensor tympani muscle,* which penetrates the auditory tube cartilage to supply this muscle with motor innervation, and the *nerve to the tensor veli palatini muscle,* which enters that muscle near its origin, supplying it with motor innervation.

Branches From the Anterior Mandibular Division. The smaller anterior division, through its branches, supplies all of the remaining muscles of mastication with motor innervation. The buccal nerve is the only branch of the anterior division that is sensory in function. Arising from this division are the deep temporal, lateral pterygoid, masseteric, and buccal nerves.

DEEP TEMPORAL NERVES. The deep temporal nerves arise from the anterior division and ascend, usually as anterior and posterior branches, between the two heads of the lateral pterygoid muscle to enter the deep surface of the temporalis muscle, which they supply. Frequently, the anterior branch arises from the buccal nerve, while the posterior branch may arise in common with the masseteric nerve.

LATERAL PTERYGOID NERVE. The lateral pterygoid nerve is very short and almost immediately enters the deep surface of the lateral pterygoid muscle. This nerve may originate from the buccal nerve as that nerve passes between the two heads of that muscle.

MASSETERIC NERVE. Passing above the lateral pterygoid muscle on its way to the mandibular notch is the masseteric nerve. As it crosses the mandibular notch to enter the masseter muscle in company with the same-named artery, it gives off a sensory twig to the temporomandibular joint.

BUCCAL NERVE. The origin of the buccal nerve is not constant. Occasionally, it may arise from the trigeminal ganglion individually, reaching its destination via a separate foramen. Alternatively, it may arise from the inferior alveolar nerve of the posterior division. The description which follows assumes origin from the anterior division. The buccal nerve ascends, passing between the two heads of the lateral pterygoid muscle. Here it may give off branches to the temporalis and/or the lateral pterygoid muscles. It then descends to ramify over the buccinator muscle, supplying innervation to the skin of the cheek. Other branches pierce the muscle to provide sensory fibers to the buccal mucosa and adjacent gingiva. The buccal nerve communicates with the facial nerve forming a complex over the buccinator muscle presumably facilitating distribution of both nerves.

Branches From the Posterior Mandibular Division. The larger posterior division of the mandibular nerve is mainly sensory in function, with the mylohyoid nerve being the only motor nerve of the division. Nerves arising from this division of the mandibular nerve are the lingual, inferior alveolar, and auriculotemporal nerves.

LINGUAL NERVE. The lingual nerve descends deep to the lateral pterygoid muscle, then courses forward between the medial pterygoid muscle and the mandible, where it is joined by the chorda tympani nerve from the facial nerve. The lingual then descends over the superior pharyngeal constrictor and styloglossus muscles to reach the lateral aspect of the tongue adjacent to the hyoglossus muscle. Here it lies between that muscle and the submandibular gland. The nerve proceeds anteriorly to the tip of the tongue lying alongside the submandibular duct just beneath the mucosa. Fibers of the lingual nerve, derived from the trigeminal nerve, provide sensory innervation to the mucous membranes of the anterior two-thirds of the tongue, the lingual gingiva, and other structures adjacent to the tongue. Fibers communicated to the lingual nerve from the facial nerve, via the chorda tympani, serve two functions: one group provides special sensory fibers for taste to the taste buds of the anterior two-thirds of the tongue, which get distributed by the lingual nerve, and the other supplies preganglionic parasympathetic fibers destined for the submandibular ganglion, which is suspended from the lingual nerve as the nerve lies between the hyoglossus muscle and the submandibular gland. The preganglionic fibers leave the lingual nerve to synapse on postganglionic cell bodies within the ganglion. The postganglionic fibers pass directly to the submandibular gland or reenter the lingual nerve for distribution to the sublingual gland and other minor salivary glands in the floor of the mouth.

INFERIOR ALVEOLAR NERVE. The inferior alveolar nerve descends along with, but lateral to, the lingual nerve in company with the inferior alveolar artery on its way to the mandibular foramen. The *mylohyoid nerve* arises from the inferior alveolar nerve just before the latter enters the mandibular foramen. The mylohyoid nerve descends in the mylohyoid groove on the mandible, then enters the mylohyoid muscle which it provides with motor innervation. A portion of this nerve continues on the superficial surface of the muscle to the anterior belly of the digastric muscle, supplying it with motor innervation.

Upon entering the mandibular foramen, the inferior alveolar nerve proceeds in the bony mandibular canal, forming a dental plexus that provides sensory innervation to the mandibular teeth and supporting structures. The nerve divides into two terminals: one, the *mental nerve,* exits the mental foramen to provide sensation to the skin of the lower lip and chin as well as to the mucous membrane of the lower lip; the other, the *incisive nerve,* continues on to supply the anterior teeth and supporting tissues with sensory innervation.

AURICULOTEMPORAL NERVE. The origin of the auriculotemporal nerve is usually two rootlets from the posterior division which surround the middle meningeal artery as it enters the foramen spinosum. The two rootlets then unite forming the nerve which courses deep to the lateral pterygoid muscle. After emerging at the neck of the mandible, the nerve turns superiorly with the superficial temporal artery within the substance of the parotid gland. It continues to ascend between the auricula and temporomandibular joint, exiting the gland to pass over the zygomatic arch to distribute sensory fibers as *superficial temporal nerves* over the skin of the temporal region. In its course, the auriculotemporal nerve sends *articular branches* to the temporomandibular joint, *anterior auricular branches* to the anterior portion of the external ear, *branches to the external acoustic meatus,* and *branches to the parotid gland.* The last named branches are postganglionic parasympathetic fibers whose cell bodies are located in the otic ganglion. These fibers, which supply secretomotor innervation to the gland, are communicated to the rootlets of the nerve from the otic ganglion for distribution to the parotid gland. Preganglionic parasympathetic fibers to the ganglion are supplied by the lesser petrosal branch of the glossopharyngeal nerve.

The auriculotemporal nerve and the facial nerve communicate freely about the parotid gland, facilitating their distribution.

VI Abducent Nerve (Fig. 18.3)

The abducent nerve arises from the brain between the pons and the medulla. On its course to the orbit, the nerve pierces the dura covering the dorsum sellae of the sphenoid bone and enters the cavernous sinus, where it receives communications from the carotid plexus. Upon entering the superior orbital fissure, the nerve courses to the lateral rectus muscle, which it supplies with motor innervation.

VII Facial Nerve (Figs. 18.8, 18.9)

The facial nerve supplies all of the muscles derived from the second branchial arch, since it is the nerve of that arch. Those muscles supplied by the motor

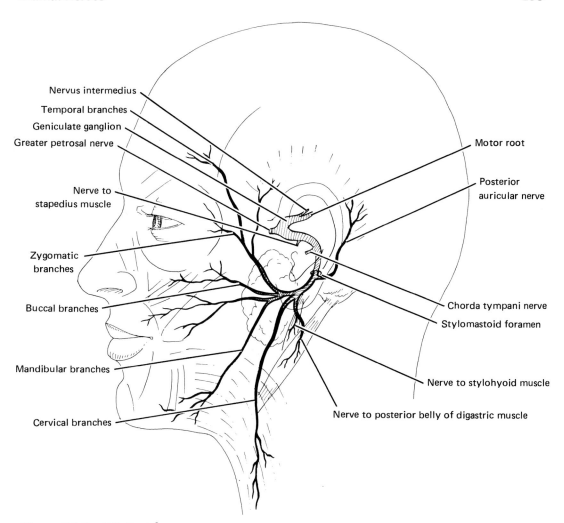

Figure 18.8. VII. Facial nerve.

component of this nerve are the muscles of facial expression, including the buccinator, platysma, and those of the scalp and external ear, and the stapedius, posterior belly of the digastric, and stylohyoid muscles. The general sensory component supplies the external acoustic meatus, soft palate, and some of the pharynx. Special sensory innervation for taste is supplied to the anterior two-thirds of the tongue. Parasympathetic fibers effecting secretomotor function are supplied to the lacrimal, nasal, palatine, submandibular, and sublingual glands.

The nerve possesses two roots, a large motor root and a smaller root, termed the *nervus intermedius*, containing the special sensory fibers for taste, parasympathetic fibers, and general sensory fibers. The two roots emerge from the brain between the pons and the inferior cerebellar peduncle. These roots enter the internal acoustic meatus along with the acoustic nerve but separate from it as the two roots enter the petrous portion of the temporal bone in a chamber of its own, the *facial canal.* Near the tympanic cavity, the nerve takes an abrupt turn inferiorly to exit the skull through the stylomastoid foramen.

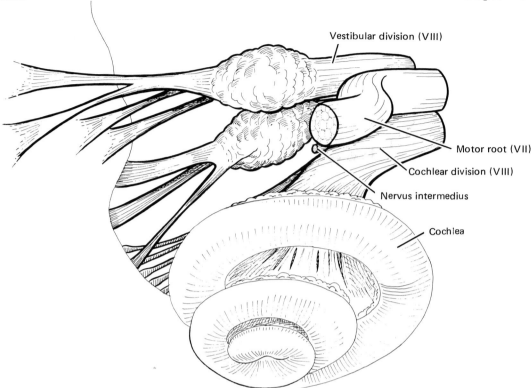

Figure 18.9. VIII. Acoustic nerve. Note the nervus intermedius and motor portion of the facial nerve accompanying the vestibular and cochlear divisions into the ear.

Located at this turn where the two roots fuse is the *geniculate ganglion,* the sensory ganglion of the facial nerve. Several branches arise from the nerve as it courses through the temporal bone. These include the greater petrosal nerve from the geniculate ganglion, the nerve to the stapedius muscle, and the chorda tympani nerve.

Greater Petrosal Nerve

Arising from the geniculate ganglion is the greater petrosal nerve, which carries preganglionic parasympathetic fibers destined for the pterygopalatine ganglion along with sensory fibers for the soft palate and pharynx. The nerve leaves the bone via the *hiatus of the facial canal* near the foramen lacerum and then enters the pterygoid canal (Vidian) joined by the *deep petrosal nerve,* a postganglionic sympathetic fiber from the carotid plexus whose cell bodies are located in the superior cervical ganglion. The *nerve of the pterygoid canal (Vidian nerve)* passes through the canal in the sphenoid bone to gain access to the pterygopalatine fossa, where it enters the pterygopalatine ganglion. The preganglionic parasympathetic fibers synapse on postganglionic parasympathetic cell bodies housed within the ganglion. Fibers of these neurons are communicated to nerves branching from the maxillary division of the trigeminal nerve for distribution to the lacrimal gland, small glands of the nasal cavity, pharynx, and palate. The sympathetic component of the Vidian nerve does not synapse in the pterygopalatine ganglion; rather, these postganglionic fibers are distributed in the same fashion as the postganglionic parasympathetic fibers.

The parasympathetic fibers are secretomotor in function, while the sympathetic fibers function mainly in vasoconstriction.

Some general sensory fibers from the geniculate ganglion travel along with the greater petrosal nerve to be distributed ultimately by branches of the maxillary division of the trigeminal nerve to the area of the soft palate.

Nerve to the Stapedius Muscle

The nerve to the stapedius muscle, arising from the facial nerve as it descends across the tympanum, provides motor fibers to that muscle.

Chorda Tympani Nerve

The chorda tympani nerve arises from the facial nerve trunk just prior to the trunk's exit from the stylomastoid foramen. The chorda tympani courses cranialward in a canal of its own, diverging away from the main nerve, bending to pass over the tympanic membrane and across the manubrium of the malleus. It leaves the tympanic cavity to enter a canal in the petrotympanic fissure, leaving the skull at the spine of the sphenoid. This nerve joins the lingual branch of the mandibular division of the trigeminal nerve for distribution to taste buds on the anterior two-thirds of the tongue and for distribution to the submandibular ganglion.

The chorda tympani nerve, which may receive a communication from the otic ganglion, contains special sensory fibers for taste and preganglionic parasympathetic fibers destined for the submandibular ganglion. The *submandibular ganglion*, suspended by short nerve filaments from the lingual nerve as it passes the hyoglossus muscle, receives the preganglionic parasympathetic fibers of the chorda tympani nerve via the parasympathetic root. Upon synapsing, postganglionic parasympathetic fibers pass to the submandibular gland or reenter the lingual nerve to be distributed to the sublingual gland and minor salivary glands in the floor of the mouth, providing them with secretomotor innervation. Sympathetic stimulation to the salivary glands is accomplished by postganglionic sympathetic fibers accompanying the arteries serving the glands. The function of this stimulation is generally to elicit vasoconstriction.

Beyond the origin of the chorda tympani nerve, the facial nerve exits the skull through the stylomastoid foramen. Thereupon, it gives rise to the posterior auricular nerve and the nerves to the posterior digastric and stylohyoid muscles. It then passes into the retromandibular fossa to enter the substance of the parotid gland to form the parotid plexus.

Posterior Auricular Nerve

As the facial nerve exits the stylomastoid foramen, the posterior auricular nerve arises from it to pass superiorly between the auricle and the mastoid process. It divides into occipital and auricular branches after communicating with the auricular branch of the vagus nerve and great auricular and lesser occipital nerves of the cervical plexus. The *auricular branch* supplies the extrinsic ear muscles as well as the few intrinsic muscles of the auricula. The *occipital branch* courses posteriorly to supply the occipitalis muscle.

Nerve to the Posterior Belly of the Digastric Muscle

The nerve to the posterior belly of the digastric muscle arises from the trunk of the facial nerve near the foramen and enters the muscle near its midbelly.

Nerve to Stylohyoid Muscle

The nerve to the stylohyoid muscle arises from the facial nerve in a similar fashion to or in common with the nerve to the posterior digastric. The nerve to the stylohyoid muscle then enters the muscle at midbelly.

Parotid Plexus

After entering the parotid gland, the facial nerve divides into temporofacial and cervicofacial divisions which form the parotid plexus, from which emerge the branches supplying motor innervation to the muscles of facial expression. These terminal branches are named for the regions they supply, usually dividing into five major branches from the plexus: *temporal, zygomatic, buccal, mandibular,* and *cervical branches.* Space does not allow for complete descriptions of each branch's distribution, nor of the muscles served by each branch, other than to state that, generally, the branch serves facial muscles originating in the area of the nerve branch.

It should be noted that branches of the facial nerve communicate freely with all of the terminal branches of the trigeminal nerve. These communications, for example that between the auriculotemporal nerve and the facial nerve, apparently serve to facilitate distribution of the sensory branches of the trigeminal nerve about the face.

VIII Acoustic Nerve (Fig. 18.9)

The nerve of hearing and balance, the acoustic nerve, is composed of two separate sets of fibers. The *vestibular nerve* for balance and the *cochlear nerve* for hearing are joined as a common nerve entering the internal acoustic meatus with the facial nerve. These two cranial nerves separate after entering the meatus as the acoustic nerve approaches the area of its destination within the inner ear. The acoustic nerve divides, sending the cochlear nerve into the laterally-oriented cochlear apparatus and the vestibular nerve medially into the vestibular apparatus.

Cochlear Nerve

The cochlear nerve has its peripheral processes in the *organ of Corti,* located in the membranous labyrinth, while its cell bodies are located in the *spiral ganglion of the cochlea* which is housed in the modiolus of the cochlea. Central processes of the spiral ganglion become the cochlear division of the nerve.

Vestibular Nerve

The vestibular nerve cell bodies are located in the *vestibular ganglion* within the internal auditory meatus. Peripheral processes of these cells divide to enter the vestibular mechanism including the three semicircular canals. Central processes of these neurons become the vestibular division of the acoustic nerve.

IX Glossopharyngeal Nerve (Fig. 18.10)

The glossopharyngeal nerve is the nerve of the third branchial arch, supplying the stylopharyngeus muscle, the only muscle developing from that arch. General visceral sensory components of this nerve supply the posterior one-third of the tongue, the fauces, the palatine tonsils, and the pharynx. Special sensory

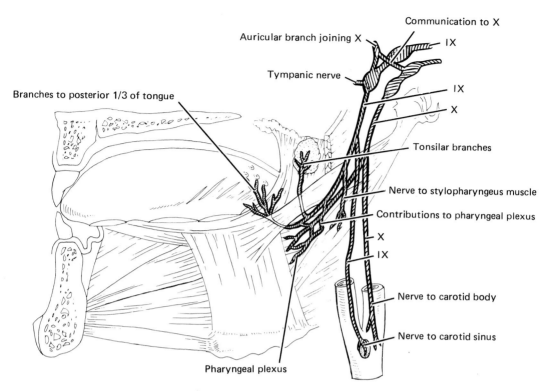

Figure 18.10. IX. Glossopharyngeal nerve. Observe the communications with the vagus nerve and the contributions of both to the pharyngeal plexus.

fibers are distributed to the taste buds located on the posterior one-third of the tongue, as well as to those located in the circumvallate papillae. Other general visceral sensory fibers supply the carotid sinus with blood pressure receptors. General visceral efferents (parasympathetic) supply the parotid gland and other minor salivary glands in the mucous membrane in and about the posterior tongue and adjacent pharynx.

The glossopharyngeal nerve leaves the brain as three or four rootlets adjacent to the vagus nerve along the medulla between the olive and the inferior cerebellar peduncle. The rootlets unite to exit the skull through the jugular foramen in company with the vagus and accessory nerves. Housed in the groove within the jugular foramen are the *superior* and *inferior ganglia* of the nerve, containing the cell bodies of the sensory fibers.

While passing through the foramen, this nerve communicates with the facial nerve, the auricular branch and superior ganglion of the vagus nerve, and the superior cervical sympathetic ganglion.

Tympanic Nerve
The tympanic nerve arises from the inferior ganglion and enters the petrous portion of the temporal bone, traveling to the tympanic cavity where it forms the *tympanic plexus* with fibers from the carotid plexus and the greater petrosal nerve. Branches from the plexus serve sensory functions to the mucous membranes of the eardrum, oval and round windows, mastoid air cells, and auditory tube.

The tympanic nerve continues on as the *lesser petrosal nerve*, providing preganglionic parasympathetic fibers to the otic ganglion, which it reaches by leaving the skull at the fissure between the petrous portion of the temporal bone and the greater wing of the sphenoid bone. The *otic ganglion*, described in the section on the mandibular division of the trigeminal nerve, lies just outside the foramen ovale, immediately behind the mandibular nerve. The ganglion receives preganglionic parasympathetic fibers from the lesser petrosal nerve and possibly some fibers from the greater petrosal nerve communicated through the tympanic plexus. Postganglionic parasympathetic fibers leave the ganglion and are communicated to the auriculotemporal nerve for distribution to the parotid gland, providing it with secretomotor innervation.

Carotid Sinus Nerve
The nerve to the carotid sinus arises as a small filament from the glossopharyngeal nerve subsequent to nerve communications at the jugular foramen. This branch descends along the internal carotid artery, ending in the bifurcation of the common carotid artery. The nerve functions as a baroreceptor within the carotid sinus.

Nerve to the Stylopharyngeus Muscle
As the glossopharyngeal nerve courses to the posterior pharyngeal wall, a nerve to the stylopharyngeus muscle arises to supply that muscle.

Pharyngeal Branches
The main trunk of the glossopharyngeal nerve terminates as several pharyngeal branches to enter the posterior pharyngeal wall. Some of these branches continue to the tongue as *lingual branches*, providing general sensation to the posterior one-third of the tongue and special sensory fibers to the taste buds on that portion of the tongue as well as to those of the circumvallate papillae. Other branches penetrate the pharyngeal wall as *tonsillar branches*, communicating with the lesser palatine nerve of the maxillary division of the trigeminal nerve, to supply the soft palate, pharynx, and fauces with general sensation. Still other fibers join with the vagus and the accessory nerves to form the *pharyngeal plexus*, which then provides most of the pharyngeal muscles with motor innervation and the adjacent mucous membrane with sensory innervation. The exact contribution of the glossopharyngeal nerve to the pharyngeal plexus is not fully understood.

X Vagus Nerve (Figs. 18.10, 18.11)

The cranial nerve having the most extensive distribution is the vagus nerve, since it serves other structures in addition to those in the head and neck. The nerve also enters the thorax to serve the heart and lungs and continues into the abdomen to supply much of the viscera.

The vagus nerve possesses four of the modalities, including somatic and visceral afferent fibers in addition to general and special visceral efferent fibers. The vagus is the nerve of the fourth branchial arch, and its recurrent laryngeal branch is the nerve of the sixth branchial arch. Consequently, it supplies muscles developed from those arches with the special visceral efferent (motor) components. Those muscles developing from the fourth arch include the pharyngeal constrictors and the cricothyroid muscles. Muscles developed from the

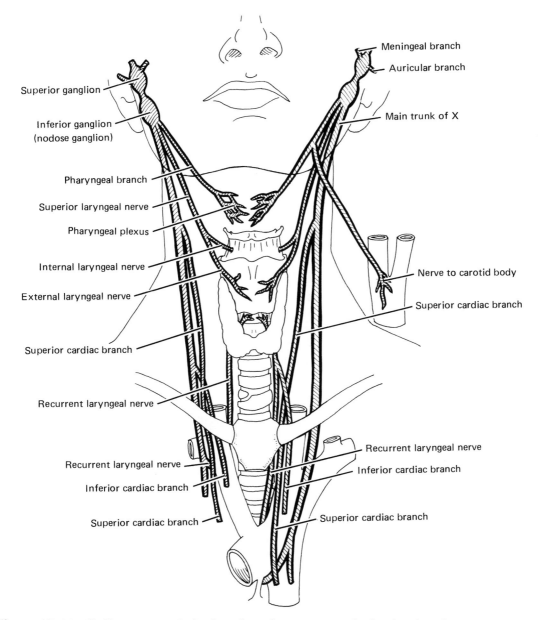

Figure 18.11. X. Vagus nerve. Only those branches arising in the head and neck are illustrated.

sixth arch include the intrinsic muscles of the larynx. General sensory fibers are provided to the skin about the ear and external acoustic meatus. The visceral sensory component supplies the mucous membranes of the pharynx, larynx, esophagus, bronchi, lungs, heart, and much of the abdominal viscera. The parasympathetic (general visceral efferent) component of the vagus nerve supplies the smooth muscles and glands of the digestive tract from the esophagus to (and including) most of the intestines plus the bronchi and trachea.

The vagus nerve exits the brain at the medulla, between the olive and the inferior cerebellar peduncle just posterior to the glossopharyngeal nerve, via a cluster of eight to ten rootlets which unite to exit the skull through the jugular foramen along with the glossopharyngeal and accessory nerves. This nerve possesses two sensory ganglia: the *superior ganglion,* housed in the jugular fossa, and the *inferior (nodose) ganglion,* appearing as a swelling on the nerve just after it exits the jugular foramen. Peripheral processes of the neurons in these ganglia are distributed with the vagus nerve as the sensory component. Several communications to these ganglia occur from the glossopharyngeal, facial, accessory, and hypoglossal nerves. The sympathetic system communicates via a filament from the superior cervical ganglion, and a communication also exists between the vagal ganglia and the first and second cervical nerves.

Prior to its exit from the jugular fossa the vagus nerve gives off two branches: the meningeal and auricular branches.

Meningeal Branch
The meningeal branch of the vagus nerve returns to the cranial vault to supply the dura in the posterior cranial fossa.

Auricular Branch
The auricular branch arises from the superior ganglion, communicates with the glossopharyngeal nerve, and then enters the mastoid canal coursing to the facial canal. Here it communicates with the facial nerve, then exits through the tympanomastoid suture to communicate with the posterior auricular nerve before distributing to the skin of the posterior aspect of the ear and the external acoustic meatus.

Vagal Branches in the Neck
The following sections describe the branches and distributions of the vagus nerve as it courses through the neck. Branches arising from the vagus in the neck include the pharyngeal, superior laryngeal, superior cardiac, and the recurrent laryngeal nerves.

Pharyngeal Branches. Pharyngeal branches of the vagus arise from the inferior ganglion and pass over the internal carotid artery to the pharyngeal constrictor muscles, providing vagal and accessory nerve input to the pharyngeal plexus. From this plexus, motor innervation is supplied to the pharyngeal muscles, with the exception of the stylopharyngeus and to all the palatal muscles except the tensor veli palatini. The mucous membranes of the pharynx are also supplied by the pharyngeal plexus.

Usually, originating from the pharyngeal branches are the *nerves to the carotid body.* These filaments descend along the internal carotid artery to terminate in the carotid body housed in the bifurcation of the common carotid artery. Chemoreceptors detect changes in oxygen tension in the blood at this site.

Superior Laryngeal Nerve. The superior laryngeal nerve arises from the vagus at the inferior end of the inferior ganglion and passes deep to the internal carotid artery descending to the thyroid cartilage, where it divides into external and internal branches. The smaller *external branch* continues to descend beneath the sternothyroid muscle to enter the cricothyroid and inferior pharyngeal constrictor muscles, which it supplies with motor innervation. The larger *internal branch* courses over and pierces the thyrohyoid membrane.

This branch supplies sensory innervation to the mucous membranes superiorly, to the base of the tongue, and to the epiglottis and the larynx as far inferiorly as the vocal folds. The internal branch also contains parasympathetic fibers to the glands associated with the mucous membranes of the regions just described. The preganglionic fibers synapse on ganglionic plexuses within the walls of the viscera served, and from there the postganglionic fibers distribute secretomotor fibers to the glands.

Superior Cardiac Branches. While the trunk of the vagus nerve descends in the neck within the carotid sheath, between and posterior to the internal jugular vein and the internal carotid artery, superior cardiac branches are given off and descend into the thorax. Their function is not described here since it is outside the realm of this text.

Recurrent Laryngeal Nerve. At the root of the neck, the recurrent laryngeal nerve arises from the vagus and ascends back into the neck. On the right side, the nerve returns around the subclavian artery, while on the left side the nerve returns around the arch of the aorta. Upon reentering the neck, each nerve follows a similar course deep to the carotid artery, along a groove between the trachea and the esophagus, to enter the larynx as *inferior laryngeal nerves,* piercing the cricothyroid membrane to supply the intrinsic muscles of the larynx with motor innervation. In the recurrent laryngeal nerve's path to the larynx, branches to the trachea and the esophagus supply those structures with sensory and parasympathetic innervation in much the same manner as the fibers of the internal branch of the superior laryngeal nerve but more distally. In addition, *pharyngeal branches* are supplied to the inferior pharyngeal constrictor muscle.

The remaining branches and distributions of the vagus nerve within the thorax and abdomen are not described here. Those interested in this subject are referred to general texts in gross anatomy and neuroanatomy as suggested in the Selected References.

XI Accessory Nerve (Fig. 18.12)

The accessory nerve arises from two sources, the brain and the spinal cord. This nerve is described as a motor nerve, serving the sternocleidomastoid and trapezius muscles, and it is regarded as the motor portions of the pharyngeal plexus and the vagus nerve.

The spinal portion arises from motor cells from the first five (or more) spinal cord segments. This portion of the nerve emerges on the surface to ascend into the skull via the foramen magnum to join or communicate with the cranial portion before exiting the jugular foramen with the vagus and glossopharyngeal nerves. The cranial portion leaves the brain very close to the vagus nerve and travels along with it to the jugular foramen. After communicating with the spinal portion, the cranial portion joins the vagus, while the spinal portion continues on to descend through the foramen. The latter descends posterior to the stylohyoid and digastric muscles to enter the sternocleidomastoid muscle, which it pierces and serves before passing obliquely over the posterior triangle to terminate in and supply the trapezius muscle. Along its way, the nerve communicates with the second, third, and fourth cervical nerves.

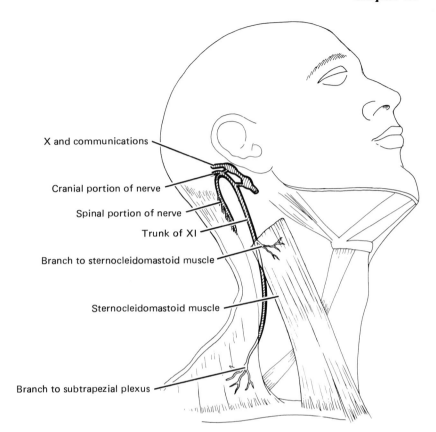

X and communications

Cranial portion of nerve

Spinal portion of nerve

Trunk of XI

Branch to sternocleidomastoid muscle

Sternocleidomastoid muscle

Branch to subtrapezial plexus

Figure 18.12.
XI. Accessory
nerve. Note the
spinal portion as-
cending into the
cranium to join the
cranial portion be-
fore exiting the
jugular foramen.

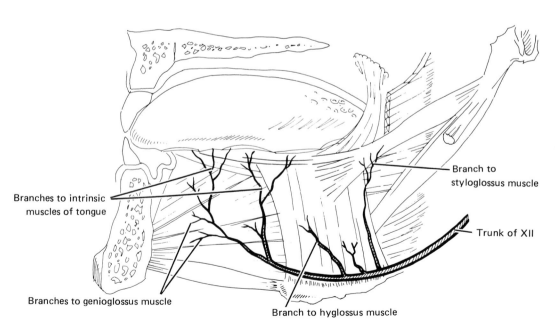

Branch to
styloglossus muscle

Branches to intrinsic
muscles of tongue

Trunk of XII

Branches to genioglossus muscle

Branch to hyglossus muscle

Figure 18.13. XII. Hypoglossal nerve.

XII Hypoglossal Nerve (Fig. 18.13)

The most caudal and the last of the cranial nerves is the hypoglossal nerve. This nerve is the motor nerve of the tongue. It arises as several rootlets from the medulla between the olive and the pyramid and, passing through the hypoglossal canal, unites to form a single nerve. It descends deep to the internal jugular vein and internal carotid artery and then becomes superficial to them as it crosses them at the mandible. It then courses over the external carotid and lingual arteries deep to the digastric and stylohyoid muscles. It enters the muscles of the tongue, which it supplies, proceeding to the ventral tip of the tongue. The nerve innervates the hyoglossus, styloglossus, genioglossus, and the intrinsic muscles of the tongue.

The hypoglossal nerve communicates with several nerves in its route, including the pharyngeal plexus, the lingual, and the first and second cervical nerves. The latter two join the hypoglossal to later exit forming the descending loop of the ansa cervicalis which innervates the infrahyoid muscles. Some fibers continue on to exit from the hypoglossal nerve near the posterior border of the hyoglossus muscle and enter the thyrohyoid and geniohyoid muscles.

CHAPTER **19**

Anatomical Basis for Local Anesthesia

Anesthesia is the loss of sensation due to injury, disease, or drug induction. Local anesthetics may be applied topically or injected either in the vicinity of the area to be anesthetized or into a conveniently accessible region in the proximity of the nerve or nerves supplying the area of interest. These anesthetic substances are pharmacologic agents that stabilize cell membranes by blocking or reducing the excitability of the membrane. When a region of a nerve fiber is exposed to an anesthetic solution, that fiber cannot relay impulses through the affected region; hence nerve conduction is blocked. Small, unmyelinated fibers are affected first, while larger, myelinated ones are blocked last. Since the effects of local anesthetics are temporary, recovery of excitability occurs in the reverse order—that is, large, myelinated fibers become conductive first and small, unmyelinated fibers last. Since pain and temperature fibers are usually small, the anesthetic can be applied in quantities which interfere mostly with these sensations, while only minimally affecting proprioception, sensation of touch, or motor functions.

Agents may be introduced to anesthetize nerve endings, which is known as *infiltration,* or to interfere with nerve conduction, known as a nerve block. Infiltration usually is restricted to mucous membranes and is of limited use in the oral cavity. *Nerve blocks,* however, are quite important and are considered in two separate categories: plexus anesthesia, restricted to a single tooth or a few teeth; and trunk anesthesia, involving blocking of pain sensation over a relatively large area. This chapter will concern itself with anesthesia of the teeth and their adnexa.

PLEXUS ANESTHESIA

Plexus anesthesia involves the delivery of anesthetic agent into the connective tissue overlying the periosteum. It is important to avoid subperiosteal injections, since such an injection causes tearing of blood vessels as the fluid detaches the periosteum from the bone, resulting in subperiosteal hematomas and considerable pain upon recovery. Plexus anesthesia may be used to advantage in regions of the oral cavity where bony tissues surrounding the roots of the teeth are relatively thin and sufficiently cancellous to permit adequate diffusion of the anesthetic agent. The maxillary buccal alveolar plate is sufficiently thin (with the exception of the first molar region), so that plexus anesthesia in this area is advantageous. Most of the mandibular cortical plate, however, is too thick for plexus anesthesia, with the exception of the canine and incisor regions. Hence, for mandibular procedures, a trunk anesthesia is the method of choice, while for maxillary procedures, plexus anesthesia is more appropriate.

Maxillary Plexus Anesthesia

The maxillary teeth are supplied by the anterior and posterior superior alveolar nerves, which are branches of the infraorbital branch and of the trunk of the maxillary division of the trigeminal nerve, respectively. A middle superior alveolar nerve, when present, assists in the sensory innervation of the teeth of the upper arch.

Proper accomplishment of plexus anesthesia should occur deep to the alveolar mucosa at or slightly above the mucogingival junction, below the fornix. Otherwise, the anesthetic agent will be injected in a region of loose connective tissue, permitting rapid dilution and removal of the anesthetic solution. Thus, the anesthetic agent will be deposited at or coronal to the apex of the tooth, permitting the drug to penetrate the periosteum and cancellous bone. Anesthesia of the three molars is achieved by injection in the region of the second molar and the second premolar. The latter site is essential only if anesthesia of the mesial buccal root of the first molar is desired, since this root is served by the middle superior alveolar nerve. When the palatal mucosa is involved in the operative procedures, the greater palatine nerve must also be blocked as it emerges from the greater palatine foramen.

Anesthesia of the two premolars (and mesial buccal root of the first molar) is achieved by depositing the anesthetic agent in the area just below the apex of the second premolar. The palatal mucosa may also be anesthetized by blocking the greater palatine nerve. It has been claimed that anterior teeth receive overlapping innervations from the right and left anterior superior alveolar nerves, necessitating blocking both sides at the level of the right and left maxillary canine. However, it is now believed that the overlapping is due to the nasopalatine nerve, whose blocking in the vicinity of the incisive papilla will usually result in complete anesthesia of this region.

Mandibular Plexus Anesthesia

Plexus anesthesia of mandibular teeth is usually accomplished only in the region of the incisors. The anesthetic solution is normally delivered into the vestibular mucosa inferior to the root of the incisors. When manipulation of the lingual gingiva is planned, block anesthesia of the lingual nerve is necessary.

TRUNK ANESTHESIA

Maxillary Teeth

Posterior Superior Alveolar Nerve
The posterior superior alveolar nerve is accessible on the maxillary tuberosity as the nerve enters the small posterior superior alveolar foramen. Anesthetic

solution should be delivered through the mucosa of the fornix at the level of the second molar, following the maxilla very closely in order to circumvent the pterygoid plexus of veins. Although the veins are easily avoided, the posterior superior alveolar artery is not. If the artery is accidentally penetrated, a large hematoma will quickly result. The bleeding may be controlled by exerting pressure on the maxilla at the anterior border of the masseter muscle, just inferior to the zygomatic arch. Block of the posterior superior alveolar nerve will anesthetize the three molars (with the exception of the mesial buccal root of the first molar) and the labial gingiva.

Infraorbital Trunk
The infraorbital nerve may be reached in the infraorbital canal, where it gives rise to the anterior (and, sometimes, middle) superior alveolar nerves. The canal is accessible via the infraorbital foramen, but caution must be exercised so that the thin bony roof of the canal is not perforated. If perforation occurs, the anesthetic solution will be deposited on the floor of the orbit in the periorbital fat, temporarily paralyzing the inferior rectus and inferior oblique muscles. The position of the foramen may be located by palpation of the orbital rim, where the zygomaticomaxillary suture is evident through the thin skin. Inferior to this suture, the bony ledge is felt to curve under, indicating the infraorbital foramen. Block of the infraorbital nerve will anesthetize the maxillary central and lateral incisors, canine, first and second premolars, and the mesial buccal root of the first molar. Frequently, anesthesia of the central incisor will not be profound, since it may receive fibers from the nasopalatine nerve.

Greater Palatine Block
The greater palatine nerve exits the same-named foramen to innervate the hard palate as far anteriorly as the canine region, where it communicates with the nasopalatine nerve. Anesthesia may be accomplished by piercing the palatal mucosa midway between the roof of the mouth and the gingival margin of the third molar. The anesthetic solution should not be deposited in the foramen or the soft palate will also be anesthetized, resulting in gagging. Should the premolars be involved, a nasopalatine block also must be performed.

Nasopalatine Block
The nasopalatine nerve supplies the anterior portion of the hard palate as well as the central incisor. The nerve exits the incisive foramen just posterior to the interdental papilla between the two central incisors. Access is very simple, since the site of injection is just deep to the incisive papilla. Since this is a painful injection, due to the sensitivity of the papilla, the solution should be delivered slowly, in advance of the needle, and in small quantities. When the premolars are involved, a greater palatine block should also be performed.

Mandibular Teeth

Inferior Alveolar and Lingual Blocks
Block of the inferior alveolar nerve, also known as a *mandibular block,* occurs at the mandibular foramen just before the inferior alveolar nerve enters it. The foramen is situated on the medial aspect of the ramus of the mandible, in close association with the lingula and the sphenomandibular ligament. The anes-

thetic agent should be delivered to this point by piercing the mucosa between the retromolar fossa and the pterygomandibular fold, at the level of the occlusal plane of the three mandibular molars. It is here that most of the anesthetic solution should be deposited. In order to anesthetize the lingual nerve, which lies close by, it is necessary to deposit solution just anterior and medial to the bony landmark. Anesthesia of the inferior alveolar and lingual nerves desensitizes the mandibular teeth and gingiva on that side. Occasionally, the buccal nerve must also be blocked to provide anesthesia of the mandibular buccal mucosa and gingiva.

Buccal Nerve Block
The buccal nerve crosses the anterior border of the ramus of the mandible at the level of the occlusal plane of the maxillary molars. Hence, this nerve may be anesthetized just lateral to the mandibular ramus. Since the tendon of the temporalis muscle may be penetrated, care must be exercised in depositing the anesthetic agent. Block anesthesia of the buccal nerve will anesthetize the buccal gingiva and mucosa of the mandibular molar and premolar regions.

Mental Nerve Block
The mental nerve exits the mandibular canal via the mental foramen, located on the lateral aspect of the mandibular body. The foramen is located just below the second premolar, halfway between the gingival margin and the inferior border of the mandible. Anesthetic solution should be introduced deep to the mucosa at the level of the second mandibular premolar, approximately at the fornix. Successful block of the mental nerve will anesthetize the mandibular premolars, canine, and incisors on one side, including adjacent gingiva.

Lymphatics of the Head and Neck

Tissue fluid is constantly being produced in excess by the circulatory system. Consequently, the interstitial spaces of the body receive more fluid from the arterial end of a capillary network than that which returns at the venous end. The excess tissue fluid, as well as proteins, fats, large particulate matter, and cells, find their way to lymphatic vessels which deliver their contents to lymph nodes located along their course. Here, foreign substances are phagocytosed and lymph is filtered. Lymph nodes are constant structures and their positions should be clearly understood by health professionals, for these structures become swollen during infections and inflammations. Since specific nodes receive lymph from specific areas of the body, the clinician should be able to deduce the general location of the infection by knowledge of lymphatic drainage. This chapter includes the names and locations of the principal lymph nodes of the head and neck, as well as the areas which they drain.

LYMPH NODES OF THE HEAD AND NECK

Head (Fig. 20.1; Table 20.1)

Lymph nodes of the head are all extracranial, since the central nervous system possesses no lymph vessels or lymph nodes. The general pattern of lymph nodes about the head is that they are regionalized into several groups to drain the posterior and anterolateral scalp as well as the superficial and deep aspects of the face.

Occipital lymph nodes (two to four in number) are located on the back of the head lying on the semispinalis capitis muscle just inferior to the attachment of the trapezius muscle. The small *mastoid (postauricular) lymph nodes* (one to three in number) are located behind the ear on the mastoid process, superficial to the insertion of the sternocleidomastoid muscle. Located anterior to the ear, are two to three *preauricular (superficial parotid) lymph nodes* lying superficial to, and sometimes deep to the capsule of the parotid gland. Those located deep to the capsule are sometimes grouped with the deep parotid lymph nodes described with those of the face.

The lymph nodes of the face are subdivided into those of the parotid, superficial face, and deep face. The *parotid lymph nodes* (ten to fifteen in number) form two groups: those lying embedded within the substance of the gland, and those lying deep to the gland adjacent the pharyngeal wall. The *superficial facial lymph nodes* (up to twelve) are disposed along the course of the facial artery and vein. These are the *maxillary (infraorbital) lymph nodes* in the vicinity of the infraorbital foramen, the *buccal lymph node(s)* on or in the buccal fat pad over the buccinator muscle, and the *mandibular lymph nodes* (two to three) along the facial artery and vein adjacent the masseter muscle. The *deep facial lymph nodes* follow the course of the maxillary artery in the infratemporal fossa superficial to the lateral pterygoid muscle.

Two additional groups of deep nodes are of importance: the *lingual lymph nodes* (numbering two to three) lying on the superficial aspect of the hyoglossus muscle; and the two to three *retropharyngeal lymph nodes* located in the buccopharyngeal fascia behind the pharynx at the level of the atlas.

Neck (Fig. 20.1; Table 20.1)

The lymph nodes of the neck are disposed in several groups; the anterior cervical, submental, submandibular, superficial cervical, and the deep cervical.

The *anterior cervical lymph nodes* are inconsistent, and are located in two groups, superficial and deep, in front of the viscera of the neck. The *superficial group* is located in an irregular row along the course of the anterior jugular vein. The *deep group* is subdivided into four small chains, the paratracheal lymph nodes of the tracheoesophageal groove; the infrahyoid lymph nodes, lying superficial to the thyrohyoid membrane; the pretracheal nodes, situated between the investing layer of the deep cervical fascia and the trachea; and the prelaryngeal nodes, which lie on the conus elasticus of the trachea.

The *submandibular lymph nodes* are located in the same-named triangle in close proximity to the submandibular gland. Although these constitute a chain of three to six lymph nodes, the only constant node is the one at the facial groove of the mandible in close association with the facial artery. *Superficial cervical lymph nodes* may be found lying adjacent the external jugular vein as it passes superficial to the sternocleidomastoid muscle.

The *deep cervical lymph nodes* are most important, since they ultimately receive all of the lymph from the head and neck. Their efferent vessels form the *jugular trunk*, which delivers the collected lymph to the right lymphatic duct, or to the thoracic duct on the left, to be returned to the circulatory system. These deep cervical lymph nodes parallel the carotid sheath along its entire length. The lymph nodes of this group may conveniently be assigned into two subgroups: the superior and inferior deep cervical lymph nodes. The *superior deep cervical lymph nodes,* some of which are large, form a chain, surrounding the internal jugular vein, extending from the mastoid process to the superior border of the subclavian triangle. The most superior node of this group is the large *jugulodigastric (tonsillar) lymph node* located between the posterior belly of the digastric muscle and the internal jugular vein. This node

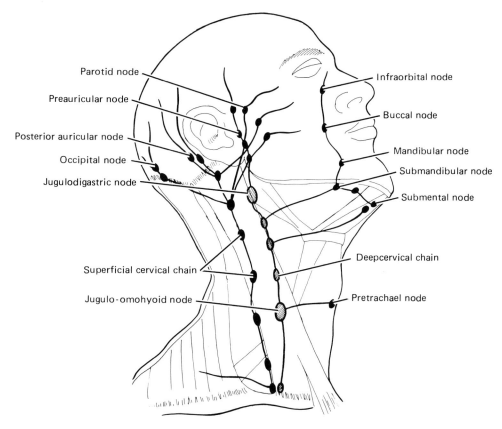

Figure 20.1. Diagrammatic representation of lymphatic drainage of the head and neck.

is of particular importance in physical diagnosis. The *inferior deep cervical lymph nodes* reside in the subclavian triangle. Nodes of this group are in close association with the brachial plexus, subclavian artery and vein, and the omohyoid muscle. A large, constant node of this group, located in the vicinity of the intermediate tendon of the omohyoid muscle, is the *jugulo-omohyoid lymph node.* (This node is located in a border zone between the superior and inferior deep cervical nodes, therefore, reference to its group association varies.)

Accompanying the deep chain in the posterior cervical triangle are the *accessory lymph nodes* (numbering two to six) lying alongside the accessory nerve and the *transverse cervical lymph nodes* (one to ten in number) accompanying the transverse cervical vessels.

LYMPHATIC DRAINAGE OF THE HEAD AND NECK

Superficial Tissues

The back of the scalp is drained by the occipital lymph nodes, whose efferent vessels empty into the superficial cervical lymph nodes. The lymph vessels of

TABLE 20.1
Lymph Nodes of the Head and Neck

Node	Location	Afferent	Efferent
Superficial Lymph Nodes of the Head			
Occipital (2–4)	Superior nuchal line between sternocleidomastoid and trapezius	Occipital part of scalp	Superficial cervical lymph nodes
Mastoid (1–3)	Superficial to sternocleidomastoid insertion	Posterior parietal scalp Skin of ear, posterior external acoustic meatus	Superior deep cervical nodes
Preauricular (2–3)	Anterior to ear over parotid fascia	Drains areas supplied by superficial temporal artery Anterior parietal scalp Anterior surface of ear	Superior deep cervical lymph nodes
Parotid (up to 10 or more)	About parotid gland and under parotid fascia Deep to parotid gland	External acoustic meatus Skin of frontal and temporal regions Eyelids, tympanic cavity Cheek, nose, (posterior palate)	Superior deep cervical lymph nodes
Facial Superficial (up to 12) Maxillary Buccal Mandibular	Distributed along course of facial artery and vein	Skin and mucous membranes of eyelids, nose, cheek	Submandibular nodes
Deep	Distributed along course of maxillary artery lateral to lateral pterygoid muscle	Temporal and infratemporal fossa Nasal pharynx	Superior deep cervical lymph nodes
Superficial Cervical Lymph Nodes			
Anterior cervical Superficial	Anterior jugular vein between superficial cervical fascia and infrahyoid fascia	Skin, muscles, and viscera of infrahyoid region of neck	Superior deep cervical lymph nodes
Deep	Between viscera of neck and investing layer of deep cervical fascia	Adjoining parts of trachea, larynx, thyroid gland	Superior deep cervical lymph nodes
Submental (2–3)	Submental triangle	Chin Medial part of lower lip Lower incisor teeth and gingiva Tip of tongue Cheeks	Submandibular lymph node to jugulo-omohyoid lymph node and superior deep cervical lymph nodes
Submandibular (3–6)	Submandibular triangle adjacent	Facial nodes Chin	Superior deep cervical lymph nodes and

314

TABLE 20.1
Continued

Node	Location	Afferent	Efferent
	submandibular gland	Lateral upper and lower lips	jugulo-omohyoid lymph nodes
		Cheeks and nose, anterior nasal cavity Maxillary and mandibular teeth and gingiva Oral palate Anterior 2/3 of tongue	
Superficial cervical (1–2)	Along external jugular vein superficial to sternocleidomastoid muscle	Lower part of ear and parotid region	Superior deep cervical lymph nodes

Deep Cervical Lymph Nodes

Node	Location	Afferent	Efferent
Superior deep cervical	Surrounding internal jugular vein deep to sternocleidomastoid and superior to omohyoid muscle	Occipital nodes Mastoid nodes Preauricular nodes Parotid nodes Submandibular nodes Superficial cervical nodes Retropharyngeal nodes	Inferior deep cervical nodes or separate channel to jugulo-subclavian junction
Jugulodigastric	Junction of internal jugular vein and posterior digastric muscle	Palatine tonsil Posterior palate Much of tongue	Inferior deep cervical lymph nodes
Jugulo-omohyoid	Above junction of internal jugular vein and omohyoid muscle	Tip of tongue, much of tongue Submandibular nodes Submental nodes	Inferior deep cervical lymph nodes
Inferior deep cervical	Along internal jugular vein below omohyoid muscle deep to the sternocleidomastoid muscle	Transverse cervical nodes Anterior cervical nodes Superior deep cervical nodes	Jugular trunk
Retropharyngeal (1–3)	Retropharyngeal space	Posterior nasal cavity Paranasal sinuses Hard and soft palate Nasopharynx, oropharynx Auditory tube	Superior deep cervical nodes
Accessory (2–6)	Along accessory nerve in posterior triangle	Occipital nodes Mastoid nodes Lateral neck and shoulder	Transverse cervical nodes
Transverse cervical (1–10)	Along transverse cervical blood vessels at level of clavicle	Accessory nodes Apical axillary nodes Lateral neck Anterior thoracic wall	Jugular trunk or Directly into thoracic duct or right lymphatic duct or independently into junction of internal jugular vein and subclavian vein

the medial surface of the ear, lateral aspects of the eyelids, the temporal region, and most of the forehead drain into the mastoid (posterior auricular), preauricular, and parotid lymph nodes. The efferents from these nodes then pass into the superior deep cervical lymph nodes. The remainder of the eye and middle ear are drained by the preauricular (parotid lymph nodes), which then drain into the superior deep cervical lymph nodes. The submandibular lymph nodes receive lymph from the nose, cheek, and lip, either directly or via the buccal lymph nodes. The lateral aspect of the cheek and the skin over the bridge of the nose are partially drained also by the parotid lymph nodes. Lymph from the mucosa over the floor of the mouth, tip of the tongue, and the central portion of the lower lip is drained into the submental lymph nodes, whence it empties into the jugulo-omohyoid lymph node of the inferior deep cervical chain. Superficial tissues of the neck are drained by the deep cervical lymph nodes directly or indirectly. Lymph from the posterior cervical triangle may first enter the superficial cervical and occipital nodes from which the lymph flows to the deep cervical lymph nodes. Lymph from the anterior cervical triangle, above the hyoid bone, is drained into the submental and submandibular lymph nodes, while that inferior to the hyoid bone drains into the anterior cervical lymph nodes whose efferents deliver it to the deep cervical lymph nodes.

Deep Tissues

Most of the lymph of the nasal cavity, paranasal sinuses, and nasopharynx drains into the retropharyngeal lymph nodes or passes directly to the deep cervical lymph chain. The thyroid gland is drained by the pretracheal, prelaryngeal, and paratracheal lymph nodes, whence lymph flows to the deep cervical lymph nodes. Frequently, some of the lymph from this endocrine gland passes directly into the deep cervical lymph nodes. The tracheal, esophageal, and laryngeal lymph in the region of the neck also passes either directly or indirectly, via the prelaryngeal or paratracheal lymph nodes, into the deep cervical chain. Tonsillar lymph is drained into the jugulodigastric lymph node of the superior deep cervical chain.

Lymph drainage from the gingiva, teeth, and tongue deserves special attention. Gingival lymph is gathered on the lingual and vestibular surfaces by submucosal plexuses of lymph vessels, which are consolidated into a series of vessels behind the molars. From here the lymph passes either to the submandibular lymph nodes or occasionally, into the deep cervical lymph nodes. However, lymph from the region of the mandibular incisors is delivered to the submental lymph nodes. The presence of lymph vessels in the pulp of the tooth has been the source of much controversy, but it is now generally agreed that these vessels are found in the pulp and that lymph vessels of the pulp and those of the periodontal ligament about the same tooth are drained by a common vessel. There is a lack of agreement concerning the precise path of lymph drainage of teeth, but a reasonable case may be made for the following description. The mandibular incisors are drained by the submental lymph nodes, while the remaining teeth are drained by the submandibular lymph nodes. Generally, lymphatic drainage is ipsilateral, though for structures near the midline, it is both ipsi- and contralateral.

Lymphatic drainage of the tongue is complex, since the tongue has a rich lymphatic plexus of vessels which is drained by three vessel groups: the marginal, dorsal, and central vessels. Additionally, drainage from the two sides is intermingled to a large extent, and the base of the tongue is drained by lymph nodes situated more cranially than those which receive lymph from the tip of the tongue. Vessels from the tip of the tongue pass to the *superior deep cervical lymph nodes,* along with those of the region of the lingual frenulum, which belong to the marginal group of vessels drained by the submental, submandibular, and jugulo-omohyoid lymph nodes. The lateral aspect of the tongue is also drained by marginal vessels, into the jugulo-omohyoid and jugulodigastric lymph nodes. The central vessels drain the medial region of the anterior two-thirds of the tongue, delivering the lymph to the jugulo-omohyoid and jugulodigastric lymph nodes. The dorsal vessels drain the region of the sulcus terminalis and the posterior one-third of the tongue, delivering lymph to the marginal lymph vessels, which are drained by the superior and inferior deep cervical lymph nodes.

The accessory lymph nodes located about the accessory nerve in the posterior cervical triangle may drain occipital and mastoid nodes in addition to areas of the lateral neck and shoulder. The transverse cervical nodes, located in the posterior cervical triangle, drain the accessory chain of nodes, the lateral neck, anterior thoracic wall, mammary gland, and occasionally the upper limb. Efferents from this group may pass into the jugular lymphatic trunk, the thoracic duct or right lymphatic duct, or they may enter the internal jugular or subclavian veins independently.

CLINICAL CONSIDERATIONS

Lymph nodes of a normal, healthy individual are soft, nonpalpable structures. However, infection, inflammation, and carcinomatous involvement of areas drained by lymph nodes cause these structures to become swollen, hard, painful, and palpable. The health professional dealing with the oral cavity should examine patients for swollen, painful lymph nodes, especially the submental, submandibular, and the superficial and deep cervical chains. The last group may be palpated with relative ease by manipulation of the relaxed sternocleidomastoid muscle. Diseased states of the oral cavity will most probably be reflected in the submental and submandibular lymph nodes. Remembering that, in the process of lymph drainage, the fluid passes through a series of lymph nodes before emptying into the thoracic or right lymphatic ducts, it becomes evident that each lymph node group is a "barrier" where the disease agent is being combatted. The first such site is known as the *primary node* which drains into a *secondary node* that may be drained by a *tertiary node.* The more nodes that are interposed in the disease agent's route of spread prior to reaching the major lymphatic channels, the better the chance of successfully combatting the disease. Hence, a knowledge of lymphatic drainage of the head and neck assists the health professional dealing with this region in determining the site of disease manifestation.

Treatment of cervical metastases may involve a radical surgery—that is, a "block resection"—of the cervical lymph nodes. It is essential that all lymph nodes of the particular side of the neck be removed. To ensure that this is the case, connective tissues, muscles, glands, and even nerves of the area are frequently sacrificed.

CHAPTER 21

Vascular Supply of the Head and Neck

The head and neck receives most of its vascular supply from branches of the external and internal carotid arteries, as well as from certain branches of the subclavian artery. The majority of the blood within the internal carotid and the vertebral branch of the subclavian artery are destined for the brain, while all of the blood carried by the external carotid artery and some branches of the subclavian artery supplies the remainder of the region. Drainage of this area is accomplished by the tributaries of the internal and external jugular veins, as well as those of the vertebral vein. The present chapter will discuss the branches and tributaries of these major vessels, their locations, sources, and destinations in a systemic fashion. However, vessels, whose primary concerns are the brain, and the internal base of the skull, will not be detailed here, instead, the reader will be referred to pertinent pages in previous chapters.

COMMON CAROTID ARTERY (Fig. 7.12, p. 142)

The *common carotid arteries* of the two sides have different origins; the right common carotid artery is a branch of the brachiocephalic trunk, while the left arises directly from the arch of the aorta. Consequently, the right common carotid artery is contained wholly within the neck, while the left begins in the upper thorax and enters the neck in the vicinity of the sternoclavicular joint. Once in the neck, both vessels are enclosed in their own compartment of the carotid sheath, and ascend approximately to the level of the thyroid cartilage (though this is quite variable), where each bifurcates into an *external* and an *internal carotid artery*. Since these vessels are considered terminal branches, the common carotid artery is said to have no branches in the neck. The common carotid artery presents a slight dilation at its bifurcation, the *carotid sinus*, a modified region of the vessel, innervated by the glossopharyngeal nerve, whose function is to monitor blood pressure. An additional structure, the *carotid body*, is also associated with the region of bifurcation. This small, oval, reddish brown structure, lying within the wall of the carotid artery and innervated by branches of the glossopharyngeal and vagus nerves, is a

319

chemoreceptor, monitoring oxygen and carbon dioxide tensions as well as the pH of the blood.

External Carotid Artery (Fig. 7.12, p. 142)

The *external carotid artery* has six collateral and two terminal branches. They will be treated in the order of their origins from an inferior to superior direction.

Superior Thyroid Artery (Fig. 7.12, p. 142)

The *superior thyroid artery* is the first branch of the external carotid artery, arising from its ventral aspect, just superior to the bifurcation of the common carotid artery. The superior thyroid artery descends in the neck, accompanied by the same named vein and the external laryngeal nerve, reaches the superior pole of the thyroid gland, and divides into its terminal branches, some of which anastomose with their counterparts of the other side and with branches of the inferior thyroid artery. The superior thyroid artery has four named branches; the infrahyoid, sternocleidomastoid, superior laryngeal, and cricothyroid arteries, as well as its terminal anterior, posterior, and occasionally lateral glandular branches serving the thyroid gland.

Infrahyoid Artery (branch).   The *infrahyoid artery* is a small vessel, passing, as its name implies, inferior to the hyoid bone to anastomose with its counterpart on the other side. Along its path, it supplies muscular branches to the infrahyoid muscles in its vicinity.

Sternocleidomastoid Artery.   The *sternocleidomastoid artery (branch)* passes ventral to the carotid sheath supplying the same-named muscle on its deep surface, and sends small twigs to structures in its vicinity.

Superior Laryngeal Artery.   To distribute to the largynx, the *superior laryngeal artery* passes superficial to the inferior constrictor muscle and pierces the thyrohyoid membrane, accompanied by the internal laryngeal nerve. Within the larynx, it serves its muscles, glands, and mucosa.

Cricothyroid Artery.   The small *cricothyroid artery* courses along the cricothyroid ligament supplying the muscle of the same name as well as additional structures in its vicinity.

Glandular Branches.   The *glandular branches* of the superior thyroid artery are the anterior, posterior, and occasionally, the lateral branches. The *anterior branch* follows the superior border of the lateral lobe, distributes to its anterior surface, and anastomoses with its opposite across the isthmus. The *posterior branch* follows a similar course on the deep aspect of the lateral lobe, ramifies on that surface, and anastomoses with the *inferior thyroid artery*, also supplying the parathyroid gland. Occasionally, a *lateral branch* is present, which supplies the lateral aspect of the lateral lobe.

Ascending Pharyngeal Artery (Fig. 7.12, p. 142)

The *ascending pharyngeal artery*, the smallest branch of the external carotid artery, arises on the medial aspect of that artery, shortly after the bifurcation of the common carotid artery. Along its ascent, between the pharynx and the internal carotid artery, it provides unnamed muscular branches to the prevertebral muscles, as well as branches to structures in the vicinity of its path. This artery has four named branches; pharyngeal, meningeal, inferior tympanic, and palatine.

Pharyngeal Branches. The *pharyngeal branches* are variable in number (two to four) and supply the stylopharyngeus and middle pharyngeal constrictor muscles as well as the region of the pharyngeal mucosa in its vicinity.

Meningeal Arteries. The *meningeal arteries* enter the cranial cavity via the jugular foramen (*posterior meningeal branch*), hypoglossal canal, and foramen lacerum to serve the dura mater.

Inferior Tympanic Artery. The *inferior tympanic artery* gains access to the tympanic cavity, via the petrous portion of the temporal bone, to vascularize that cavity's medial wall. It is accompanied by the tympanic branch of the accessory nerve.

Palatine Artery. The *palatine artery* courses along the superior pharyngeal constrictor muscle and supplies branches to the tonsils, auditory tube, and soft palate, anastomosing with other arteries of this region.

Lingual Artery (Fig. 15.1, p. 237)

The *lingual artery* often arises in common with the facial artery, becoming then the lingofacial trunk. The lingual artery originates near the posterior extent of the greater cornu of the hyoid bone, passes deep to the hypoglossal nerve, then between the middle pharyngeal constrictor and hyoglossus muscle. The artery enters the deep surface of the tongue and extends as far anteriorly as its apex. The lingual artery has four named branches; the suprahyoid, dorsal lingual, sublingual, and deep lingual arteries.

Suprahyoid Artery. The slender *suprahyoid artery* courses along the superior border of the hyoid bone, serving the muscles in its vicinity, and anastomoses with its counterpart on the other side.

Dorsal Lingual Artery. The *dorsal lingual artery* arises deep to the hyoglossus muscle. It ascends to the posterior dorsum of the tongue to supply the palatoglossal arch, mucous membrane of the tongue, palatine tonsil, and some of the soft palate, freely anastomosing with other arteries in its vicinity.

Sublingual Artery. The *sublingual artery* arises at the border of the hyoglossus muscle, to course between the genioglossus and mylohyoid muscles on its way to the sublingual gland, which it supplies along with adjacent muscles in addition to the mucous membrane of the floor of the mouth and gingiva. Branches of this artery anastomose with the submental branch of the facial artery.

Deep Lingual Artery. The terminus of the lingual artery, known as the *deep lingual artery*, passes along the ventral aspect of the tongue, immediately deep to the mucous membrane accompanied by the lingual nerve, to its apex, where it anastomoses with its counterpart of the other side.

Facial Artery (Fig. 7.12, p. 142; 8.2, p. 158)

The *facial artery* arises just above (or in common with) the lingual artery and ascends, deep to the stylohyoid and posterior belly of the digastric muscles, to lie in a groove on the posterior aspect of the submandibular gland. The vessel enters the face by crossing the base of the mandible, just anterior to the masseter muscle, in the groove for the facial artery. In the face, the artery travels superficially, just under the cover of the platysma muscle. It passes, via a tortuous path deep to the zygomaticus major, risorius, and levator anguli oris muscles, to the corner of the mouth. Here, it ascends lateral to the nose to terminate as the angular artery at the medial corner of the eye. The branches of the facial artery are the ascending palatine, tonsillar, glandular, and submental arteries in the neck; and inferior labial, superior labial, lateral nasal, and angular arteries, in the face.

Ascending Palatine Artery.   The *ascending palatine artery* originates near the tip of the styloid process. It ascends between that process and the superior pharyngeal constrictor muscle, then between the stylopharyngeus and styloglossus muscles, to supply the levator veli palatini, superior pharyngeal constrictor and neighboring muscles, the soft palate, tonsils, and auditory tube, finally anastomosing with other arteries in its vicinity.

Tonsillar Artery.   The *tonsillar artery* passes between the styloglossus and medial pterygoid muscles and pierces the superior pharyngeal constrictor muscle to supply the palatine tonsil and the posterior tongue.

Glandular Arteries.   The *glandular arteries* distribute as three or four vessels to the submandibular gland to supply it and the adjacent area.

Submental Artery.   The *submental artery* arises from the facial artery near the anterior border of the masseter muscle. It follows the base of the mandible in an anterior direction and turns onto the chin at the anterior border of the depressor anguli oris muscle. The submental artery supplies the muscles it encounters along its passage, and anastomoses with several arteries in its vicinity.

Inferior Labial Artery.   The *inferior labial artery* originates near the corner of the mouth, passes deep to the depressor anguli oris muscle and pierces the orbicularis oris muscle. The artery courses superficial to that muscle, supplying it as well as the substance of the lip. It anastomoses with its counterpart of the other side as well as with branches of the mental and submental arteries.

Superior Labial Artery.   The *superior labial artery* arises just above and follows the same pattern as the inferior labial artery. It passes superficial to the orbicularis oris muscle in the upper lip to serve that muscle as well as the substance of the upper lip. It sends a small twig, the septal branch into the nasal septum, and another one, the alar branch, into the wing of the nose. The terminus of the vessel anastomoses with its counterpart of the opposite side.

Lateral Nasal Artery.   The *lateral nasal artery* is a small branch arising at and passing into the wing and bridge of the nose, which it supplies. This vessel anastomoses with various other arteries in its vicinity.

Angular Artery.   The *angular artery* is the terminal continuation of the facial artery, supplying the tissues in the vicinity of the medial corner of the eye, and anastomosing with arteries of that region.

Occipital Artery (Fig. 7.12, p. 142)

The *occipital artery* originates on the posterior aspect of the external carotid artery, approximately at the same level as the origin of the facial artery. It passes deep to the hypoglossal nerve, the sternocleidomastoid muscle, and the posterior belly of the digastric muscle and lodges in the groove for the occipital artery on the medial aspect of the mastoid process. It passes between the splenius capitis and semispinalis capitis muscles and pierces the superficial layer of the deep cervical fascia at the region of attachment of the trapezius and sternocleidomastoid muscles, just inferior to the superior nuchal line. The artery ramifies in the superficial fascia of the scalp, serving the back of the head. The occipital artery has the following branches; sternocleidomastoid, mastoid, auricular, muscular, descending, meningeal, and occipital arteries.

Sternocleidomastoid Artery.   The *sternocleidomastoid artery* originates near or at the origin of the occipital artery, or occasionally directly from the external carotid artery. It courses across the hypoglossal nerve and enters the deep aspect of the sternocleidomastoid muscle, which it serves. Frequently, this artery exists as two separate upper and lower branches, where the latter accompanies the accessory nerve into the muscle.

Mastoid Artery.   The *mastoid artery* is a small branch that gains access to the cranial cavity via the mastoid foramen. Along its path, it supplies the mastoid air cells, dura mater, and additional structures in its vicinity.

Auricular Artery.   The *auricular branch* passes superficial to the mastoid process to reach and supply the back of the auricle.

Muscular Branches.   The several unnamed *muscular branches* of the occipital artery distribute to the digastric, stylohyoid, longissimus and splenius capitis muscles.

Descending Artery.   The *descending artery*, the longest of all of the branches, originates while the occipital artery is still deep to the splenius capitis muscle. Shortly after its origin, the descending artery bifurcates into a superficial and a deep branch, serving the trapezius muscle and the deep muscles of the back of the head, respectively. The superficial branch anastomoses with the transverse cervical artery while the deep portion anastomoses with the vertebral and deep cervical arteries, providing a collateral circulation between the subclavian and external carotid systems of arteries.

Meningeal Artery.   The *meningeal branches* gain access to the cranial vault via the condyloid canal and jugular foramen to vascularize the dura mater and the bones of the posterior cranial fossa.

Occipital Branches. *Occipital branches* which are usually two in number (medial and lateral) follow the course of the greater occipital nerve to serve the muscles and tissues of the scalp. Small branches may traverse the parietal foramen to supply the parietal meninges.

Posterior Auricular Artery
The *posterior auricular artery* arises from the posterior aspect of the external carotid artery near the level of the distal end of the styloid process. In passing through the substance of the parotid gland, it provides glandular branches, as well as muscular branches to several muscles along its course. Its three named branches are the stylomastoid, auricular, and occipital arteries.

Stylomastoid Artery. The *stylomastoid artery* ascends to enter the stylo-mastoid foramen, accompanying the facial nerve, where it provides a twig, the *posterior tympanic artery*, that will follow the chorda tympani nerve to vascularize the tympanic membrane. The stylomastoid artery serves the mastoid air cells, stapedius muscle, and structures in its vicinity.

Auricular Artery. The *auricular branch* reaches the back of the auricle to supply it, as well as its anterior aspect either by piercing the cartilage or by coursing around its free edge.

Occipital Artery. The *occipital artery* crosses superficial to the insertion of the sternocleidomastoid muscle to supply it as well as the scalp in the vicinity. Its branches anastomose with branches of the superficial temporal and occipital arteries.

Superficial Temporal Artery (Figs. 8.2, p. 158; 11.4, p. 196; 12.6, p. 210)
The *superficial temporal artery*, one of the terminal branches of the external carotid artery, arises near the level of the earlobe within the substance of the parotid gland, which it supplies. The vessel branches profusely at its cranial-most aspect to supply the region superficial to the zygomatic arch as far medially as the lateral corner of the eye as well as the temple and the lateral aspect of the scalp. The branches of the superficial temporal artery include the transverse facial, middle temporal, zygomatico-orbital, anterior auricular, frontal, and parietal arteries.

Transverse Facial Artery. The *transverse facial artery* arises near the level of the mandibular condyle within the substance of the parotid gland. It accompanies, and supplies, the parotid duct in its path across the masseter muscle. Additionally, it sends branches to the parotid gland, masseter muscle, and other tissues in its vicinity.

Middle Temporal Artery. The *middle temporal artery* pierces the temporalis fascia near its origin to supply the temporalis muscle and anastomoses with branches of the deep temporal arteries.

Zygomatico-Orbital Artery. The *zygomatico-orbital artery*, occasionally a branch of the middle temporal artery, follows the zygomatic arch to the lateral corner of the eye. Subsequent to supplying the orbicularis oculi muscle, it anastomoses with branches of the ophthalmic artery.

Anterior Auricular Branches.   The *anterior auricular branches* serve the anterior aspect of the ear, the ear lobe, and the proximal region of the ear canal. This vessel anastomoses with branches of the posterior auricular artery.

Frontal Branch.   The *frontal branch* follows a tortuous path deep to the integument of the forehead, where it ramifies, supplying the frontalis and orbicularis oculi muscles, as well as additional tissues of the region. It anastomoses with branches of the supraorbital and supratrochlear arteries.

Parietal Branch.   The *parietal branch* passes posterosuperiorly behind the auricle, supplying it, and the side and back of the scalp. It anastomoses with branches of the occipital and posterior auricular arteries, as well as its counterpart of the other side.

Maxillary Artery (Figs. 12.5, p. 209; 12.6, p. 210)
The *maxillary artery*, the large terminal branch of the external carotid artery, originates deep within the body of the parotid gland. It courses anteriorly, medial to the ramus of the mandible near the level of the condylar process, but superficial to the sphenomandibular ligament. Passing on the superficial or deep surface of the lateral pterygoid muscle, the maxillary artery reaches and enters the pterygopalatine fossa, where it divides into its terminal branches. The maxillary artery is described as consisting of three portions as it courses through the mandibular, pterygoid, and pterygopalatine regions. The first, or *mandibular portion* courses deep to the mandible between the ramus and the sphenomandibular ligament. Its branches are the deep auricular, anterior tympanic, inferior alveolar, middle meningeal, and accessory meningeal arteries. The course of the second, or *pterygoid portion*, of the maxillary artery is inconsistent, since it may be either superficial or deep to the lateral pterygoid muscle, and the artery enters the pterygopalatine fossa by passing between the two heads of this muscle. Branches of the pterygoid portion are the deep temporal, pterygoid, masseteric, and buccal arteries. The third, or *pterygopalatine portion*, of the maxillary artery gains access to the pterygopalatine fossa via the pterygomaxillary fissure. Branches of the pterygopalatine portion are the posterior superior alveolar, infraorbital, greater palatine, artery of the pterygoid canal, pharyngeal, and sphenopalatine arteries.

Branches of the Mandibular Portion.

DEEP AURICULAR ARTERY.   The small, *deep auricular artery* passes medial to the temporomandibular joint, which it supplies to penetrate the wall of the external acoustic meatus, serving its lining and the tympanic membrane.

ANTERIOR TYMPANIC ARTERY.   The *anterior tympanic artery* is also small and may arise as a common trunk with the deep auricular artery. It ascends to enter the petrotympanic fissure to reach the tympanic cavity, where it serves the tympanic membrane and associated structures.

INFERIOR ALVEOLAR ARTERY.   The *inferior alveolar artery* arises from a point between the condylar process of the mandible and the sphenomandibular ligament. It passes inferiorly, to enter, along the inferior alveolar nerve and vein, the mandibular foramen. Within the mandibular canal, in the vicinity of the first premolar tooth, it bifurcates to form the *incisive* and *mental arteries*. Additional branches of the inferior alveolar artery are the mylohyoid and dental arteries. The *mylohyoid artery* arises from its parent vessel before that artery enters the mandibular foramen. It passes along the mylohyoid groove, accompanied by the mylohyoid nerve, to serve the muscle of the same name. *Dental branches* enter the roots and periodontal ligaments of the molar and premolar teeth. The *incisive branch* continues anteriorly within the mandible, to serve the lateral and central incisor teeth and to anastomose with its counterpart of the other side. The *mental artery*, accompanied by the mental nerve and veins, exits the mandibular canal via the mental foramen, to vascularize the chin and lower lip. Its branches anastomose with those of the inferior labial and submental arteries.

MIDDLE MENINGEAL ARTERY. The *accessory* and *middle meningeal arteries* arise from the superior aspect of the maxillary artery or by a common trunk from the same artery. As the middle meningeal artery ascends to enter the foramen spinosum, it is engirdled by the two branches of the auriculotemporal nerve. The *accessory meningeal artery* traverses the foramen ovale. The distribution of these arteries is detailed in a previous chapter (p. 170).

Branches of the Pterygoid Portion.

DEEP TEMPORAL ARTERIES. The *anterior* and *posterior deep temporal arteries* pass superiorly, deep to the temporalis muscle which they supply. They anastomose with the middle temporal and lacrimal arteries.

PTERYGOID ARTERIES. The short *pterygoid arteries* arise from this portion to vascularize the medial and lateral pterygoid muscles.

MASSETERIC ARTERY. The *masseteric artery*, accompanied by the same-named nerve, passes through the mandibular notch to serve the masseter muscle. Some of its branches anastomose with branches of the transverse facial and facial arteries.

BUCCAL ARTERY. The *buccal artery* accompanies the buccal nerve and passes in close association to the tendon of the temporalis muscle. It arborizes on the buccinator muscle to supply it and the mucous membrane of the mouth. Branches of the buccal artery anastomose with those of the infraorbital and facial arteries.

Branches of the Pterygopalatine Portion.

POSTERIOR SUPERIOR ALVEOLAR ARTERY. The *posterior superior alveolar artery* branches from the maxillary artery as that vessel enters the pterygomaxillary fissure. It travels along the maxillary tuberosity and enters the posterior superior alveolar foramen in conjunction with the like-named nerve. The vessel ramifies within the maxilla to serve the maxillary sinus, molar and premolar teeth, as well as the neighboring gingiva.

INFRAORBITAL ARTERY. The *infraorbital artery*, the continuation of the maxillary artery, enters the floor of the orbit through the inferior orbital fissure, lies in the infraorbital groove, then leaves the orbit via the infraorbital canal to enter the face by way of the infraorbital foramen. Branches of the infraorbital artery are the *orbital branches,* serving the inferior oblique and inferior rectus muscles, as well as the lacrimal gland. The *anterior superior alveolar branches* vascularize the maxillary sinus, maxillary canine, and incisor teeth as well as their respective gingiva. The *facial branches* enter the face via the infraorbital foramen deep to the levator labii superioris muscle, where they provide *labial, nasal,* and *palpebral branches* to serve the lacrimal sac, nose, and upper lip. The various branches anastomose with branches of the angular, dorsal nasal, buccal, transverse facial, and facial arteries.

GREATER PALATINE ARTERY (**Fig. 16.1, p. 246).** The *greater palatine artery* and its branch, the *lesser palatine* artery, pass through the pterygopalatine (greater palatine) canal to gain entrance to the palate via the greater palatine and lesser palatine foramina, respectively. The greater palatine artery courses in an anterior direction on the lateral aspect of the hard palate to supply the palatal mucosa, gingiva, and glands and then proceeds to anastomose with the nasopalatine artery in the incisive canal. The lesser palatine artery vascularizes the soft palate and tonsil. It anastomoses with the ascending palatine branch of the facial artery as well as the tonsillar branches of the facial, lingual, and ascending pharyngeal arteries.

ARTERY OF THE PTERYGOID CANAL. The small *artery of the pterygoid canal* passes through the posterior wall of the pterygopalatine fossa by way of the pterygoid canal. It supplies part of the auditory tube, pharynx, middle ear, and sphenoidal sinus.

PHARYNGEAL BRANCH. The small *pharyngeal branch* passes dorsally, through the pharyngeal canal, to vascularize the auditory tube, sphenoidal sinus, and portions of the pharynx.

SPHENOPALATINE ARTERY. The *sphenopalatine artery* leaves the pterygopalatine fossa via the sphenopalatine foramen on its medial wall to enter the nasal fossa, where it vascularizes portions of the nasal conchae and meatuses by its *posterior lateral nasal branches* as well as the posterior segment of the median nasal septum by its *posterior septal branches.* The longest branch of this vessel is the *nasopalatine artery* that descends along the vomer bone to enter the incisive canal. It is here that it anastomoses with branches of the greater palatine artery.

Internal Carotid Artery (Fig. 7.12, p. 142)

The *internal carotid artery* has no branches in the neck. It ascends deep to the parotid gland, digastric muscle, and muscles attached to the styloid process, in its own compartment of the carotid sheath. The internal carotid artery gains access to the cranial cavity via the carotid canal of the petrous temporal bone, to vascularize the part of the brain, orbit, portions of the nasal cavity, and the forehead. Associated with the artery is the carotid plexus of nerves, composed of postganglionic sympathetic nerve fibers, derived from the superior cervical sympathetic ganglion. The internal carotid artery is described as having four portions; cervical, petrous, cavernous, and cerebral, referring to its termination in the vicinity of the lateral cerebral fissure. The *cervical portion* of the artery has no branches. The *petrous portion*, located entirely within the carotid canal of the petrous temporal bone has four branches; the caroticotympanic, artery of the pterygoid canal, cavernous, and hypophyseal arteries. The *cavernous portion*, located within the cavernous sinus (but isolated from the cavernous blood by the endothelially lined fibrous sheaths), gives rise to the ganglionic, anterior meningeal, ophthalmic, as well as the anterior and middle cerebral arteries. The *cerebral portion* is the terminal region of the internal carotid artery, whose terminal branches are the posterior communicating and anterior choroidal arteries.

Petrous Portion

Since the arteries of the petrous portion are quite small, they will be treated as a single unit. The *caroticotympanic branch* leaves the carotid canal to gain access to the tympanic cavity, part of which it vascularizes. The *artery of the pterygoid canal* is not always present, when it is, it anastomoses with the same-named branch of the maxillary artery within the pterygoid canal. The several *cavernous* and *hypophyseal branches* supply the trigeminal ganglion, pituitary gland, as well as the dura mater in their vicinity.

Cavernous Portion

The small *ganglionic* and *anterior meningeal branches* supply the trigeminal ganglion and the dura mater of the anterior cranial fossa, respectively.

OPHTHALMIC ARTERY. The *ophthalmic artery* originates a few millimeters dorsal to the optic foramen (canal) through which it gains access to the orbit accompanied by the optic nerve, which is superior and medial to it. Within the orbit, the artery crosses superior to the nerve, but inferior to the superior rectus muscle, to reach the medial wall of the orbit. The ophthalmic artery serves the orbit as well as the orb and its muscles and its branches are described accordingly. The *orbital group* consists of the lacrimal, supraorbital, posterior and anterior ethmoidal, medial palpebral, supratrochlear, and dorsal nasal arteries. The *ocular group* is composed of the central artery of the retina, short and long posterior ciliary, anterior ciliary, and muscular arteries.

LACRIMAL ARTERY. The *lacrimal artery* arises on the lateral aspect of the ophthalmic artery, and passes, accompanied by the lacrimal nerve, to the lacrimal gland, which it supplies. The *lateral palpebral branches* of the lacrimal artery serve the upper and lower eyelids. Additional named branches include the *zygomatic* and *recurrent branches*. The former, passing through the zygomaticotemporal and zygomaticofacial foramina serve the contents of the temporal fossa and the substance of the cheek, while the latter supplies the dura mater, reaching it via the superior orbital fissure.

SUPRAORBITAL ARTERY. The *supraorbital artery* courses forward in the orbit on the medial margin of the superior rectus muscle and then travels with the frontal nerve, superficial to the levator palpebrae superioris muscle (serving both muscles), to reach and enter the supraorbital foramen. The artery distributes on the forehead, and anastomoses with branches of the superficial temporal and supratrochlear arteries, as well as with its counterpart of the other side.

POSTERIOR ETHMOIDAL ARTERY.   The small *posterior ethmoidal artery* leaves the orbit via the same-named foramen, accompanying the same-named nerve, supplies the posterior ethmoidal air cells, the dura mater of the cribriform plate, and regions of the nasal cavity.

ANTERIOR ETHMOIDAL ARTERY.   The *anterior ethmoidal artery* is larger than the previous vessel. It leaves the orbit by way of the anterior ethmoidal foramen, accompanying the same-named nerve. It vascularizes the frontal sinus, all of the ethmoidal air cells (except for the posterior) and a region of the dura mater of the anterior cranial fossa. Its large *nasal branch* enters the nasal cavity along a hiatus by the crista galli, to serve the walls of the nasal cavity. A cutaneous twig of the nasal branch, serves the bridge of the nose.

MEDIAL PALPEBRAL ARTERIES.   The *superior* and *inferior medial palpebral arteries* each form an arch in the upper and lower eyelids, respectively. The inferior palpebral artery also sends a twig to the nasolacrimal sac and duct. These vessels form extensive anastomoses with other arteries of the region and with each other.

SUPRATROCHLEAR ARTERY.   The *supratrochlear artery*, a terminal branch of the ophthalmic artery, leaves the orbit medial to the supraorbital foramen. It serves the forehead and anastomoses with the supraorbital artery and its counterpart of the other side.

DORSAL NASAL ARTERY.   The *dorsal nasal artery*, the inferiorly positioned terminal branch of the ophthalmic artery, leaves the orbit at its medial angle to serve the bridge and side of the nose. Its lacrimal branch supplies the nasolacrimal sac and duct.

CENTRAL ARTERY OF THE RETINA.   The small *central artery of the retina* passes within the optic nerve to supply it as well as the retina of the bulb.

SHORT POSTERIOR CILIARY ARTERIES.   The several *short posterior ciliary arteries* pass to the orb around the periphery of the optic nerve. They pierce the sclera to serve it and the ciliary processes.

LONG POSTERIOR CILIARY ARTERIES.   The two *long posterior ciliary arteries* pass lateral and medial to the optic nerve to supply the ciliary muscle and iris, subsequent to piercing the sclera.

ANTERIOR CILIARY ARTERIES.   The *anterior ciliary arteries* pass deep to the conjunctiva and penetrate the sclera just posterior to the corneoscleral junction to serve the ciliary muscles.

MUSCULAR BRANCHES.   The *superior* and *inferior muscular branches* serve all of the extrinsic muscles of the orb, as well as the levator palpebrae superioris.

The *anterior cerebral, middle cerebral, posterior communicating,* and *anterior choroidal arteries* are discussed on page 276, and the reader is referred to that page.

SUBCLAVIAN ARTERY (Fig. 7.10, p. 138)

The *subclavian artery* is a short vessel extending as far laterally as the outer border of the first rib. The origins of the right and left subclavian arteries differ in that the left one arises directly from the arch of the aorta, while the right is one of the terminal branches of the brachiocephalic trunk.

The right subclavian artery originates deep to the sternoclavicular joint, and the left originates behind the common carotid artery around the third or fourth thoracic vertebra. Both right and left arteries travel superiorly to the root of the neck and posterior to the anterior scalene muscle, emerging into the posterior triangle through the interval between the anterior and middle scalene muscles on their way to the lateral border of the first rib, where each artery becomes known as the axillary artery. This passage, deep to the anterior scalene muscle, permits a convenient division of the subclavian artery into three parts. The first part is from the origin of the vessel to the medial border of the anterior scalene muscle; the second part lies deep to this muscle; while the third part extends from the lateral border of the anterior scalene to the lateral border of the first rib. The branches of the subclavian artery are the vertebral artery, internal thoracic artery, and thyrocervical trunk from the first part, the costocervical trunk from the second part, and the dorsal scapular artery from the third part.

First Part of the Subclavian Artery

Vertebral Artery

The *vertebral artery* takes its origin from the posterosuperior aspect of the first part of the subclavian artery. It ascends behind the anterior scalene muscle, along the transverse process of the seventh cervical vertebra, and enters the foramen transversarium of the sixth cervical vertebra. The artery travels through the foramina transversaria of the upper six cervical vertebrae, enters the suboccipital triangle, from where it traverses the foramen magnum. Branches of the vertebral artery are described according to the region occupied by the vessel, namely cervical and cranial branches. The cervical branches are the spinal and muscular arteries, while the cranial branches are five in number; the meningeal, posterior spinal, anterior spinal, posterior inferior cerebellar, and medullary arteries. Only the cervical branches will be discussed here, since the cranial branches were treated in an earlier chapter (p. 276) in a systemic manner.

Cervical Branches.

SPINAL ARTERIES. The numerous *spinal arteries* gain access to the vertebral canal via the intervertebral foramina to serve the spinal meninges, spinal cord, as well as the bony vertebral column.

MUSCULAR BRANCHES.   The unnamed *muscular branches* provide numerous twigs to supply the deep muscles of the neck. Branches of these vessels anastomose with other vessels in their vicinity.

Internal Thoracic Artery

The *internal thoracic artery* originates from the inferior aspect of the first part of the subclavian artery. This artery passes directly inferiorly on the internal anterior thoracic wall just lateral to the margin of the sternum to the sixth or seventh rib, where it bifurcates to form the medially placed *superior epigastric* and laterally positioned *musculophrenic arteries*. Since the internal thoracic artery is a vessel whose distribution is limited to the thorax and abdomen, its branches will not be discussed.

Thyrocervical Trunk

The *thyrocervical trunk* is a short vessel arising from the superior aspect of the first part of the subclavian artery. This trunk lies just medial to the anterior scalene muscle, where it trifurcates to form three major branches; the suprascapular, transverse cervical, and inferior thyroid arteries.

Suprascapular Artery.   The *suprascapular artery* travels obliquely across the anterior surface of the anterior scalene and deep to the sternocleidomastoid muscles, which it supplies. It passes deep to the inferior belly of the omohyoid muscle to reach the scapular notch. Occasionally, the suprascapular artery is a branch of the third part of the subclavian artery.

Transverse Cervical Artery.   The *transverse cervical artery* crosses the neck in a fashion similar to, but above, the suprascapular artery. It crosses the floor of the subclavian triangle, accompanied by the spinal accessory nerve, to burrow under the anterior border of the trapezius muscle, supplying it and other muscles in the vicinity.

Inferior Thyroid Artery.   The *inferior thyroid artery* travels superiorly in front of the medial border of the anterior scalene muscle. It then passes deep to the carotid sheath and approaches the inferior aspect of the thyroid gland, which it supplies. The inferior thyroid artery has several small branches, including the *ascending* and *descending branches* ending in the body of the thyroid gland, as well as *muscular branches* and the *ascending cervical artery* supplying anterior vertebral muscles of the neck. Additionally, branches are also distributed to larynx (the *inferior laryngeal artery*), trachea (*tracheal*), and esophagus. (portion

Second Part of the Subclavian Artery

Costocervical Trunk

The *costocervical trunk* has different origins on the two sides of the body. On the left, it springs from the posterior aspect of the first part of the subclavian artery, while on the right it springs from the posterior aspect of the second part of that artery. This trunk has two terminal branches; the superior intercostal and deep cervical arteries.

Superior Intercostal Artery. The *superior intercostal artery* serves the first and second intercostal spaces.

Deep Cervical Artery. The *deep cervical artery* is interposed between the first rib and the transverse process of the seventh cervical vertebra. It passes between the semispinalis cervicis and semispinalis capitis muscles, supplying these as well as adjacent muscles, finally anastomosing with the occipital and vertebral arteries.

Third Part of the Subclavian Artery

Dorsal Scapular Artery
The *dorsal scapular artery* is the only branch arising from the third part of the subclavian artery, though frequently it is a branch of the second part. The dorsal scapular artery passes among the trunks of the brachial plexus, anterior to the middle scalene muscle, to reach the superior angle of the scapula, where it supplies muscles in the vicinity.

VEINS OF THE HEAD AND NECK

The veins serving the region of the head and neck are subdivided, for descriptive purposes, into three major groups: the veins of the face, cranium, and neck. Most of the veins of the cranium are detailed in an earlier chapter (pp. 170–173) and will not be treated at this point.

Veins of the Face (Fig. 8.2, p. 158)

The veins of the face are subdivided into two categories, namely superficial and deep veins. The named superficial veins are the facial, superficial temporal, posterior auricular, occipital, and retromandibular veins, while the named deep veins are the maxillary and pterygoid plexus of veins.

Facial Vein
The *facial vein* serves as the principal venous vessel of the superficial face. It begins in the medial corner of the eye as the *angular vein*, the confluence of the frontal and supraorbital veins, passes inferiorly following the course of the facial artery deep to the zygomaticus major and zygomaticus minor muscles, where it parts company with the artery to empty into the internal jugular vein. The facial vein communicates with the pterygoid plexus of veins as well as with the ophthalmic veins, both of which present possible passageways to the cavernous sinus due to lack of directional valves. Tributaries of the facial vein include the *deep facial vein* which connects it to the pterygoid plexus of veins, the *frontal vein* which drains a region of the forehead, and the *supraorbital* and *supratrochlear veins*. Additionally, the superior palpebral, external nasal, masseteric, anterior parotid, superior and inferior labial, and submental veins also join the facial vein.

Superficial Temporal Vein

The *superficial temporal vein* follows the course of the same-named artery to drain the scalp, temple, and part of the forehead and ear. This vessel begins as a plexus of small veins on the side and top of the head. Among the tributaries of the superficial temporal vein are: the *transverse facial vein, middle temporal vein,* and *anterior auricular veins.*

Posterior Auricular Vein

The *posterior auricular vein,* one of the two veins participating in the formation of the *external jugular vein,* begins as a plexus of small veins behind the ear and courses in an anteroinferior direction, passing superficial to mastoidal attachment of the sternocleidomastoid muscle. Its tributaries include the *stylomastoid vein.*

Occipital Vein

The *occipital vein* enters the suboccipital triangle to join a plexus of veins drained by the vertebral vein. Tributaries of the occipital vein include the *mastoid emissary vein.* Occasionally, the occipital vein joins either the internal jugular or the posterior auricular veins.

Retromandibular Vein

The *retromandibular vein,* one of the two veins participating in the formation of the *external jugular vein,* is frequently formed within the substance of the parotid gland. It is formed when the maxillary vein joins the superficial temporal vein. Tributaries of this short vessel include the common facial, middle temporal, and anterior auricular veins.

Maxillary Vein

The relatively short *maxillary vein* follows the mandibular portion of the same-named artery deep to the mandibular ramus to participate in conjunction with the superficial temporal vein, in the formation of the *retromandibular vein.* The maxillary vein arises from the pterygoid plexus of veins.

Pterygoid Plexus of Veins

The *pterygoid plexus of veins* is a massive network of venous channels lying on or about the surfaces of the lateral and medial pterygoid muscles and extending into the spaces of the deep face within the infratemporal fossa. This plexus is in direct or indirect communication with a vast area, including the cranial cavity and cavernous sinus, the nasal cavity, orbit, paranasal sinuses, and superficial face. Some of its tributaries include the middle meningeal veins, posterior superior and inferior alveolar veins, veins that serve the muscles of mastication, infraorbital vein, buccal veins, and sphenopalatine vein. Additionally, it receives emissary veins and a communication from the inferior ophthalmic vein. Moreover, numerous smaller named and unnamed veins join the pterygoid plexus of veins.

Veins of the Cranium

Although most of the *veins of the cranium* were detailed elsewhere (pp. 170–173), the superior and inferior ophthalmic veins of the orbit will be treated in this section.

Superior Ophthalmic Vein

The *superior ophthalmic vein* is formed by the confluence of the *angular* and *nasofrontal* (derived from the supraorbital and supratrochlear) *veins*. It enters the cranial cavity via the superior orbital fissure and empties its contents into the *cavernous sinus*. Its tributaries include; the posterior and anterior ethmoidal, lacrimal, ciliary, and a branch of the inferior ophthalmic veins. Additionally, numerous smaller named and unnamed veins join the superior ophthalmic vein.

Inferior Ophthalmic Vein

The *inferior ophthalmic vein* is formed by the confluence of several small veins in the anterior floor of the orbit, among which are unnamed inferior muscular branches and the *anterior ciliary vein*. The inferior ophthalmic vein bifurcates into a superior portion that usually joins the superior ophthalmic vein (or drains directly into the cavernous sinus), and an inferior portion that becomes a tributary of the pterygoid plexus of veins, which it reaches through the inferior orbital fissure.

Veins of the Neck

The veins of the neck include the external jugular, internal jugular, vertebral, and subclavian veins.

External Jugular Vein (Fig. 7.2, p. 115)

The *external jugular vein* is formed by the union of the *posterior auricular* and *retromandibular veins* just posterior to the angle of the mandible, sometimes within the body of the parotid gland. It passes straight down the neck, under the cover of the platysma muscle and associated superficial fascia, superficial to the fleshy belly of the sternocleidomastoid muscle. Along its path, it crosses this muscle at an oblique angle. Once it reaches the subclavian triangle, the external jugular vein pierces the investing fascia, parallels the posterior border of the sternocleidomastoid muscle, and dives deep to the clavicle to deliver its blood into the *subclavian vein*, which it joins. The external jugular vein has two pairs of incompetent valves just before it empties into the subclavian vein. Several tributaries join the external jugular vein, namely the *posterior external jugular vein*, which drains the superficial aspect of the back of the neck, and two others, the *transverse cervical* and *suprascapular veins*. The last two veins drain the region of the shoulder. Another superficial vessel, the *anterior jugular vein*, occasionally empties into the external jugular vein, but usually it joins the subclavian vein directly. The anterior jugular vein is quite variable, but normally it begins at the level of the body of the hyoid bone and descends parallel to the anterior midline of the neck. Inferiorly, near the origin of the medial head of the sternocleidomastoid muscle, the vein pierces the superficial lamina of the investing layer and turns laterally, pierces the posterior lamina, and joins the subclavian (or occasionally, the external jugular) vein. While it is between the two laminae of the investing facia, the anterior jugular vein communicates with its corresponding vein of the other side via a venous connection, the *jugular arch*, which occupies the suprasternal space.

The external jugular, posterior external jugular, and anterior external jugular veins have numerous smaller named and unnamed tributaries, which drain the areas in their immediate vicinity.

Internal Jugular Vein (Figs. 7.10, p. 138; 11.4, p. 196)

The *internal jugular vein* is the main vessel responsible for collecting blood from the brain, superficial aspects of the face, and the neck. The vessel extends from its dilated origin, the *superior jugular bulb* housed in the jugular foramen, to its inferior dilation, the *inferior jugular bulb* terminating in the brachiocephalic vein. The internal jugular vein is enclosed in the carotid sheath as it travels the length of the neck, and its tributaries pierce this fascia to deliver their blood to the vessel. The internal jugular vein receives blood from the following tributaries: dural venous sinus drainage from with the cranium; the facial vein from the superficial face; the lingual vein from the tongue and floor of the mouth; pharyngeal, superior and middle thyroid, and occasionally the occipital veins from the neck. The dural venous sinuses and their drainage into the superior bulb of the internal jugular vein were described in an earlier chapter (pp. 170–173). The facial and occipital veins were detailed in this chapter under the heading "Veins of the Face", therefore, only the lingual, pharyngeal, and superior and middle thyroid veins will be discussed below. The *lingual vein* receives several tributaries which drain the tongue and floor of the mouth. These are the *sublingual, dorsal lingual,* and *deep lingual veins*, and they follow the paths of their corresponding arteries. The small *pharyngeal veins* communicate with the pharyngeal plexus of veins, and sometimes deliver their blood to the superior thyroid, lingual or facial veins, instead of the internal jugular vein. The *superior* and *middle thyroid veins* both drain the thyroid gland and join the internal jugular vein at its superior and inferior aspects, respectively. Both vessels receive smaller named and unnamed tributaries.

Vertebral Veins

Unlike their arterial counterpart, the *vertebral veins* do not traverse the foramen magnum, instead they are formed from the confluence of many small tributaries within the suboccipital triangle. The vertebral veins enter the foramen transversarium of the axis and form a plexus of veins surrounding the vertebral artery and descend with it within the foramina transversaria of the remaining cervical vertebrae but the last. They end in the brachiocephalic vein or occasionally in the subclavian vein. Tributaries of the vertebral veins include the *anterior* and *accessory vertebral veins*, and the *deep cervical vein*.

Subclavian Vein (Fig. 7.10, p. 138)

The *subclavian vein* is quite short, since it is the continuation of the auxiliary vein, and it joins the internal jugular vein to form the large brachiocephalic vein. Thus, the subclavian vein extends from the external border of the first rib to the junction with the internal jugular vein, passing anterior to the anterior scalene muscle which separates it from the subclavian artery. Here it lies in front of the subclavius muscle, which acts as a cushion, protecting the underlying vessels and nerves.

The main tributary of the subclavian vein is the *external jugular vein*, though frequently the subclavian may receive the *dorsal scapular* and *anterior jugular veins*. The left subclavian vein receives lymph from most of the body via the *thoracic duct*, while lymph from the right upper quadrant of the body is delivered to the right subclavian vein by the *right lymphatic duct*. These ducts pierce the superior aspects of the subclavian veins, just before these are joined by the internal jugular veins.

CHAPTER 77

Fasciae of the Head and Neck

Fasciae are thickened condensations of fibroelastic connective tissue that separate various moveable structures from one another. Spaces between layers of fascia are filled with a loose type of connective tissue which permits infection to spread from one locale to another with relative ease. Since infection may travel along these fascial sheets, the clinician should possess a working knowledge of their locations, extent, and intercommunications. Armed with this knowledge, one can anticipate possible complications that may arise from the various procedures that were performed, and develop a sound therapeutic program for their prevention and treatment.

Since fasciae are merely sheets of connective tissue of various thicknesses, considerable controversy surrounds their limits, attachments, and their interrelationships. Compounding these problems is that different authors frequently assign different names for the same fascial layer, or suggest that some of the flimsier connective tissue sheets are not deserving to be classified as fascia. The goal of this chapter is to present fascia and fascial spaces from a standpoint of boundaries and communications so that varying terminologies will be less confusing, thus providing a foundation for the clinician.

CERVICAL FASCIA (Figs. 22.1, 22.2)

Superficial Cervical Fascia

The fascia of the neck is subdivided into superficial and deep layers. The *superficial cervical fascia* (tela subcutanea) surrounds the neck in a cylindrical fashion. It contains the platysma anterolaterally as well as the cutaneous branches of the cervical plexus. Inferiorly, the fascia is continuous with that over the pectoral and deltoid region anteriorly, while posteriorly it blends with the fascia over the back, where it becomes firmly attached to the deep fascia. This thin fascia is freely attached anteriorly, thus facilitating movement unlike that in its thick attached posterior region.

Superiorly, the superficial cervical fascia passes into the head posteriorly

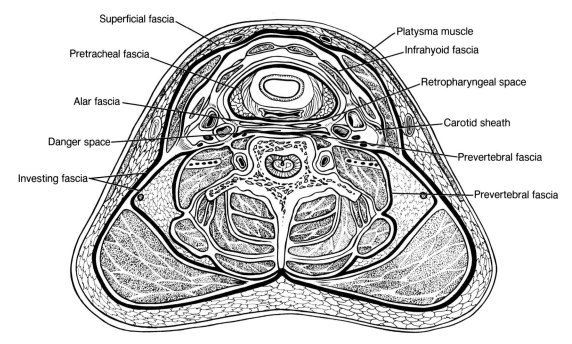

Figure 22.1. Cervical fascia and spaces. The view is approximately at the level of the seventh cervical vertebra.

and over the mandible anteriorly to cover the face and skull, wherein lie the muscles of facial expression as well as nerves and vessels serving the structures located there.

Deep Cervical Fascia

The *deep cervical fascia* is, for descriptive purposes, usually divided into three layers: investing, pretracheal, and prevertebral, although this is not a completely accurate division. Actually, there are several other named fascial layers of anatomical and clinical importance in the cervical region.

Investing Fascia

The *investing fascia,* known also as *superficial* or *anterior cervical* layer of the *deep fascia,* surrounds the neck as a cylinder covering the anterior and posterior cervical triangles and investing the muscles forming the boundaries of these triangles. This fascia arises from the spinous processes of the cervical vertebral column and ligamentum nuchae then encircles the neck. As it passes anteriorly, it divides into two laminae enveloping the trapezius muscle. The two layers unite before crossing over the posterior cervical triangle to form a single sheet. While there, it splits to surround the inferior belly of the omohyoid muscle and forms a ligament that fixes the intermediate tendon of that muscle in a constant position relative to the clavicle. At the posterior border of the sternocleidomastoid muscle, the investing fascia divides once more to encompass that muscle. The two layers fuse again prior to passing superficial to the anterior triangle as a single layer. As this fascia encounters the infrahyoid muscles, it envelops each muscle with a thin fascial covering that is attached

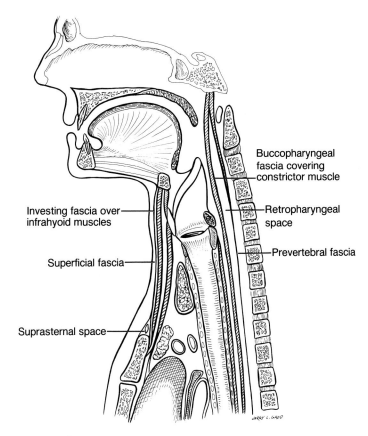

Figure 22.2. Cervical fascia. Sagittal view.

superiorly to the hyoid bond. Inferiorly, the fascia is attached to the acromion of the scapula and the clavicle, subsequently it divides to become attached to the anterior and posterior surfaces of the manubrium creating a space between the two layers known as the *suprasternal space* which usually contains the jugular arch, a venous connection between the two anterior jugular veins, and an occasional lymph node embedded in adipose tissue.

The superior extent of the investing layer of the deep cervical fascia attaches to the external occipital protuberance, superior nuchal line, and the mastoid process of the temporal bone. Here it splits to enclose the adjacent parotid gland and continues superiorly as the *parotid fascia*. The superficial lamina of the fascia attaches to the inferior margin of the zygomatic arch and the deep lamina continues along the temporal bone to the carotid canal. It is from this deep lamina that the *stylomandibular ligament* is formed coursing from the styloid process to the inferior border of the angle of the mandible. Thus, this ligament effectively separates the parotid from the submandibular gland.

Pretracheal Fascia

Another layer of the deep fascia is the *pretracheal fascia* or middle layer of the cervical fascia. Since most of the viscera of the neck is encased by this layer, it is sometimes referred to as the visceral fascia.

The thin, filmy anterior lamina of this fascia lies deep to, but makes contact and blends with, the deep layer of the investing fascia covering the infrahyoid muscles. Because of this intimate relationship, it is sometimes described as being derived from the deep layer of the investing fascia. The remainder of the pretracheal fascia completely invests the thyroid gland and its deeper layer encircles the larynx and trachea as a tubular structure while being well developed on the pharynx and lateral aspects of the esophagus. The posterior lamina, that separating the esophagus from the prevertebral fascia, is called the *buccopharyngeal fascia* whose superior attachment is the pharyngeal tubercle of the occipital bone. Upon covering the superior pharyngeal constrictor muscle, it continues laterally over the buccinator muscle and attaches to the pterygoid hamulus and pterygomandibular raphe. The portion blanketing the medial pharyngeal constrictor muscle continues anteriorly with the fascia covering the hyoglossus and genioglossus muscles. Additional superior attachments include the hyoid bond and the stylohyoid ligament.

Inferiorly, the pretracheal fascia begins with the oblique line of the thyroid cartilage and descends to merge with the fascia covering the aorta and the fibrous pericardium, and to the fascia of the posterior thoracic wall.

Prevertebral Fascia

The third major layer of the deep cervical fascia is the prevertebral fascia which encases the layers of musculature about the vertebral column. This fascia is described as originating from the ligamentum nuchae and the spinous processes of the cervical vertebrae. It covers those muscles of the back that extend the neck, and therefore, lies deep to the trapezius muscle and the investing fascia. Laterally, it blankets the scalene muscles then turns medially to attach to the transverse processes, where it splits, forming a double lamina that fuses with its two layered counterparts of the opposite side. In its position, it forms the floor of the posterior cervical triangle. Superiorly, it is in contact with the investing fascia covering the trapezius muscle. Inferiorly, this fascia continues into the thorax to cover the muscles of the neck as they insert into the rim of the superior thoracic aperature.

A fascial space is evident in the posterior triangle housing the accessory nerve and a few lymph nodes. Near the base of the posterior triangle, the fascial space is enlarged as the prevertebral fascia passes over the scalene muscles. This permits passage of parts of the subclavian and external jugular veins, the transverse cervical and suprascapular vessels, supraclavicular and suprascapular nerves, and the inferior belly of the omohyoid muscle.

As the roots of the brachial plexus emerge from between the anterior and middle scalene muscles, the prevertebral fascia is reflected onto them which blends with the axillary sheath. In covering the anterior scalene muscle, the fascia also overlies the phrenic nerve as it courses superficial to that muscle on its way to the thoracic cavity.

Additionally, as the prevertebral fascia approaches the anterior tubercles of the vertebrae where it attaches, it also contributes to the formation of the posterior portion of the carotid sheath and covers the cervical sympathetic trunk. In continuing on its medial course from the anterior tubercle, the fascia splits into two laminae as it crosses the midline immediately deep to the buccopharyngeal fascia of the posterior visceral wall. The anterior lamina is called the *alar fascia* while the posterior lamina, lying against the body of the vertebrae, remains known as the prevertebral fascia. Thus, the space formed between these two laminae is referred to as the *"danger space"* or *"Space 4"*, not to be confused with the retropharyngeal space or the prevertebral space, both of which will be discussed later. The danger space is continuous for the base of the skull through the neck into the thorax to end at the diaphragm.

Carotid Sheath

The fascial covering that surrounds the common carotid artery, internal jugular vein, vagus nerve, and the internal carotid artery is the *carotid sheath*. This cylindrical structure lies between the investing and pretracheal fasciae anteromedially and between the investing and prevertebral fasciae posteromedially. The anterolateral portion of the sheath is formed by the investing fascia with some contribution from the pretracheal fascia. The posterior wall is derived from a medial lamina of the investing fascia, thus the medial wall of the sheath is formed as the two leaves of the forming sheath unite. Additionally, the medial wall of the sheath is attached to the prevertebral fascia. Superiorly, the sheath is attached to the skull around the jugular foramen while inferiorly it is continuous with the fasciae of the great vessels and heart. The interior of the sheath is compartmentalized to separate the artery, vein, and nerve.

CERVICAL FASCIAL SPACES

Potential spaces, spaces, and fascial clefts between fascial layers and the structures they cover are of clinical importance since these may afford passageways for the spread of infection. Though many of these spaces are inconsequential, several are worthy of description.

Visceral Compartment

The visceral compartment of the neck includes the area bounded anteriorly by the deep layer of the infrahyoid fascia and the loose connective tissue surrounding the thyroid gland, trachea, and esophagus; laterally by the medial portion of the carotid sheath; and posteriorly by the buccopharyngeal fascia superiorly, blending with the visceral fascia inferiorly. The anterior portion of this compartment surrounding and anterior to the trachea has been termed the pretracheal space while that posterior to the trachea and surrounding the esophagus is termed the retrovisceral space often referred to as the retropharyngeal space. It should be remembered that the retropharyngeal space is continuous inferiorly with the retroesophageal space, thus the term retrovisceral space is the more accurate and inclusive term.

Pretracheal Space

The *pretracheal space,* one of those located in the visceral compartment of the neck surrounds the trachea as it lies against the esophagus. It is limited superiorly by the infrahyoid attachments to the thyroid cartilage and hyoid bone and inferiorly it continues into the mediastinum.

Retropharyngeal Space

The *retropharyngeal space* lies in the posterior portion of the visceral compartment between the pharynx/esophagus and the prevertebral fascia. It is not restricted to the neck, however, since it extends superiorly to the base of the skull and inferiorly, into the mediastinum. This space is of particular importance to the clinician since it is the pathway for the transmission of infections from the head and neck into the mediastinum.

Danger Space (Space 4)

The *danger space* is often described as being synonymous with that of the retropharyngeal (retrovisceral) space when, in fact, it is not. The danger space lies posterior to the retropharyngeal space which is bounded posteriorly by the alar fascia, and anterior leaf of the prevertebral fascia, extending across the midline from the anterior tubercles of transverse processes of the cervical and thoracic vertebrae. The danger space lies behind this alar fascia in the pocket formed between the alar fascia and the posterior leaf of the prevertebral fascia passing just anterior to the vertebral bodies from one transverse process across the midline to the other transverse process. This space extends from the base of the skull to the diaphragm and is a closed space. It appears, therefore, that infections located in the danger space result from infectious dissections through the alar fascia from the retropharyngeal (retrovisceral) space.

FASCIAE OF THE FACE AND DEEP FACE ══════════════════════════════

The fasciae about the face, deep face, and the remainder of the head are continuation of the fasciae of the neck and in some areas are further specializations of the deep fasciae covering certain regions and structures of the deep face.

Superficial Fascia

The *superficial fascia* (tela subcutanea) of the face and scalp lies immediately deep to the skin and contains the muscles of facial expression, nerves, arteries, and veins. This layer of fascia is closely applied except around the eyelids, about the buccal fat pad, and near the galea aponeurotica of the scalp. Except for a danger space in this fascia about the scalp and the other areas mentioned, the fascia is without spaces.

Deep Fascia

The superficial layer of the deep cervical fascia (investing fascia) extends superiorly over the mandible from its attachment to the hyoid bone anteriorly, and from the vicinity of the sternocleidomastoid laterally, to reach the zygomatic area. In coursing across this region, the fascia covers the muscles forming the floor of the mouth; namely, the mylohyoid and anterior belly of the digastric muscles. As the fascia reaches the mandible, it forms two leaflets to attach to the medial and lateral aspects of this bone. Along its way also the fascia splits and fuses to encapsulate the submandibular gland and to enclose the insertions of the masseter and the medial pterygoid muscles. Laterally, that portion of the fascia covering the masseter muscle also blankets the angle and ramus of the mandible in addition before inserting on the zygomatic arch. The other leaf of this fascia covers the inferior surface of the medial pterygoid muscle then inserts on the medial surface of the lateral pterygoid plate. Further posteriorly that portion of the investing fascia surrounding the insertion of the sternocleidomastoid muscle separates to pass to the zygomatic arch and in so doing forms a capsule (parotid fascia, parotideomasseteric fascia) surrounding the parotid gland.

This splitting of the superficial layer of the deep cervical fascia (investing fascia) as it passes superiorly from its attachment to the hyoid bone forms numerous potential spaces, however, since most are closed they do not communicate. As the fascia encompasses the submandibular gland it becomes the capsule of the gland. This fascia is thicker on the lateral than on the medial aspect, thus dissecting infections in this area usually progress in a medial direction.

Masticator Space (Fig. 22.3)

The *masticator space* is formed as the investing fascia splits at the inferior border of the mandible to cover the medial pterygoid and masseter muscles as they attach to the inferior border of the mandibular ramus. Further superiorly the fascia covers the inferior border of the temporalis muscle blending with its fascial covering. The space is closed posteriorly as the two laminae of the

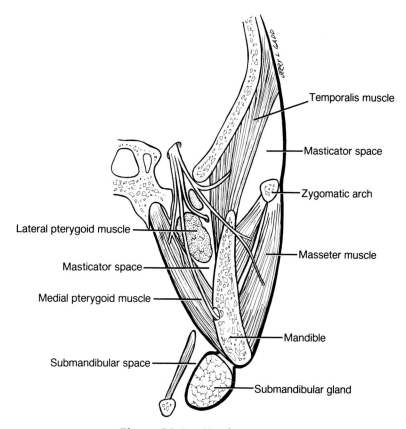

Figure 22.3. Masticator space.

fasciae fuse with each other. Anteriorly, the investing fascia fuses to the mandible in front of the masseter and temporalis muscles then passes medially across the buccal fat pad to attach to the maxilla and to blend with the fascia covering the buccinator muscle. The masticator space contains the lateral pterygoid muscle, the maxillary artery and its branches, the mandibular nerve and its branches, connective tissue, and much of the buccal fat pad.

The space of the parotid gland contains the gland, several lymph nodes, the facial nerve and several of its branches that will exit the space to supply the muscles of facial expression.

Submandibular Space

The *submandibular space* is larger than the space enclosed by the fascia covering the submandibular gland. Indeed, it is bounded superiorly by the tongue and mucous membrane of the floor of the mouth and inferiorly, by the superficial layer of the cervical deep fascia (investing fascia) covering the anterior belly of the digastric muscle, as well as the mylohyoid muscle and its attachment at the hyoid bone. The placement of the mylohyoid muscle divides the submandibular space into the *sublingual space,* superiorly and the *submaxillary space,* inferiorly. These two spaces communicate with each other at the posterior margin of the mylohyoid muscle.

The submandibular space contains the submandibular gland and part of its duct, as well as structures housed in the floor of the oral cavity including the sublingual gland, geniohyoid and genioglossus muscles, the lingual and hypoglossal nerves, the lingual artery and some of its branches.

Although the submandibular space is described as being bilateral, its position in the vicinity of the midline and its relations to the mylohyoid muscle, communication normally occurs between the two sides. Additionally, the submandibular space communicates with the peripharyngeal spaces.

Peripharyngeal Spaces

Surrounding the pharyngeal wall posteriorly and laterally and communicating anteriorly with the submandibular space is a common space that is further subdivided into the *peripharyngeal spaces.* This space, encircling the perimeter of the pharynx, lies deep to all laminae of the superficial cervical deep fascia (investing fascia) and freely communicates with several other spaces. The peripharyngeal spaces, because of their relationships with other fascial spaces and the masticator space, are accessible avenues for the spread of infection by way of perforations through other fascial layers. Infections which may break into the peripharyngeal spaces include those of the teeth, nose, throat, mandible, maxillae, etc.

Retropharyngeal Space

The *retropharyngeal space* was described earlier during the discussion of fascial spaces in the neck. The reader should recall that the retropharyngeal space lies behind the pharynx/esophagus and extends from the base of the skull into the mediastinum. It is bounded posteriorly by the alar fascia, anteriorly by the pharyngeal fascia, and laterally by loose connective tissue separating it rather incompletely from the lateral pharyngeal space. The retropharyngeal space is regarded as the primary route of the spread of infection from lesions in the head and neck into the thorax, since it is accessible to dissecting or perforating infections originating from numerous neighboring fascial spaces.

Lateral Pharyngeal Space

The retropharyngeal space extends laterally around the pharynx with only loose connective tissue intervening between it and the space lateral to it, the *lateral pharyngeal space* (known also by various other names including parapharyngeal, peripharyngeal, pharyngomaxillary, pterygomandibular, pterygopharyngeal, etc.). The lateral pharyngeal space is bounded medially by the pharyngeal fascia and laterally by the pterygoid muscles and the sheath of the parotid gland. Its superior extent is similar to that of the retropharyngeal space, in that it reaches the base of the skull; however, inferiorly it extends only as far as the hyoid bone, being limited by the fascia of the submandibular gland, stylohyoid muscle and posterior belly of the digastric muscle. Coursing through this space are the two other muscles originating from the styloid process; the styloglossus and stylopharyngeus muscles. The lateral pharyngeal space extends to the pterygomandibular raphe and, above the submandibular gland, it communicates with the floor of the oral cavity. Because of its extent and association about the structures of the oral region, it is the most frequently infected secondary area from the primary areas of the masticator space, teeth, tongue, salivary glands, and the tonsillar region. Since infections perforating into this space readily gain access to the retropharyngeal space and thus pass into the mediastinum, the lateral pharyngeal space is of utmost importance to the clinician.

Glossary

Abducent nerve. Sixth cranial nerve.

Abduction. A motion that moves a structure away from the body centerline.

Accessory bone. A bone formed when ossification centers fail to unite during development.

Acoustic nerve. Eighth cranial nerve.

Adam's apple. Laryngeal prominence. A prominent protuberance of the thyroid cartilage in the anterior midline of the neck, especially in adult males.

Adduction. A motion that moves a structure closer to the body centerline.

Adenoids. Hypertrophy of the pharyngeal tonsil due to infection.

Aditus. An opening or inlet.

Afferent. Leading toward a specific area, as toward the central nervous system or a lymph node.

Agonists. Muscles whose contractions produce a desired motion.

Alveolar arch. Bony portions on the maxillae and mandible that surround the teeth.

Alveolus. A small cavity. The socket of a tooth.

Anastomosis. Direct communication between blood vessels and between nerves.

Anatomy. The science of the structure of the body.

Anesthesia. Loss of sensation due to injury, disease, or induction by drugs.

Ankyloglossia. Tongue tied. Lingual frenulum attached too far anteriorly on the tongue impeding speech.

Anomaly. Deviation from the normal.

Ansa cervicalis. Nerve loop derived from C1, C2, and C3 to supply the infrahyoid muscles.

Ansa subclavia. Loop around the subclavian artery connecting the middle and inferior cervical sympathetic ganglia.

Antagonists. Muscles that act in opposition to agonists.

Anterior. Front of the body.

Anterior triangle. Triangular area of the neck bounded by the sternocleidomastoid muscle, the anterior midline of the neck, and the inferior border of the mandible.

Aponeurosis. A flat sheet-like tendinous muscle attachment.

Appendicular skeleton. Bony skeleton composed of the bones comprising the superior and inferior extremities.

Arachnoid. Intermediate layer of the meninges covering the brain and spinal cord.

Arachnoid granulations. Modified elements of the arachnoid which filter cerebrospinal fluid from the subarachnoid space into the lacunae lateralis.

Arrector pili. Involuntary smooth muscles arising in the dermis and inserting into the hair follicle. Contractions produce "goose bumps."

Articular disk. Meniscus. Disk intervening between the mandibular condyle and the temporal bone.

Atlas. First cervical vertebra. Articulates with the occipital bone of the skull.

Auditory tube. Eustachian tube. Opening of the middle ear cavity into the pharynx.

Autonomic nervous system. A functional system controlling cardiac and smooth muscles and glandular activity.

Axial skeleton. Bony skeleton composed of the skull, vertebral column, hyoid bone, ribs, and sternum.

Axis. The second cervical vertebra.

Basal ganglia. Subcortical nuclei associated with somatic motor functions.

Blind spot. Optic disk. The light-insensitive region of the retina where the optic nerve exits the bulb of the eye.

Blood-brain barrier. Pial-glial elements surrounding blood vessels of the central nervous system that control the entry of materials into the intercellular spaces of the CNS.

Bolus. A masticated chunk of food ready for deglutition.

Bony depressions. Intervals between bony elevations. Descriptions include: pits, foveae, and fossae.

Bony elevations. Sites of attachment of structures to bone. Descriptions include: lines, crests, ridges, processes, tubercles, tuberosities, and spines.

Brachial plexus. Plexus of nerves formed by the ventral primary rami of C5, C6, C7, C8, and T1, with contributions from C4 and T2.

Brainstem. The oldest part of the central nervous system mainly responsible for vital functions.

Branchial arches. Pharyngeal arches.

Branchial grooves. Pharyngeal clefts.

Buccal glands. Minor salivary glands located in the mucosa of the buccal vestibule.

Buccopharyngeal fascia. Posterior lamina of the pretracheal fascia.

Bursae. Fluid-filled sacs overlying joints functioning in lubrication.

Canal. A passageway or tunnel in bone.

Cardiac muscle. Heart muscle. A special striated involuntary muscle.

Carotid body. Structure located at the bifurcation of the common carotid artery to monitor oxygen tension in the bloodstream.

Carotid plexus. Postganglionic sympathetic fibers derived from the superior cervical ganglion, traveling on the internal carotid artery.

Carotid sheath. Fascial sheath, derived from the deep cervical fascia, enveloping the major neurovascular bundle of the neck.

Carotid sinus. Structure located in the wall of the carotid artery at its beginning, monitoring blood pressure.

Carotid triangle. One of the subdivisions of the anterior triangle of the neck bounded by the posterior belly of the digastric, superior belly of the omohyoid, and the sternocleidomastoid muscles.

Cartilaginous joint. A bony union or joint with cartilage interposed between the bones.

Caudal. Inferior. Toward the tail.

Cavernous sinus. A large, labyrinthine dural venous sinus located lateral to the sella turcica.

Central nervous system. CNS. Composed of the brain and spinal cord.

Cephalic. Rostral. Toward the rostral end of the organism.

Cerebellum. Portion of the brain derived from the metencephalon. Responsible for balance and spatial orientation.

Cerebral arterial circle. Circle of Willis. Arterial anastomosis around the base of the brain.

Cerebral hemispheres. Largest portion of the brain, derived from the prosencephalon.

Cerebrospinal fluid. A clear, colorless, acellular fluid, produced by the choroid plexus. Circulates in the ventricles of the brain, the central canal of the spinal cord, and the subarachnoid space.

Cervical plexus. Plexus of nerves formed by the ventral primary rami of C1, C2, C3, C4, and (sometimes) C5.

Cervical sympathetic trunk. Cervical continuation of the thoracic sympathetic trunk.

Chain ganglia. Sympathetic ganglia located along the vertebral column.

Choanae. Apertures of the nasal cavities opening into the nasopharynx.

Choroid plexus. Modified pial/ependymal elements located in the ventricles of the brain which function to elaborate cerebrospinal fluid.

Ciliary body. A portion of the middle coat of the eye, including the ciliary muscle and ciliary process.

Circle of Willis. Cerebral arterial circle.

Collateral ganglia. Sympathetic ganglia located away from the vertebral column, usually near the viscera along major blood vessels.

Computed tomography. A radiographic procedure whereby cross-sectional images of the body are visualized.

Conchae. Turbinate bones. Three, mucosa-covered, scroll-like bones on the lateral nasal wall which jut into the nasal fossa.

Condyle. The rounded articular end of a bone.

Cones. Light-sensitive cells of the retina specialized for color vision.

Confluence of sinuses. A region of dural sinuses, located at the internal occipital crest, receiving several major venous sinuses of the dura mater.

Cornea. Anteriorly placed, modified transparent portion of the sclera of the eye.

Coronal plane. Frontal plane. A vertical plane at right angles to the sagittal plane.

Coronal suture. A skull suture located in the frontal plane, from temple to temple.

Cranial. Superior. In the direction of the head, craniad.

Cranial fossa. A deep depression in the internal base of the skull, consisting of three regions, anterior, middle, and posterior.

Cranial outflow. Parasympathetic outflow from the brain in cranial nerves III, VII, IX, X.

Craniosacral outflow. The combined parasympathetic outflow regions of origin for the entire body.

Crenated tongue. Indentations along the lateral margins of the tongue indicating impressions from the teeth.

Cricothyrotomy. A relatively safe emergency procedure for opening the airway by incising the cricothyroid membrane to relieve dyspnea.

Deep. Relative position from the surface of the body from any direction.

Deep cervical lymph nodes. Chain of lymph nodes following the carotid sheath. These ultimately receive all of the lymph from the head and neck.

Deep fascia. Connective tissue sheath surrounding and compartmentalizing many of the structures of the body including the muscles.

Deglutition. The act of swallowing.

Dendrite. One of the cell processes of a neuron which conducts impulses toward the cell body.

Depress. To pull down or lower.

Dermal papillae. Projections of the dermis that interdigitate with epidermal pegs at the epidermis/dermis interface.

Dermis. Deep layer of the skin beneath the epidermis.

Developmental anatomy. The study of the growth and development of an organism from conception to birth.

Diaphragma sella. An incomplete covering composed of meningeal dura that acts as a membraneous lid over the sella turcica.

Diencephalon. Rostralmost portion of the brainstem.

Diploic veins. Veins traveling in and draining the diploë of the skull.

Distal. 1. Away from the origin. 2. Term used in describing relative positions of the teeth. Away from the midline anteriorly.

Dorsal. Equal to *posterior* but usually reserved for quadrupeds.

Dorsal horn. Gray matter of spinal cord containing cell bodies receiving sensory axons from the dorsal root.

Dorsal root. Sensory root carrying axons from dorsal root ganglion to the spinal cord.

Dorsal root ganglion. Sensory ganglion located on the dorsal root of each spinal nerve.

Duct of Bartholin. Large sublingual duct of the sublingual gland opening very near or with the submandibular duct at the sublingual caruncula.

Ducts of Rivinus. Small sublingual ducts of the sublingual gland opening along the surface of the plica sublingualis below the tongue.

Dura mater. The outer layer of the meninges covering the brain and spinal cord.

Efferent. Leading away from a specific area, as away from the central nervous system or a lymph node.

Elastic cartilage. Type of cartilage located in external ear, auditory tube, epiglottis, and parts of the larynx.

Elevate. To lift up.

Emissary veins. Veins originating on the scalp then emptying into the dural venous sinuses through like-named foramina in the skull.

Endochondral bone formation. Type of bone development upon a cartilaginous template.

Epidermal pegs. Projections of the epidermis that interdigitate with the dermal papillae at the epidermis/dermis interface.

Epidermis. Surface layer of the skin.

Epiglottis. An unpaired, leaf-shaped piece of elastic cartilage of the larynx projecting above and anterior to the superior laryngeal aperture.

Eustachian tube. Auditory tube.

Extension. A motion that increases the joint angle.

External. Away from the center of the body.

External acoustic meatus. Opening in the temporal bone leading into the middle ear.

Extrinsic muscles of the eye. Muscles attached to and responsible for movement of the eyeball.

Facial nerve. Seventh cranial nerve.

Falx cerebelli. Meningeal reflection of the dura mater, on the caudal surface of the tentorium cerebelli, intervening between the two cerebellar hemispheres.

Falx cerebri. Sickle-shaped meningeal reflection of the dura mater intervening between the right and left cerebral hemispheres.

Fascia. Collagenous connective tissue which encloses structures and separates them into various groups.

Fibrocartilage. Type of cartilage in intervertebral discs, pubic symphysis, and mandibular symphysis, as well as on certain regions of the temporomandibular joint.

Fibrous joint. A bony joint connected by fibrous connective tissue.

Fissured tongue. Excessive fissures in the dorsum of the tongue.

Fixators. Muscles that act to stabilize a structure.

Flexion. A motion that reduces the joint angle.

Foramen. An opening or hole in bone.

Foramen cecum. Shallow pit-like depression on tongue, just posterior to the sulcus terminalis, indicating the opening of the embryological thyroglossal duct.

Fordyce's granules. Ectopic sebaceous glands incorporated into the vestibular mucosa during development.

Frontal plane. Coronal plane. A vertical plane at right angles to the sagittal plane.

Ganglion. An accumulation of neuron cell bodies outside the central nervous system.

General somatic afferent. Sensation traveling to the central nervous system from the body.

General somatic efferent. Motor innervation from the central nervous system to the skeletal muscles.

General visceral afferent. Sensation traveling to the central nervous system from the viscera.

General visceral efferent. Motor innervation from the central nervous system to the smooth muscles of the viscera.

Gingiva. The gums. Specialized mucosa overlying the alveolar bone of each dental arch.

Glands of Blandin–Nuhn. Minor salivary glands located on either side of the lingual frenulum.

Glands of von Ebner. Minor serous salivary glands which empty into the vallate papillae.

Glaucoma. Condition of increased pressure in the anterior chamber of the eye.

Glossopharyngeal nerve. Ninth cranial nerve.

Gray matter. Region of the central nervous system consisting mainly of cell bodies.

Gray rami communicantes. Unmyelinated fibers (postganglionic) entering spinal nerve from a sympathetic ganglion.

Groove. A linear depression on a bone housing a structure.

Gross anatomy. Macroscopic anatomy. Study of the body with the unaided eye.

Gyrus. Convoluted elevation of the cerebral hemispheres, bounded by sulci.

Histology. The study of tissues. Used interchangeably with "microscopic anatomy."

Horizontal plane. Transverse plane. Plane passing through body at right angles to sagittal and frontal planes.

Hyaline cartilage. Type of cartilage found on articular surfaces of bones. Forms a template for endochondral bone formation.

Hyoid arch. Second pharyngeal arch giving rise to the muscles of facial expression in addition to some other structures.

Hypoglossal nerve. Twelfth cranial nerve.

Hypophysis. Pituitary gland.

Inferior. Tailward or caudal.

Inferior cervical ganglion. Inferiormost ganglion of the cervical sympathetic trunk. Located at the level of the seventh cervical vertebra.

Infrahyoid muscles. Strap muscles. Several muscles attached to the inferior aspect of the hyoid bone.

Infratemporal fossa. A region inferior to the zygomatic arch and deep to the mandible.

Insertion. Site on the bone or in skin where the muscle inserts.

Internal. Closer to the center of the body.

Intramembranous bone formation. Type of bone development within mesenchyme and without a cartilaginous model.

Intrinsic muscles of the eye. Smooth muscles located within the eyeball responsible for accommodation and pupil size.

Intrinsic muscles of the tongue. Four muscles, wholly within the tongue, responsible for altering its shape.

Investing fascia. Superficial layer of the deep cervical fascia.

Involuntary muscle. Smooth or non-striated muscle and striated cardiac muscle. Contraction occurs without conscious control.

Iris. Colored, anteriorly placed portion of the intermediate tunic of the eye.

Isthmus faucium. Oropharyngeal isthmus.

Jugulodigastric lymph node. A large lymph node of the deep cervical chain located between the posterior belly of the digastric muscle and the internal jugular vein.

Jugulo-omohyoid lymph node. A large node of the deep cervical chain located near the intermediate tendon of the omohyoid muscle.

Kiesselbach's area. Anteroinferior region of the nasal septum, a common site of nosebleed.

Labial commissure. Lateral connection of the upper and lower lip.

Labial frenula. Folds of tissue attaching the lips to the gingiva.

Labial glands. Minor salivary glands located in the mucosa of the labial vestibule.

Lacrimal puncta. Orifice of the lacrimal canaliculus located on each eyelid in the vicinity of the medial commissure.

Lacuna lateralis. Meninx-lined depressions on either side of the superior sagittal sinus. These house the arachnoid granulations.

Lambdoidal suture. A suture of the skull separating the occipital bone from the parietal bones.

Lamina. A flat membranous or osseous plate.

Langer's lines. Cleavage lines in skin utilized in surgery.

Laryngeal pharynx. Most inferior region of the pharynx surrounding the larynx.

Lateral. Away from the midline of the body.

Lingual frenulum. Tissue fold attaching ventral surface of tongue to the floor of the oral cavity.

Lingual tonsils. Tonsillar tissue located on the base of the tongue.

Lymphatic ring of Waldeyer. Clumps of lymphatic tissue surrounding the oropharynx.

Lymph nodes. Filtering bodies located along the lymphatic vessels. Lymphocytes are also propagated here.

Macroglossia. Large tongue.

Macroscopic anatomy. Study of the human body with the unaided eye.

Mandibular arch. First pharyngeal arch to form which gives rise to the maxilla and mandible among other structures.

Mandibular fossa. Glenoid fossa. A concavity in the temporal bone that is the area of articulation with the mandible.

Mandibular torus. Bony exostosis on the lingual aspect of the mandible protruding into the floor of the oral cavity proper.

Masticator compartment. A fascia-enclosed space on the lateral aspect of the face containing the muscles of mastication.

Maxillary process. Superiormost developing segment of the mandibular arch in pharyngeal arch formation.

Meatus. A passageway or tunnel in bone.

Meatuses. Tunnels deep to the turbinate bones of the nasal cavity.

Meckel's cartilage. A cartilage developed in the mandibular arch which later nearly disappears.

Medial. Toward the midline of the body.

Median lingual sulcus. A shallow groove on the dorsum of the tongue.

Median plane. Plane passing through body from anterior to posterior through the midline. Midsagittal plane.

Median rhomboid glossitis. An area devoid of papillae on the dorsum of the tongue.

Medulla. Medulla oblongata. The caudalmost portion of the brainstem. It contains the fourth ventricle.

Meninx. Meninges (plural). Membranes covering the central nervous system: the dura mater, arachnoid, and pia mater.

Meniscus. Articular disk. Disk intervening between the mandibular condyle and the temporal bone.

Mental symphysis. Mandibular symphysis. Area of fusion of the right and left halves of the mandible.

Mesencephalon. Midbrain. A short segment of the brainstem located between the diencephalon and the pons. It contains the third ventricle.

Mesial. Term used to describe relative positions of teeth nearest the midline, anteriorly.

Metencephalon. Part of the brainstem between the mesencephalon and myelencephalon surrounding the cerebral aqueduct.

Metopic suture. An inconstant suture, which may persist, between the developing halves of the frontal bone.

Microglossia. Small tongue.

Microscopic anatomy. Specialized study of cells, tissues, and organs of the body utilizing a microscope.

Middle cervical ganglion. A small, inconstant cervical sympathetic ganglion located at the level of the sixth cervical vertebra.

Midsagittal plane. Median plane passing through the body from anterior to posterior through the midline.

Minor salivary glands. Small salivary glands located in the oral, palatal, and lingual mucosae.

Motor end-plate. An axon terminal which participates in the formation of a myoneural junction.

Mucogingival junction. A sharp, scalloped line separating the gingival mucosa from alveolar mucosa.

Muscle fascicle. A bundle of muscle fibers surrounded by perimysium.

Muscles of facial expression. Muscle mass developed in second branchial arch. These muscles arise in hypodermis or on bone and insert into the dermis of the face, scalp, and neck.

Muscles of mastication. Four muscles responsible for masticatory motions: the masseter, temporalis, external pterygoid, and internal pterygoid.

Muscular triangle. One of the subdivisions of the anterior triangle of the neck bounded by the sternocleidomastoid and superior belly of the omohyoid muscles and the midline of the neck.

Nasal septum. Vertical midline structure of the nasal cavity comprised of the perpendicular plate of the ethmoid and vomer bones along with cartilage.

Nasopharyngeal tonsil. Tonsillar tissue located behind the lip of the auditory tube on the posterior pharyngeal wall.

Nasopharynx. Most superior region of the pharynx ending inferiorly at the soft palate.

Neuroanatomy. The specialized study of the structure and function of the nervous system.

Neuron. Specialized cell of the nervous system able to perceive stimuli and conduct them along its processes.

Neurovascular bundles. Nerves and vessels traveling together enwrapped in connective tissue.

Nodose ganglion. Inferior ganglion of the vagus nerve.

Notch. A greatly depressed region on a bone functioning as a passageway.

Nucleus. An accumulation of neuron cell bodies located within the central nervous system.

Occipital triangle. One of the subdivisions of the posterior triangle of the neck bounded by the inferior belly of the omohyoid, the sternocleidomastoid, and trapezius muscles.

Oculomotor nerve. Third cranial nerve.

Olfactory bulb. An extension of the olfactory tract located on the cribriform plate of the ethmoid bone. It receives olfactory filaments.

Olfactory nerve. First cranial nerve.

Optic chiasma. Region of decussation of the two optic nerves resting on the chiasmatic groove of the sphenoid bone.

Optic nerve. Second cranial nerve.

Oral cavity proper. Area internal to the dental arches.

Origin. Site on a bone from which muscle arises.

Oropharyngeal isthmus. Posterior boundary of the oral cavity. Muscular aperture guarding pharynx.

Oropharynx. Middle portion of the pharynx extending from the soft palate to the larynx.

Ossicles of the ear. Three small bones of the middle ear: the malleus, incus, and stapes.

Otis media. Infection of the middle ear cavity.

Palatine torus. Bony exostosis of the palate protruding into the oral cavity.

Palpebral fissure. Space between upper and lower eyelids.

Panniculus adiposus. Areas of the body containing large deposits of fat in the superficial fascia.

Paranasal sinuses. Four mucosa-lined cavities in the bones of the face. They communicate with the nasal fossae.

Parasympathetic nervous system. Division of the autonomic nervous system originating in the brain and sacral spinal cord. System returns the body to homeostatic state.

Parotid fascia. Cranial continuation of the investing fascia which encloses the parotid gland.

Parotid papilla. Opening of the parotid duct (Stenson's duct) in the buccal vestibule opposite the second maxillary molar.

Passavant's bar. A ridge of tissue on the posterior wall of the pharynx representing the contact zone between pharynx and palate when the pharynx is sealed off.

Peripheral nervous system. The portion of the nervous system located outside the skull and vertebral canal including the 12 pairs of cranial nerves and the 31 pairs of spinal nerves.

Pharyngeal arches. Branchial arches. Bulging bars of mesoderm observed in the head/neck of the developing embryo. Each gives rise to certain structures.

Pharyngeal clefts. Branchial grooves. Grooves on the surface of the developing head/neck region of an embryo between the pharyngeal arches.

Pharyngeal plexus. A plexus of nerves, derived from cranial nerves IX, X, and XI, responsible for innervation of much of the pharynx.

Pharyngeal pouches. Branchial pouches. Outpocketings of the pharynx during development.

Pia mater. Innermost delicate layer of the meninges covering the brain and spinal cord.

Posterior. Back of the body.

Posterior triangle. Triangular area of the neck bounded by the sternocleidomastoid and trapezius muscles and the middle one-third of the clavicle.

Postganglionic. Visceral motor neurons whose cell bodies are located in one of the autonomic ganglia.

Preganglionic. Visceral motor neurons of the autonomic system that have not yet synapsed in one of the autonomic ganglia.

Pretrachial fascia. Deep layer of the deep cervical fascia surrounding the viscera of the neck.

Prevertebral fascia. Deep layer of the deep cervical fascia enveloping the vertebrae and the deep cervical muscles of the neck.

Principal lymph node of the tongue. A large lymph node of the deep cervical chain responsible for draining the tip of the tongue and the region of the lingual frenulum.

Protrusion. A motion that juts away from its normal resting place, such as the motion possible with the mandible.

Proximal. Closer to the origin.

Pterygopalatine fossa. Small pyramid-shaped space enclosed by the maxilla, sphenoid, and palatine bones.

Pupil. Circular orifice in the middle of the iris through which light enters the eye.

Rathke's pouch. A diverticulum of oral ectoderm in the roof of the developing oral cavity destined to give rise to a portion of the pituitary gland.

Reflex arc. The simplest form of functional neurological pathway bypassing many connecting neurons.

Regional anatomy. Study approach in which individual anatomical regions of the body are considered as units.

Reichert's cartilage. A cartilage developed in the second pharyngeal arch which later becomes obscured.

Retraction. A motion that causes a structure to be drawn back, such as the motion possible with the mandible.

Right lymphatic duct. Major vessel of the lymphatic system delivering lymph to the right subclavian vein.

Rods. Light-sensitive cells of the retina concerned with vision in dim light.

Rostral. Cephalad. Toward the cephalic end of the organism.

Rotation. To move about an axis.

Rotatory motion. One of the motions possible at the temporomandibular joint, involving the mandibular condyle and articular disk.

Sacral outflow. Parasympathetic outflow to the viscera of the pelvic region from the sacral spinal cord.

Sagittal suture. A suture of the skull, located in the midline, which separates the parietal bones.

Sclera. White of the eye.

Sesamoid bones. Bones developed in tendons providing extra leverage or reducing friction at the joint.

Sialography. Radiologic examination of salivary glands and their ducts subsequent to introduction of a radioopaque dye.

Sinusitis. Inflammation of the mucosa of the paranasal sinuses.

Special somatic afferent. Sensation traveling to the brain from the special senses of vision and hearing.

Special visceral afferent. Sensation traveling to the brain via cranial nerves from the special visceral senses of taste and smell.

Special visceral efferent. Motor innervation from the brain via cranial nerves to the muscles of branchiomeric origin.

Spinal accessory nerve. Eleventh cranial nerve.

Stellate ganglion. Fused inferior cervical and first thoracic sympathetic ganglia.

Stenson's duct. Parotid duct.

Striated muscle. Skeletal muscle. Voluntary muscle.

Subarachnoid space. Space between the arachnoid and pia mater containing the cerebrospinal fluid.

Subclavian triangle. One of the subdivisions of the posterior triangle bounded by the inferior belly of the omohyoid muscle, the sternocleidomastoid muscle, and middle one-third of the clavicle.

Subcutaneous connective tissue. Hypodermis. Loose connective tissue deep to the dermis. Superficial fascia.

Subdural space. Potential space between the dura mater and the arachnoid layers of the meninges.

Sublingual caruncula. Opening of the submandibular duct at the base of the lingual frenulum.

Submandibular triangle. One of the subdivisions of the anterior triangle of the neck bounded by both bellies of the digastric muscle and the inferior border of the mandible.

Submental triangle. The only unpaired subdivision of the neck. It is bounded by the anterior bellies of the digastric muscles and the hyoid bone.

Suboccipital triangle. A triangular area in the back of the neck circumscribed by three muscles: rectus capitis posterior major, obliquus capitis superior and inferior.

Sulcus. 1. A depression on the bone housing a structure. 2. A depression or groove located between gyri on the surface of the cerebral hemispheres.

Sulcus terminalis. A posteriorly directed V-shaped groove separating the anterior two-thirds and posterior one-third of the tongue.

Superficial. Relative position near surface of the body from any respect.

Superficial cervical lymph nodes. Chain of lymph nodes aligned along the external jugular vein.

Superficial fascia. Subcutaneous connective tissue deep to the dermis.

Superior. Toward the head or cranial.

Superior cervical ganglion. The superiormost ganglion of the cervical sympathetic trunk, located at the level of the second and third cervical vertebrae.

Superior laryngeal aperture. The superior inlet of the larynx.

Suture. Type of fibrous joint found in bones of the skull.

Sympathetic nervous system. Division of the autonomic nervous system originating in thoracic and first few lumbar spinal cord segments. System prepares for "fight or flight."

Sympathetic trunk. The sympathetic chain ganglia and their connections.

Symphysis. A cartilaginous bony joint between two continuous bones.

Synapse. A place where one nerve cell communicates with another cell.

Synchondrosis. Temporary cartilaginous joint that will be ossified later.

Syndesmosis. Bony joint with fibrous connective tissue union permitting little movement.

Synovial fluid. Fluid produced within the synovial sheath to bathe the muscle tendon joint and bursa, thus reducing friction.

Synovial joint. A bony joint surrounded by synovial cavities.

Synovial sheath. A sac-like covering over a muscle tendon or joint producing synovial fluid to bathe the tendon and joint, thus reducing friction.

Systemic anatomy. Study approach in which each system of the body is considered separately.

Temporal fossa. A depression on the lateral aspect of the skull containing the temporalis muscle and its fascia, vessels, and nerves.

Tentorium cerebelli. Meningeal reflection of the dura mater intervening between the cerebellum and the occipital lobe of the cerebrum.

Terminal ganglia. Parasympathetic ganglia usually located very near the viscera or glands to be innervated.

Thalamus. Largest portion of the diencephalon. Functions to relay sensory impulses to the cerebral cortex.

Thoracic duct. Major vessel of the lymphatic system delivering lymph to the left subclavian vein.

Thoracolumbar outflow. Region of spinal cord from which sympathetic system originates.

Thyroglossal duct. Remnants of the embryological origins and migratory path of the tissue destined to be the thyroid.

Tracheotomy. A surgical procedure whereby an incision is made in the anterior aspect of the trachea to provide an airway passage to relieve dyspnea.

Translatory motion. One of the motions possible at the temporomandibular joint, involving the temporal bone and the articular disk (a sliding motion).

Transverse plane. Horizontal plane at right angles to sagittal and frontal planes.

Trigeminal nerve. Fifth cranial nerve.

Trochlear nerve. Fourth cranial nerve.

Turbinate bones. Conchae. Three mucosa-covered, scroll-like bones on the lateral nasal wall jutting into the nasal fossa.

Tympanic plexus. Plexus of nerves derived from cranial nerve IX and the sympathetic plexus. It serves the mucous membranes of the middle ear.

Tympanum. Middle ear cavity; also eardrum.

Vagus nerve. Tenth cranial nerve.

Vallate papillae. Circumvallate papillae. A row of large mushroom-shaped papillae anterior to the sulcus terminalis on the tongue.

Venous pterygoid plexus. A venous plexus receiving tributaries from many areas of the head. It is located between the temporalis and the pterygoid muscles.

Venous sinus. Large venous channel not possessing the normal histologic complement of veins.

Ventral. Equal to *anterior* but usually reserved for quadrupeds.

Ventral horn. Gray matter of the spinal cord containing motor neurons.

Ventral root. Motor axons exiting the ventral root of the spinal cord.

Vermilion zone. Red area of the lips.

Vestibule. Cleft or space between lips and cheeks and the teeth and gingiva.

Vidian nerve. Nerve of the pterygoid (Vidian) canal. It is composed of the greater petrosal nerve (of cranial nerve VII) accompanied by the deep petrosal nerve (of the carotid plexus) as they pass through the pterygoid canal.

Vocal cord. A fold of mucous membrane on the lateral wall of the larynx responsible for the formation of sound.

Voluntary muscle. Striated or skeletal muscle. Contraction occurs by conscious control.

Wharton's duct. Duct of the submandibular gland.

White matter. Region of the central nervous system consisting mainly of fiber tracts.

White rami communicantes. Myelinated fibers (preganglionic) connecting spinal nerves with a sympathetic ganglion.

Wormian bones. Additional bones which may be found in suture lines of the skull.

Zygomatic arch. Malar arch. The arch formed by the temporal process of the zygoma and the zygomatic process of the temporal bone.

Suggested Readings

Gross Anatomy Textbooks

Anson BJ (ed): *Morris' Human Anatomy,* 12th ed. New York: McGraw-Hill, 1966.

Basmajian JV: *Grant's Method of Human Anatomy,* 10th ed. Baltimore: Williams & Wilkins, 1980.

Crafts RC: *A Textbook of Human Anatomy,* 3rd ed. New York: Wiley, 1985.

DiDio LJ: *Synopsis of Anatomy.* St. Louis: C.V. Mosby Co., 1970.

Gardner, E, Gray DJ, O'Rahilly R: *Anatomy. A Regional Study of Human Structure,* 5th ed. Philadelphia: Saunders Co., 1986.

Clemente CD (ed): *Gray's Anatomy,* 30th ed. Philadelphia: Lea & Febiger, 1985.

Hamilton WJ (ed): *Textbook of Human Anatomy,* 2nd ed. St. Louis: C.V. Mosby Co., 1976.

Hollinshead WH, Rosse C: *Textbook of Anatomy,* 4th ed. Hagerstown: Harper & Row, 1985.

Lachman E: *Case Studies in Anatomy,* 2nd ed. New York: Oxford University Press, 1971.

Leeson RC, Leeson, TS: *Human Structure. A Companion to Anatomical Studies.* Philadelphia: Saunders Co., 1972.

Moore KL: *Clinically Oriented Anatomy,* 2nd ed. Baltimore: Williams & Wilkins, 1985.

Scheider L: *Anatomical Case Histories.* Chicago: Year Book Medical Publishers, 1976.

Snell RS: *Clinical Anatomy for Medical Students,* 3rd ed. Boston: Little, Brown & Co., 1986.

Warwick R, Williams PL (eds): *Gray's Anatomy,* 36th British ed. Philadelphia: Saunders Co., 1980.

Woodburne RT: *Essentials of Human Anatomy,* 7th ed. London: Oxford University Press, 1983.

Developmental Anatomy Textbooks

Arey LB: *Developmental Anatomy,* 7th ed. Philadelphia: Saunders Co., 1965.

Corliss LE: *Patten's Human Embryology.* New York: McGraw-Hill, 1976.

Hamilton WJ, Mossman HW: *Hamilton, Boyd and Mossman's Human Embryology,* 4th ed. Baltimore: Williams and Wilkins, 1972.

Kraus BS, Kitamusa H, Latham RA: *Atlas of Developmental Anatomy of the Face.* New York: Harper & Row, 1966.

Sadler TW: *Langman's Medical Embryology,* 5th ed. Baltimore: Williams & Wilkins, 1985.

Moore KL: *The Developing Human: Clinically Oriented Embryology,* 3rd ed. Philadelphia: Saunders Co., 1982.

Patten BM: *Human Embryology,* 3rd ed. New York: McGraw-Hill, 1968.

Snell RS: *Clinical Embryology for Medical Students,* 3rd ed. Boston: Little, Brown & Co., 1984.

Torrey TW: *Morphogenesis of the Vertebrates.* New York: Wiley, 1962.

Tuchmann-Duplessis H, David G, Haegel P: *Illustrated Human Embryology*, 3 vols. New York: Springer Verlag, 1972.

Neuroanatomy Textbooks

Afifi AK, Bergman RA: *Basic Neuroscience*, 2nd ed. Baltimore: Urban and Schwarzenberg, 1985.

Barr ML, Kiernan JA: *The Human Nervous System. An Anatomic Viewpoint*, 4th ed. Hagerstown: Harper & Row, 1983.

Carpenter MB: *Core Text of Neuroanatomy*. 3rd ed. Baltimore: William & Wilkins, 1985.

Carpenter MB, Sutin J: *Human Neuroanatomy*. 8th ed. Baltimore: William & Wilkins, 1983.

Clark RG (ed): *Manter and Gatz's Clinical Neuroanatomy and Neurophysiology*, 5th ed. Philadelphia: Davis, 1975.

Dunkerley GB: *A Basic Atlas of the Human Nervous System*. Philadelphia: Davis, 1975.

Noback CR: *The Human Nervous System*, 2nd ed. New York: McGraw-Hill, 1975.

Noback CR, Demarest RJ: *The Nervous System: Introduction and Review*. New York: McGraw-Hill, 1972.

Werner JK: *Neuroscience: A Clinical Perspective*. Philadelphia: Saunders, 1980.

Willis WJ, Grossman, RG: *Medical Neurobiology*. 2nd ed. St. Louis: C.V. Mosby Co., 1977.

Head and Neck Anatomy Textbooks

Berkowitz BK, Holland GR, Moxham BJ: *A Colour Atlas and Textbook of Oral Anatomy*. London: Wolfe Medical Publications, Ltd., 1978.

Brand RW, Iselhard DE: *Anatomy of Orofacial Structures*. 2nd ed. St. Louis: C.V. Mosby Co., 1982.

DuBrull EL: *Sicher's Oral Anatomy*, 7th ed. St. Louis: C.V. Mosby Co., 1980.

Fried LA: *Anatomy of the Head, Neck, Face and Jaws*, 2nd ed. Philadelphia: Lea & Febiger, 1980.

Hollingshead WH: *Anatomy for Surgeons: Volume I The Head and Neck*, 3rd ed. Hagerstown: Harper & Row, 1982.

Paff GH: *Anatomy of the Head and Neck*. Philadelphia: Saunders, 1973.

Sarnat GG, Laskin DM (eds): *The Temporomandibular Joint*. Springfield, IL: Thomas, 1979.

Zarb GA, Carlsson GE (eds): *Temporomandibular Joint Function and Dysfunction*. St. Louis: C.V. Mosby Co., 1979.

Atlases

Anderson JE: *Grant's Atlas of Anatomy*, 8th ed. Baltimore: Williams & Wilkins, 1983.

Carter G, Moorehead J, Wolpert S, et al: *Cross Sectional Anatomy: Computed Tomography and Ultra-sound Correlation*. New York: Appleton, 1977.

Clemente CD: *Anatomy. A Regional Atlas of the Human Body*. 2nd ed. Baltimore: Urban and Schwarzenberg, 1981.

Langman J, Woerdeman MW: *Atlas of Medical Anatomy*. Philadelphia: Saunders, 1978.

Lopez-Antunez L: *Atlas of Human Anatomy*. Philadelphia: Saunders, 1971.

McMinn RH, Hutchings RT: *Color Atlas of Human Anatomy*. Chicago: Year Book Medical Publishers, 1977.

Netter FH: *The CIBA Collection of Medical Illustrations. Vol. III. Digestive System Part I*. Summit, NJ: CIBA, 1959.

Snell RS: *Atlas of Clinical Anatomy*. Boston: Little, Brown & Co., 1978.

Wolf-Heidegger G: *Atlas of Systematic Human Anatomy*. New York: Hafner Publishing Co., 1962.

Index

Page numbers in italics denote figures.

Abducent nerve, 174,
    184, 294, 317
Abduction, 14, 317
Accessory nerve, 283,
    303, *304*
Accessory sinus, 229
Acoustic nerve, 174, 188,
    283, 298, 317
    destruction of, 189
Adam's apple. *See* Larynx
Adduction, 14, 317
Adenoids, 263, 317
Aditus, defined, 317
Afferent
    defined, 317
    somatic, 27, 279, 280,
        327
    visceral, 27, 279, 280,
        328
Agonists, 15, 317
Air cells, posterior
    ethmoid, 76
Ala (wing), 31
Alcamaeon, 1
Alveolar artery
    inferior
        incisive branch, 212
        mental branch, 212
    superior
        anterior, 225
        posterior, 212, 225
Alveolar mucosa, 36
Alveolar nerve
    inferior, 215
        incisive branches,
            215
    superior
        anterior, 291
        middle, 291
        posterior, 215, 226,
            291
Alveolar processes, 44

Alveolus, 44, 317
Anastomosis, defined,
    317
Anatomical variation,
    7–8
Anatomy, 5, 317
    concepts of, 5–8
    developmental, 5
    founder of, 1
    gross, 5
    histology, 5
    macroscopic, 5, 324
    microscopic, 5, 324
    neuro-, 5
    regional, 327
    systemic, 329
Anesthesia, 317
    anatomical basis for
        local, 307–310
    plexus, 307–308
        mandibular, 308
        maxillary, 308
    of posterior superior
        alveolar nerve,
            308–309
    trunk, 308
        mandibular trunk,
            309–310
        maxillary, 308
Ankyloglossia, 53, 69,
    317
Anomaly, defined, 317
Ansa cervicalis, 135, 317
Ansa subclavia, 148, 317
Antagonists, 15, 317
Anterior, defined, 5, 317
Aorta, 22
Aperture
    laryngeal, superior, 328
    nasal
        anterior, 75
        posterior, 75

Aponeurosis, 14, 318
Aqueous humor, 179
Arachnoid, 28, 266, 318
    granulations, 266, 275,
        318
Arch(es)
    alveolar, 97, 317
    dental, 76
    mandibular, 59–61,
        324
    pharyngeal, 58, 59, 62,
        326
    superciliary, 74
    vertebral, posterior,
        110
    zygomatic, 94–96, 330
Arch defects, 68
Archicerebellum, 271
Areolar tissue, loose, 10
Aristotle, 1
Arrector pili, 12, 318
Arterioles, 22
Artery(ies)
    alveolar
        anterior superior,
            225, 327
        inferior, 212, 325
        posterior superior,
            212, 225, 326
    angular, 163, 323
    ascending palatine,
        144, 254, 322
    ascending pharyngeal,
        143, 195, 249, 254,
        320
    auricular, 144, 196,
        323, 324
        anterior, 325
        deep, 196, 325
        posterior, 144, 155,
            192, 193, 196, 324
    basilar, 276

363

Artery(ies) (*continued*)
brachiocephalic trunk, 319
buccal, 163, 212, 326
caroticotympanic, 328
carotid
common, 141, 195, 319
external, 141, 192, 193, 195, 254, 320
internal, 141, 195, 327
cerebellar
anterior inferior, 276
posterior inferior, 276
superior, 276
cerebral
anterior, 276
middle, 276
posterior, 276
cervical
ascending, 139, 331
deep, 139, 332
transverse, 138, 139, 331
choroidal, anterior, 276
ciliary, 329
Circle of Willis, 276
communicating
anterior, 276
posterior, 276
costocervical trunk, 139, 331
cricothyroid, 143, 320
deep temporal, 212
anterior, 212
posterior, 212
dorsal lingual, 242, 331
dorsal nasal, 164
dorsal scapular, 139, 332
ethmoidal
anterior, 232, 329
posterior, 232, 329
facial, 143, 162, 243, 322
transverse, 163, 324
frontal, 325
inferior tympanic, 143
infrahyoid, 143, 320
infraorbital, 163, 225, 326

intercostal, superior, 139, 332
internal thoracic, 138, 331
labial
inferior, 162, 322
superior, 162, 322
labyrinthine, 276
lacrimal, 328
laryngeal, superior, 143, 320
lateral nasal, 163, 323
lingual, 143, 212, 239, 242, 321
deep, 239, 242, 321
dorsal, 242, 321
masseteric, 212, 326
maxillary, 144, 163, 192, 196, 211, 225, 232, 325
mandibular portion, 212, 325, 326
pterygoid portion, 212, 326
pterygopalatine portion, 212, 225, 326, 327
meningeal
accessory, 170, 212, 326
anterior, 170, 328
middle, 170, 212, 326
of occipital, 144, 323
posterior, 170
mental, 163, 212
musculophrenic, 331
mylohyoid, 212
nasal
dorsal, 329
lateral, 232
nasopalatine, 227, 249, 327
occipital, 144, 155, 195, 196, 323, 324
ophthalmic, 164, 185, 276, 328
palatine, 321
greater, 225, 249, 327
lesser, 225, 249, 327
palpebral, 328, 329
pharyngeal, 143, 225, 321, 327
pontine, 276
pterygoid, 212, 326

retinal, central, 329
septal, 232
sphenopalatine, 226, 327
sternocleidomastoid, 143, 144, 320, 323
stylomastoid, 196, 324
subclavian, 137, 330
sublingual, 242, 321
submental, 144, 243, 322
superficial, temporal, 144, 155, 163, 193, 196
superior epigastric, 331
suprahyoid, 242, 321
supraorbital, 155, 164, 328
suprascapular, 138, 331
supratrochlear, 155, 164, 329
temporal, deep, 212, 326
anterior, 212
middle, 324
posterior, 212
temporal, superficial, 163, 192, 193, 324
thoracic, internal, 138, 331
thyrocervical trunk, 138, 331
thyroid
inferior, 139, 146, 255, 261, 331
superior, 143, 146, 254, 261, 320
thyroidea ima, 146
tonsillar, 144, 254, 322
transverse cervical, 138, 139, 331
transverse facial, 193, 197, 324
tympanic anterior, 325
vertebral, 137, 276, 330
zygomaticofacial, 164
zygomaticoorbital, 324
Articular coverings, 218
Aryepiglottic fold, 253
Arytenoid, transverse, 260
Atlas, 110, *111*, 318
anterior arch, 110
lateral masses, 112
posterior arch, 112

Atresia, congenital, 233
Atrium, left, 22
Auditory tube, 50, 318
  ostium of, 250
Auricular artery, 144,
    196, 323, 324
  deep, 196, 325
  posterior, 144, 155,
    192, 196, 324
Auricular nerve
  great, 117, 195
  posterior, 197
Auricular vein, posterior,
    114, 164, 333, 334
Auriculotemporal nerve,
    161, 193, 294
  articular branches, 294
  external acoustic
    meatus, branches
    to, 294
  parotid gland, branches
    to, 294
Autonomic nervous
    system, 28–30, 318
  parasympathetic, 30
  sympathetic, 29–30
Avicenna, 2
Axis, *111*, 112, 318
  cylinder, 25
  dens of, facet for, 110
Axon, 25
Axon, hillock, 25

Bartholin, duct of, 38, 240
  Basilar artery, 276
Basophils, 22
Bell's Palsy, 165, 199
Bifid nose, 234
Bifid tongue, 69
Blind spot, 180, 318
Block(s)
  buccal nerve, 310
  greater palatine, 309
  inferior alveolar and
    lingual, 309–310
  mental nerve, 310
  nasopalatine, 309
Blood–brain barrier, 266,318
Blood platelets, 22
Body systems, 9–30
Bolus, defined, 318
Bone(s)
  accessory, 17, 317
  cancellous, 20
  classification of, 17–18

compact, 20
development, 19–20
ethmoid, 73
  cribriform plate of,
    101
  crista galli of, 101
  perpendicular plate
    of, 76
flat, 17
formation
  endochondral, 19, 20,
    321
  intramembraneous,
    19, 323
frontal, 73, 74
hyoid, 109, *110*
  body (corpus), 109
  cornua (horns), 109
of inferior extremity,
    17
irregular, 17
lacrimal, 73
long, 17
marrow, 16
  red, 20
nasal, 73, 75
occipital, 73
  basilar portion of, 98
  jugular notch of, 99
palatine, 73
  horizontal plates of,
    75
  pyramidal process of,
    98
parietal, 73
sesamoid, 17, 327
sphenoid, 73
  ethmoidal spine, 101
  lateral pterygoid
    plates of, 98
  medial pterygoid
    plates of, 98
  spine of, 99
structure, *21*
of superior extremity,
    17
sutural, 96
temporal, 73, 218
  articular eminence
    of, 217
  jugular notch of, 99
  petrous portion of,
    98
  zygomatic process of,
    94

turbinate, 329
Wormian, 17, 96, 330
zygomatic, temporal
    process of, 94
Bone shaft, characteristics
    of, 17
  canals, 17
  crests, 17
  foramina, 17
  fossae, 17
  foveae, 17
  lines, 17
  meatuses, 17
  notches, 17
  pits, 17
  processes, 17
  ridges, 17
  smooth area, 17
  spines, 17
  tubercles, 17
  tuberosities, 17
Bony ossicles and their
    associations, 187
Brain, 266–276
  arachnoid, 167
  blood supply, 275–276
  divisions of, 266–274
  dura mater, 167
  lateral view of, *267*
  midsagittal section of,
    268
  pia mater, 167
  and spinal cord,
    265–277
  spinal nerves and,
    26
  venous drainage, 276
  ventral view and its
    major arterial
    supply, *269*
Brainstem, *268, 271, 272,
    273,* 318
  dorsal view of, *273*
  ventral view of, *272*
Branchia, 57
Branchial arches, 318
Branchial grooves, 58,
    318
Buccal glands, 34, 318
Buccal nerve, 161, 293
  block, 310
Buccal vestibule, 33
Buccinator muscle, 160
Buccopharyngeal fascia,
    253, 318

Buccopharyngeal
    membrane, 58
Bursae, 11, 14, 318

Calvaria, internal surface
    of, 100
Canal(s), 17, 318
    carotid, 98
    facial, 102, 295
    hiatus of, 102
    hypoglossal, 99, 102
    incisive, 76, 98, 230
    infraorbital, 75
    mandibular, 76, 105
    nasolacrimal, 75, 76
    pharyngeal, 98
    pterygoid, 94, 98
    pterygopalatine, 94
    vertebral, 110
    vidian, 98
Canine, 42
    eminence, 33
    fossa, 33
Capillaries, 22
Capillary bed, 22, *23*,
    24
Capsule, 218–220
Cardiovascular system,
    22–24, *23*
Carotid artery(ies), 141,
    142, 143, 144, *193*,
    194, 195, 196, 254,
    319, 320, 327
    common, 141, 195, 319
    external, 141, 142–143
    192, *193*, 195, 254,
    320
        ascending
            pharyngeal, 143,
            195, 249, 254, 320
        facial, 143, 162, 243,
            322
        lingual, 143, 212,
            239, 242, 321
        occipital, 144, 155,
            195, 196, 323, 324
        posterior auricular,
            144, 155, 192, 193,
            196, 324
        superficial temporal,
            155, 163, 192, 193,
            324
        superior thyroid,
            143, 146, 254, 261,
            320

internal, 98, 141, 195,
    276, 327
    supraorbital, 155,
        164, 328
    supratrochlear, 155,
        164, 329
    and vessels in neck, 24
Carotid body, 24, 141,
    319
    nerves to, 302
Carotid plexus, 148, 319
Carotid sheath, 117,
    120–121, 319
Carotid sinus, 24, 141, 319
    nerve, 300
    syndrome, 151
Carotid triangle, 131, 319
Cartilage, 21, 257–258
    arytenoid, 258
    corniculate, 258
    cricoid, 113, 257–258
    cuneiform, 258
    elastic, 21, 321
    epiglottic, 258
    fibrous, 21
    greater alar, 228
    hyaline, 18, 20, 21
    lateral nasal, 228
    median nasal septal, 228
    Reichert's, 327
    thyroid, 257
Caruncula, sublingual, 240
Cataract, 185
Cauda equinae, 277
Caudal, defined, 5, 319
Cavernous sinus, 172, 319
    infection of, 165
Cell(s), 9
    connective tissue, 9
    epithelium, 9
    muscle, 9
    nerve, 9
    neuroglial, 25
Cell body, 25
Cellulitis, orbital, 234
Cementum, 44
Central nervous system
    (CNS), 15, 28, 264,
    319
Cephalic, defined, 319
Cerebellar artery(ies)
    inferior
        anterior, 276
        posterior, 276
    superior, 276

Cerebellar cortex, 271
Cerebellar vein(s), 276
    inferior, 276
    superior, 276
Cerebelli, tentorium, 101
Cerebelli, terminal, 329
Cerebellum, 271, 319
Cerebral aqueduct, 272,
    275
Cerebral arterial circle,
    319
Cerebral artery(ies)
    anterior, 276
    middle, 276
    posterior, 276
Cerebral edema, 165
Cerebral vein, great, 276
Cerebrospinal fluid, 275,
    319
Cervical artery
    ascending, 139, 331
    deep, 139, 332
Cervical nerve(s)
    first. *See* Suboccipital
        nerve
    transverse, 117
Cervical region
    muscle involvements,
        149–150
    nerve involvements,
        150
    thyroid gland
        involvements,
        151–152
    vascular involvements,
        151
Cervical plexus, 319
    branches of, 135
Cervical sinus, 62
Cervical sympathetic
    trunk, *136*, *147*,
    148, 319
Cervical triangles,
    boundaries of, 130
Cervical vein, transverse,
    115
Cheek, muscle of, 160
Chiasma, optic, 280, 325
    groove for, 101
Choana (ae), 75, 229, 319
Chondroblasts, 20
Chondroclasts, 20
Chondrocytes, 20
Chondroglossus muscle,
    239

Chorda tympani nerve, 241, 297
Choroid, 179
Choroidal artery, anterior, 276
Choroid plexus, 266, 275, 319
Ciliary body, 179, 319
Ciliary gland, 176
Ciliary muscle, 182
Ciliary nerve(s)
long, 184, 289
short, 184
Circle, cerebral arterial, of Willis, 276, 319
Circulatory system, 21–24
Circumvallate papillae, 37
Cisterna cerebelo-medullaris. *See* Cisterna magna
Cisterna magna, 275
Cisterns, 275
cisterna interpeduncularis, 275
superior, 275
Cleft, 58
lip, 69–71, *70*
bilateral, 71
median, 71
palate, 70–71, *70*, 262
anterior, 71
bilateral, 71
posterior, 71
surgically repaired, 37
unilateral, 71
pharyngeal, 58, 326
Clivus, 102
CNS. *See* Central nervous system
Cochlea, 188
Cochlear nerve, 298
Cock's comb, 101
Colliculus(i)
facial, 274
inferior, 274
brachium of, 274
superior, 274
brachium of, 274
Column
dorsal gray, 277
intermediolateral cell, 277

Columna, 227
Commissural lip pit, 31
Commissure, anterior, 271
Communicating artery
anterior, 276
posterior, 276
Concha(ae), of nasal cavity, 229, 319
inferior, 73, 76, 229, 230
middle, 76, 229, 230
superior, 76, 229
Conduction, 25
Condyle(s), 17, 319
mandibular, 105
occipital, 98, 99
Cones, 320. *See also* Rods and cones
elastic, 258
Connective tissue (hypodermis), subcutaneous, 10
Conus medullaris, 277
Cornea, 177, 179, 320
Cornu(a)
greater, 109
inferior, 257
lesser, 109
superior, 257
Corpora quadrigemina, 274
Corpus callosum, 271
Corrugator muscle, 159
Corti, spiral organ of, 188, 298
Costocervical trunk, 139
Cranial, defined, 5
Cranial fossa, 167–174, 320
Cranial nerve(s), *169*, 173–174, 279–305
abducent, 174, 184, 294
accessory, 283, 303, *304*
acoustic, 174, 188, 283, 298
eighth (VIII). *See* Acoustic nerve
eleventh (XI). *See* Accessory nerve
facial, 158, 161, 162, 165, 174, 188, 192, 193, 197, 226, 282–283, 294–296

fifth (V). *See* Trigeminal nerve
first (I). *See* Olfactory nerve
fourth (IV). *See* Trochlear nerve
glassopharyngeal, 174, 195, 283, 298–300
hypoglossal, 136, 174, 198, *237*, 242, 283, *304*, 305
ninth (IX). *See* Glossopharyngeal nerve
oculomotor, 173, 182, 282, 284–285
olfactory, 101, 173, 280, *281*, 282
optic, 173, 179, 182, 280, *281*, 282
second (II). *See* Optic nerve
seventh (VII). *See* Facial nerve
sixth (VI). *See* Abducent nerve
tenth (X). *See* Vagus nerve
third (III). *See* Oculomotor nerve
trigeminal, 173, 174, 184, 193, 226, 241, 282, 285–286
trochlear, 282, 285, 287–288
twelfth (XII). *See* Hypoglossal nerve
vagus, 146–147, 174, 302–303, 329
Cranial outflow, 30, 320
Craniosacral outflow, 30, 320
Crest(s), 17
alveolar
lateral, 105
medial, 105
buccal, lateral, 105
frontal, 100
infratemporal, 99
occipital
external, 96
internal, 103
zygomaticoalveolar, 96
Cretinism, 152

Cricoarytenoid muscle
  lateral, 259
  posterior, 260
Cricoid cartilage, 113
Cricothyroid artery, 143,
  320
Cricothyroid muscle, 259
Cricothyrotomy, 263, 320
Cuneus, 271
Cupid's bow, 31
Cusps, 44
Cysts, cervical, 68

"Danger space," 120,
  149, 153
da Vinci, Leonardo, 2
Deep, defined, 320
Deglutition, 261–262
Dendrites, 25, 320
Dens, 112
Dental anatomy
  distal aspect, 43, 44
  mesial aspect, 43, 44
Dental arch(es), 43
  mandibular, 40
  maxillary, 40
Denticulate ligaments,
  277
Dentition
  deciduous, 46
  mixed, 47
  permanent, 47
Depress, 320
Depressions, bony, 318
Depressor anguli oris, 159
Depressor labii inferioris,
  159
Dermal papillae, 10, 320
Dermis, 10, 320
  layers of, 10
Developmental anatomy,
  320
Diaphragma sella, 170, 320
Diaphysis, 20
Diencepahlon, 271–274,
  320
Digastric muscle, 198,
  236, 297
  anterior belly, 236
  posterior belly, 236
  nerve to, 297
Dilatator pupillae
  muscles, 182

Diploë, 97
Diploic veins, 172–173
Disk, articular, 18, 217,
  218, 318
Distal, defined, 6, 320
Distal aspect, in dental
  anatomy, 44
Dorsal, defined, 5, 320
Dorsal horn, defined, 320
Dorsal root ganglion, 27, 320
Dorsum sellae, 102
Duct(s)
  of Bartholin, 38, 321
  lacrimal, 177, 178
  lymphatic, right, 139, 327
  nasolacrimal, 65
  parotid, 191, 199
  of Rivinus, 321
  Stenson's, 328
  sublingual, 240
  submandibular, 38, 240
  thoracic, 24, 139, 329
  thyroglossal, 37, 69,
    145, 329
  Wharton's, 38, 330
Dural reflections,
  167–168, 169
Dura mater, 28, 167, 321
  blood supply of, 170
  meningeal layer, 167
  periosteal layer, 167
  venous drainage of, 170
  venous sinuses of, 168,
    169, 170–172
Dyspnea, 263

Ear
  development, 185–186
  external, 186–187
    nerve supply, 187
  inner, 188
    nerves, 188
    vestibule, 188
  middle, 186, 187
    vessels and nerves
      of, 187–188
    muscles of, 158
    ossicles of, 326
Eardrum, 186
Edinger–Westphal
  nucleus, 284
Efferent, 321
  visceral, 27, 279, 280

Elevate, defined, 321
Elevations, bony, defined,
  318
Embryo at 4–5 weeks, 58
Embryology of head and
  neck, 57–72
Eminence
  arcuate, 102
  articular, 218
  canine, 76
  cruciate, 103
  parietal, 97
Emissary veins, 173, 321
Endolymph, 188
Endomysium, 13
Endosteum, 20
Eosinophils, 22
Ependyma, 266
Epicranius muscle, 154
  frontal belly, 154
  occipital belly, 154
Epidermal pegs, 10, 321
Epidermis, 10, 321
Epidural fat, 265
Epiglottic vallecula, 253
Epiglottis, 50, 252, 321
Epimysium, 13
Epiphyses (ends), 20
Epithalamus, 272
Eponychium (cuticle), 12
Erector spinae, 121
Erythrocytes, 22
Esophagus, 252, 255
  vascular supply of, 255
Ethmoid, uncinate
  process of the, 230
Ethmoidal bulla, 230
Ethmoidal nerve(s), 184
  anterior, 184, 288
  posterior, 184, 288
Eustachian tube, 50, 321
Exophthalmos, 185
Exostoses, bony, 55
Extension, 14, 321
External, defined, 6, 321
Eye, 175
  external anatomy of,
    178
  muscles of 178, 180,
    181, 182
    extrinsic, 178, 321
    intrinsic, 182
  ptosis of, 165

refractive media of,
  180
Eyelid, 175–176

Face, 76–77
  deep, 201–216
    innervation, 213–215
    muscles and fascia,
      202–211
    vascular supply, 211
  development of, *60,*
    65–68
  formation of, *67*
  superficial, 153–165
    blood supply of, *158,*
      162–164
    danger area of, 165
    motor innervation,
      162
    muscles of, 155–160
    sensory innervation
      of, *158,* 160
    surface anatomy, 153
    vascular and nerve
      supply of, *158*
    venous drainage of,
      164
Facets
  articular, 110
    inferior, 112
    superior, 112
Facial artery, 143–144,
    162–163, 197, 243,
    332
  glandular branches,
    243
  groove for, 105
  labial, 162
  transverse, 163, 197
Facial canal, 102, 295
Facial component
    derivatives, *68*
Facial nerve, 158, 161,
    162, 165, 174, 188,
    192, 193, 197, 226,
    282–293, 294–296
  branches of, 163
  buccal branch, 162,
    192, 193
  cervical branch, 162,
    192, 193
  damage to, 165
  digastric branch, 197

mandibular branch,
    162, *192,* 193
  posterior auricular
      branch, 162
  stylohoid branch, 197
  temporal branches, 162
  zygomatic branches,
    161
Facial vein, 164, 243, 322
  common, 243
Falx cerebelli, 168, 321
Falx cerebri, 100, 168,
    321
Fascia, 321
  buccopharyngeal, 120
  cervical, midsaggital
      view, 119
  deep, 13, 320
  investing, 323
  masseteric, 203
  parotid, 119, 326
  parotideo-masseteric,
    203
  pretracheal, 120, 327
  prevertebral, 119–120,
    327
  pterygoid, 203
  superficial, 10, 114
  temporal, 203
Fascial layers, 149
  investing, 117–119
  pretracheal, 117, 120
  prevertebral, 117,
    119–120
Fatty region, 40
Fauces, 36
  anterior. *See*
      Palatoglossal fold
  pillars of, 36, 50
  posterior. *See*
      Palatopharyngeal
      fold
Fenestra cochleae, 187
Fenestra vestibuli, 187
Fibrocartilage, 321
Filum terminale, 277
Fissure
  longitudinal, 270
  orbital, superior, 102
  palpebral, 177, 326
  petrosquamous, 99
  petrotympanic, 99
  posterior median, 274

pterygomaxillary, 94
  ventral median, 277
Fistula
  branchia, 68
  tracheoesophageal, 262
Fixators, 15, 321
Flexion, 14, 321
Foramen (foramina), 17,
    321
  cecum, 37, 64, 101, 322
  condylar, 99
  ethmoidal, 75
  hypoglossal, 102
  incisive, 76, 98, 230
  infraorbital, 75, 76
  interventricular, 271,
    272, 275
  intervertebral, 110
  jugular, 99, 102
  lacerum, 98, 102
  of Luschka, 275
  of Magendie, 275
  magnum, 96, 99, 102
  mandibular, 105
  mastoid, 96, 100
  mental, 76, 103
  olfactory, 101
  optic, 75
  ovale, 77, 99, 102
  palatine
    greater, 98
    lesser, 98, 225
  parietal, 97
  rotundum, 94, 102, 226
  of skull, 106–109
  sphenopalatine, 94
  spinosum, 77, 99, 102
  stylomastoid, 96, 100
  supraorbital, 74
  transversarium, 110
  vertebral, 110
  zygomaticofacial, 96
  zygomaticoorbital, 96
  zygomaticotemporal, 96
Fordyce's granules, 34,
    35, 322
Fornix, 33
Fossa(ae), 17
  canine, 76
  cerebellar, 103
  condylar, 99
  cranial, 167–174
    anterior, 100, 101

Fossa(ae) (*continued*)
  cranial (*continued*)
    middle, 100,
      101–102
    posterior, 100,
      102–103
  glenoid, 95, 99
  hypophyseal, 101
  incisive, 33, 76, 98, 103
  infratemporal, 77, 202,
    203, 323
    communications, 202
  interpenduncular, 274
  mandibular, 95, 99, 324
  nasal, 228–229, 230
  pterygoid, 98
  pterygopalatine, 94,
    225, 327
  retromolar, 105
  submandibular, 105
  temporal, 77, 201–202
Foveae, 17
Fovea centralis, 179
Frederick II, 2
Frenulum, superior
  labial, *53*
Frontal plane, defined,
  322
Frontal nerve, 184, 287
Frontonasal prominence,
  65

Galea aponeurotica, 153,
  154
Galen, 2
Ganglion, 25, 322
  cervical, middle, 325
  of cochlea, spiral, 298
  dorsal root, 27
  geniculate, 296
  inferior cervical, 148,
    149, 323
  middle cervical, 148,
    149
  otic, 300
  pterygopalatine, 226,
    227, 288
  semilunar. *See*
    Ganglion,
    trigeminal
  stellate, 148
  submandibular, 241,
    297

superior cervical, 148
  trigeminal, 174, 285
  vestibular, 298
Ganglia
  basal, defined, 318
  chain, 30, 319
  collateral, 30, 319
  terminal, 30
General somatic afferent,
  25, 322
General somatic efferent,
  25, 322
General visceral afferent,
  25, 322
General visceral efferent,
  25, 27, 322
Geniculate bodies, 273
  lateral, 273
  medial, 273
Genioglossus, 239
Geniohyoid, 237
Gingiva, 36, 322
Gingival mucosa, 36
Glabella, 74
Glands, 12
  of Blandin–Nuhn, 38,
    322
  buccal, 34
  ciliary, 176
  incisive, 40
  labial, 34
  lacrimal, 177, 178
  mammary, 12
  palatine, 40
  parathyroid, 146
  parotid, 191, *192, 193,*
    194
  salivary, minor, 325
  sublingual, 240, 241
  sweat, 12
  thyroid, 145
  of von Ebner, 37,
    322
Glandular artery, 144
Glandular region, 40
Glaucoma, 185, 322
Globular process, 65
Glossitis, median
    rhomboid, *55*
Glossoepiglottic folds,
    252–253
  lateral, 252–253
  median, 252–253

Glossopharyngeal nerve,
    174, 195, 283,
    298–300, 322
  ganglia of, 299
    inferior, 299
    superior, 299
Goiter, 151–152
Gracilis
  nucleus, 274
  tuberculum, 274
Granularis, fovea, 100
Gray commissures, 277
  dorsal, 277
  ventral, 277
Gray rami
    communicantes,
    30, 322
Groove, 36, 58, 322
  infraorbital, 75
  mylohyoid, 105
  nasolacrimal, 65
Gross anatomy, 322
Growth
  appositional, 20
  interstitial, 20
Gum, 36
Gyrus, defined, 322
  cingulate, 271
  postcentral, 270
  precentral, 270
  rectus, 271

Habenular trigone, 272
Hair, 11–12
  root, 12
  shaft, 12
Hamulus, pterygoid, 98
Harvey, William, 2
Head, 17
  lymph nodes, 311, *312*
  movements of, 15
  parasympathetic
    ganglia of, 286
  posterior–anterior
    radiograph of, *95*
Head and neck,
    embryology of,
    57–72
Helicotrema, 188
Hemispheres
  cerebellar, 271
  cerebral, 266, *267, 268,*
    269, 270–271, 319

Herophilus, 1
Hiatus, semilunar, 230
Histology, defined, 5, 322
Hoarseness, 263
Horner's Syndrome, 150
Horns
  dorsal, 277
  ventral, 277
Human figure, 6
Hyaline cartilage, 322
Hyoid arch, 61, 322
Hyoid bone, 113
Hyoglossus, 239
Hyperopia, 185
Hyperthyroidism, 152
Hypodermis, 10, 114
Hypoglossal nerve, 136, 174, 198, *237*, 242, 283, *304*, 305
Hypophysis, 273, 322
Hypothalamus, 273
Hypothyroidism, 152

Iliocostalis cervicis, 121
Impression, trigeminal, 102
Incisal edge, 44
Incisive canal, 76, 98, 230
Incisive foramen, 76, 98, 230
Incisive fossa, 33, 76, 98
Incisive glands, 40
Incisors, 42
Incus, 186
Inferior, defined, 5, 322
Inferior alveolar nerve, 294
Infiltration, defined, 307
Infrahyoid artery, 143, 320
Infrahyoid muscles, 140–141, 323
Infraorbital artery, 225, 326
  orbital branches, 225, 226
Infraorbital groove, 75
Infraorbital nerve, 161, 226, 291
Infraorbital trunk, anesthesia of, 309

Infratrochlear nerve, 161, 184, 288
Infundibulum, 273
Insula, 270
Integumentary system, 9–12
  structure of, 10–12
Intercalated discs, 13
Internal, defined, 323
Interspinales, 126
Intertransversarii, 126
Intercavernous sinuses, 172
  anterior, 172
  posterior, 172
Intercostal artery, superior, 139, 332
Internal, 6
Internal thoracic artery, 138, 331
Involuntary nervous system, 28
Iris, 179, 323
Irritability, 25
Isthmus faucium, 31, 323

"Jaw Opener," 211
Jaws, panographic radiograph of, *44*
Joint(s), 18–19
  cartilaginous, 18, 319
    symphyses, 18
    synchondroses, 18
  fibrous, 18, 321
    sutures, 18
    syndesmoses, 18
  synovial, 18
  types, *18*
Jugular arch, 116, 119
Jugular notch, 113
Jugular vein
  anterior, 115, 334, 336
  external, 114, 193, 333, 334, 336
  posterior, 115, 334
  internal, 145, 171, 335
    superior bulb of, 171

Kiesselbach's area, 234, 323

Labial commissures, 31
Labial frenula, 34

Labial glands, 34
Labial tubercle, 31
Labial vestibule, 33, *35*
  superior, 33
Labiomental groove, 31
Labyrinth
  bony, 188
  membranous, 188
Labyrinthine artery, 276
Lacrimal ducts, 177, *178*
Lacrimal fossa, 75
Lacrimal gland, 177, *178*
Lacrimal nerve, 161, 184, 287
Lacrimal sac, 177, *178*
Lacteals, 24
Lacunae, 20
Lacunae lateralis, 171
Laminae, posterior, 110
Langer's lines, 114
Laryngeal aperture, superior, 256
Laryngeal artery, superior, 143, 320
Laryngeal nerves
  inferior, 303
  recurrent, 303
  superior, 147, 302–303
    external branch of, 302
Laryngeal prominence, 113
Laryngopharynx, foreign material in, 263
Larynx, 113, *252*, 255–257
  arterial supply of, 261
  classification of muscles, 259–260
  infraglottic cavity, 256
  intrinsic muscles of, 259
  sensory innervation of, 261
  ventricle, 256
  vestibule, 256
Lateral, defined, 7
Leucocytes, 22
Levator anguli oris, 160
Levator labii superioris alaque nasi, 159–160

Levator palpebrae
  superioris, 175,
  180
Levator scapulae, 134
Levator thyroideae, 145
Levator veli palatini, 246
Ligament(s), 221
  capsular, 221
  cricothyroid, median,
    258
  denticulate, 266, 277
  lateral, 221
  periodontal, 44
  pterygospinous, 203
  sphenomandibular,
    203, 221
  stylohoid, 198
  stylomandibular, 221
  temporomandibular,
    221
  vocal, 258
Ligamentum nuchae, 117
Limb(s)
  upper
    arterial insufficiency
      of, 150
    uncontrollable
      bleeding in, 151
Line(s), 17
  mylohyoid, 105
  nuchal
    highest, 97
    inferior, 96
    median, 96
  temporal
    inferior, 77
    superior, 77
Linea alba, 52
Lingual artery, 143, 242,
  321
  deep, 242, 321
  dorsal, 242, 321
Lingual frenulum, 37
Lingual nerve(s), 241,
  293, 300
Lingual tonsils, 37
Lingual vein, deep, 243,
  325
Lingula, 102, 271
Lip(s), 31–33, 51
  anatomy of, 32
  and buccal vestibule,
    32
  cleft, 51

depressors of, 159
elevators of, 159–160
pits, congenital
  commissural, 51
Lobe
  occipital, 270
  temporal, 270
Longissimus capitis, 124
Longissimus cervicis, 124
Longus capitis, 149, 150
Longus colli, 149, 150
Lumbar cistern, 277
Lymph, 24
Lymphatic drainage,
  313–314
  deep tissue, 314
  superficial tissues, 313
Lymphatic duct, right, 139
Lymphatic ring of
  Waldeyer, 56
Lymphatic System, 24
Lymph nodes, 24,
  311–313
  anterior cervical, 312,
    314
  buccal, 311, 314
  deep cervical, 195,
    312–313, 315, 320
  infrahyoid, 313
  infraorbital, 311
  jugulodigastric, 313,
    315, 323
  jugulo-omohyoid, 313,
    315, 323
  mandibular, 311, 314
  mastoid, 311, 314
  maxillary, 311, 314
  occipital, 311, 314
  paratracheal, 313
  parotid, 311, 314
  posterior auricular, 311
  prelaryngeal, 313, 314
  pretracheal, 313, 314
  primary, 315
  retropharyngeal, 311,
    315
  secondary, 315
  submandibular, 312,
    315
  submental, 312, 314
  superficial, 195, 311
  tertiary, 315
  of tongue, 314, 315
Lymphocytes, 22

Macroglossia, 53, 69, 324
Macroscopic anatomy,
  324
Macula, 179
Malformations,
  congenital, 149
Malleus, 186
Mammillary bodies, 273
Mandible, 73, 103–109,
  217–218
  angle, 77, 105
  body, 103
  condyle of, 105
  dislocation of, 223
  external surface, 103
  internal surface, 105
  lateral aspect, *104*
  medial aspect, *104*
  neck of, 105
  oblique line, 77, 103
  rami, 103
  superior aspect, *104*
Mandibular arch, 59–61,
  324
Mandibular fossa, 324
Mandibular nerve,
  291–292
  mandibular division,
    292–293
    anterior, 292–293
    posterior, 293–294
Mandibular process, 60
Mandibular torus(i), 53,
  324
Mandibular trunk, main,
  292
  medial pterygoid nerve,
    292
  recurrent meningeal
    nerve, 292
Massa intermedia, 272
Masseteric nerve, 293
Masseter muscle, 197,
  204, 206
Mastication, 215–216
  muscles of, 202, 204,
    215
  process of, 215
Masticator compartment,
  203, 324
Mastoidectomy, 263
Matter
  gray, 270, 322
  white, 270

Maxilla, 73
  zygomatic process of, 76
Maxillary artery, 196, 225–226, 325
  branches of, 163–164, 325–327
  nasal branch, posterior lateral, 232
  pterygopalatine portion, 225, 326–327
Maxillary nerve(s), 226
  greater palatine nerve, 290
    nasal branches, posterior inferior, 290
  lesser palatine nerve, 290
    nasal branches, posterior inferior, 226
    superior, 226, 291
  orbital branches, 290
  pharyngeal branch, 291
Maxillary ostium, 231
Maxillary process, 59, 324
Maxillary sinus, 231
Maxillary tuberosity, 34
Meatus, 17, 76, 324
  acoustic
    external, 96, 321
    internal, 102
  auditory, internal, 102
  inferior, 76
  middle, 76, 230
  superior, 76, 229
Meckel's cartilage, 60, 324
Meckel's cave, 170, 285
Medial, 7, 324
Median lingual sulcus, 324
Median rhomboid glossitis, 53, 324
Median plane, 324
Median sulcus, 36
Medulla, 324
Medulla oblongata. *See* Myelencephalon
Melanin, 12
Membrane(s)
  buccopharyngeal, 58
  cricotracheal, 259

quadrangular, 258
synovial, 19
thyrohyoid, 259
Meningeal artery
  accessory, 170, 212, 326
  anterior, 170, 328
  middle, 170, 326
  posterior, 170
Meningeal nerve, middle, 290
Meninges, 265–266
Meninx, 324
Meniscus, 217, 218, 324
Mentalis muscle, 159
Mental nerve, 162, 294
Mental symphysis, 324
Mesencephalon, 274, 324
Mesial, defined, 6, 324
Mesial aspect, in dental anatomy, 44
Metastases, cervical, 315
Metencephalon, 274, 324
Metopic suture, 16, 324
Microglossia, 53, 324
Micrognathia, 69
Microscope, invention of, 2
Microscopic anatomy, 324
Midbrain. *See* Mesencephalon
Middle cervical ganglion, 325
Midsaggital plane, 325
Minor salivary glands, 325
Modiolus, 188
Molars, 42
Monocytes, 22
Motor end-plate, 15, 27, 325
Motor neuron, 27
Mouth
  anterior floor of, 39
  development of, 66
  floor of, *41*, 53
  muscles surrounding, 159
  submandibular region and floor of, 235–244
    contents and boundaries, 235
    muscles and fascia vascular supply to, 242

Movements of head, 15
  depression, 15
  elevation, 15
  protusion, 15
  retraction, 15
  rotation, 15
Mucobuccal, 33
Mucogingival junction, 36, 325
Mucolabial folds, 33
Multifidus spinae, 125
Mumps, 199
Muscle(s)
  action of, 14, 15
  aryepiglotticus, 256
  arytenoid, 259, 260
  attachment of, 14
  auricular, 156, 158
  bipennate, 14
  buccinator, 156, 160
  cardiac, 13
  chondroglossus, 239
  ciliary, 182
  constrictors, pharyngeal, 248, 253, 254
  corrugator, 156, 159
  cricoarytenoid, 259, 260
  cricothyroid, 259
  deep prevertebral, 149, 150
  depressor
    anguli oris, 156, 159
    labii inferioris, 156, 159
    septi, 156, 158
  digastric, 198, 223, 236
  dilatator pupillae, 182
  epicranius, 153, 154
  erector spinae, 117
  fasicle, 13
  fibers
    involuntary, 12
    voluntary, 12
  form of, 14
  frontalis, 154, 156
  genioglossus, 239
  geniohyoid, 223, 237
  hyoglossus, 239
  inferior oblique, 180
  inferior pharyngeal constrictor, 248, 254

Muscle(s) (*continued*)
infrahyoid, 140, 141
insertion of, 14
intrinsic
of the eye, 182, 183
of the tongue, 238
involuntary, 12
levator anguli oris,
156, 160
levator glandulae
thyroideae
levator labii superioris,
156, 159, 160
levator labii superioris
alaque nasi, 156
levator palpebrae
superioris, 180,183
levator scapulae, 132,
134
levator veli palatini,
246, 248
longissimus capitis,
122
masseter, 197, 204,
206, 223
mentalis, 156, 159
middle pharyngeal
constrictor, 248,
254
multipennate, 14
mylohyoid, 223, 237
nasalis, 156, 158
nerve control of, 15
oblique
inferior, 180
superior, 180
obliquus capitis, 124
occipitalis, 154, 155
occipitofrontalis, 153,
154
omohyoid, 132, 133,141
orbicularis oculi, 156,
158
orbicularis oris, 156,
159
origin of, 14
palatoglossus, 247, 248
palatopharyngeus, 248,
249
pennate, 14
pharyngeal
constrictors, 248
inferior, 248, 254
middle, 248, 254
superior, 160, 248,253

platysma, 132, 156,
159
prime movers, 15
procerus, 156, 158
pterygoid
lateral, 204, 208, 223
medial, 204, 207, 223
pupillary, 182
recti, 180, 183
risorius, 156, 159
scalpingopharyngeus,
248, 254
scalene
anterior, 132, 134
middle, 132, 134
posterior, 132, 134
semispinalis capitis,
122
skeletal, 13
smooth, 13
sphincter pupillae, 182
splenius capitis, 122,
132
stapedius, 186
sternocleidomastoid,
132
sternohyoid, 140
sternothyroid, 140
striated, 13
structure of, 13
styloglossus, 198, 239
stylohoid, 198, 223,
236
stylopharyngeus, 198,
248, 254
subclavius, 139
suboccipital, 126, 127
superior oblique, 180
superior pharyngeal
constrictor, 160,
248, 253
suprahyoid, 223, 236,
237, 238
synergists, 15
temporalis, 204, 205,
223
temporoparietalis, 155,
156
tensor tympani, 187
tensor veli palatini,
246, 248
thyroarytenoid, 259,260
thyrohyoid, 141
transversospinal group,
125, 126

trapezius, 121, 122
of uvula, 247, 248
vocalis, 259, 260
voluntary, 12
zygomaticomandibularis,
207
zygomaticus
major, 156, 160
minor, 156, 160
Muscular system, 12–15
Muscular triangle, 131,
325
Musculus uvulae, 247
Myelencephalon, 274
Myelin sheath, 25
Mylohyoid muscle, 237
Mylohyoid nerve, 241,
294
Myofibrils, 13
Myopia, 185

Nails, 12
Naris, (nares), 227, 229
Nasal artery, dorsal, 164
Nasal cavity, 75–76, *227,*
228–229
lateral wall of, 76
nerve supply of,
232–233
vascular supply of, 232
Nasal concha(ae), 73, 76,
229
inferior, 73, 76, 229,
230
middle, 76, 229, 230
superior, 76, 229
Nasal fossa, 228–229,
230
floor of, 230
lateral wall of, 229
medial wall of, 229
roof of, 230
Nasal nerve(s)
external, 161, 184
internal, 184
Nasal septum
defined, 325
deviation of, 234
median, 228
Nasociliary nerve, 184,
288–289
Nasolabial groove, 31
Nasolacrimal duct, 177,
178, 230
Nasopalatine nerve, 291

Nasopharyngeal tonsil, 50, 325
Nasopharynx, 50, 325
Neck, 113–152, *312*, 313
  cross section, *118*
  deep fascia, 117–120
  deep prevertebral muscles of, 149, 150
  lymph nodes, 312–313
  nerve supply to, *147*
  posterior, 131–139
  root of, *138*
  sensory innervation of, 116–117
  superficial structures of, 114
  superficial venous drainage, 114–116
  surface anatomy of, 113
  triangles of, 128–131
  vagal branches in, 302–303
Neocerebellum, 271
Nerve(s)
  abducent, 174, 184, 188, 281, 294
  accessory, 132, 174, 282, 303
  accessory phrenic, 137
  acoustic, 174, 282, 298
  alveolar
    inferior, 215, 294
    anterior superior, 291
    middle superior, 291
    posterior superior, 215, 226, 291
  ansa cervicalis, 135
  ansa subclavia, 148
  auricular
    great, 117, 135, 187, 195
    posterior, 162, 197, 297
    of vagus, 187, 302
  auriculotemporal, 155, 161, 187, 193, 195, 214, 294
    anterior auricular branches, 214, 294
    articular branches, 214, 294
  autonomic, 28, 29, 30

brachial plexus, 116, 134
buccal
  of facial, 162, 298
  of mandibular, 161, 213, 293
cardiac, 303
carotid plexus, 148, 195
  of carotid sinus, 300
cervical branch (of facial), 162, 193, 298
  of cervical plexus, 116, 135
cervical, transverse, 117, 135
chorda tympani, 188, 214, 241, 293, 297
ciliary
  long, 184, 289
  short, 184, 289
cochlear, 298
cranial. (*See* by name)
cutaneous (cervical), 116, 135
deep temporal, 214, 292
descending hypoglossal, 135
ethmoidal
  anterior, 184, 288
  posterior, 184, 288
facial, 162, 174, 188, 193, 197, 281, 294
frontal, 184, 287
glossopharyngeal, 174, 188, 195, 282, 298
hypoglossal, 174, 239, 242, 282, 305
incisive, 215, 294
infraorbital, 161, 291
infratrochlear, 161, 184, 288
intermedius (nervus), 295
lacrimal, 161, 184, 287
laryngeal
  external, 147, 261
  inferior, 303
  internal, 147, 261
  recurrent, 148, 261, 303
  superior, 147, 302
lingual, 214, 241, 293

mandibular, 161, 291
  anterior division of, 213, 292
  posterior division of, 214, 293
mandibular branch (facial), 162, 193, 298
masseteric, 213, 293
maxillary, 161, 226, 232, 289
meningeal
  trigeminal, 213, 290, 292
  vagal, 302
mental, 162, 215, 294
mylohyoid, 215, 241, 294
nasal
  external, 161, 184, 288, 291
  lateral
  posterior superior, 226, 291
nasociliary, 184, 288
nasopalatine, 226, 291
occipital
  greater, 116
  lesser, 116, 135, 187
  third, 116
oculomotor, 173, 182, 281, 284
olfactory, 173, 280, 281
ophthalmic, 161, 232
optic, 173, 182, 280, 281
orbital, 290
palatine
  greater, 226, 290
  lesser, 226, 290
parotid plexus, 162, 198
petrosal
  deep, 296
  greater, 296
  lesser, 300
pharyngeal
  of maxillary, 226, 290
  of glossopharyngeal, 300
  of vagus, 147, 302, 303
pharyngeal plexus, 148, 255

Nerve(s) (*continued*)
  phrenic, 137
  phrenic, accessory, 137
  pterygoid
    lateral, 214, 293
    medial, 213, 292
  of pterygoid canal, 296
  pterygopalatine, 226, 290
  recurrent laryngeal, 148, 303
  spinal accessory, 132, 174, 282, 303
  to stapedius, 188, 297
  suboccipital, 126, 128
  supraclavicular, 117, 135
  supraorbital, 155, 161, 184, 288
  supratrochlear, 155, 161, 184, 288
  sympathetic cervical trunk, 148
  temporal
    deep, 214, 292
    of facial, 162, 193, 298
    superficial, 214, 294
  to tensor tympani, 213
  to tensor veli palatini, 213
  tonsillar, 300
  transversus coli, 117, 135
  trigeminal, 174, 184, 213, 241, 281, 285
    mandibular, 174, 213, 241, 291
    maxillary, 174, 215, 289
    ophthalmic, 174, 184, 286
  trochlear, 173, 184, 281, 285
  tympanic plexus, 187, 299
  vagus, 146, 174, 282, 300
  vertebral, 148
  vestibulocochlear, 174, 282, 298
  Vidian, 296
  visceral, 28

zygomatic
  of facial, 162, 193, 298
  of maxillary, 226, 290
zygomaticofacial, 161, 290
zygomaticotemporal, 155, 161, 290
Nervous system, 24–30
  central (CNS), 25
  functional components of, 25–27
  parasympathetic, 326
  peripheral, (PNS), 25, 27–28, 326
  structure of, 25
Nervus intermedius, 295
Neuralgia, trigeminal, 165
Neurilemma sheath, 25
Neuroanatomy, 5, 325
Neurocirculatory compression, 150
Neuroglial cells, 25
Neuron(s), 25, 325
  connecting, 25
  intercalary, 25
  motor, 25
  sensory, 25
Neurovascular bundles, 15, 325
Neutrophils, 22
Nissl bodies, 25
Nodes of Ranvier, 25
Nodose ganglion, 147, 325
Nose
  bleeding from, 234
  development of, 65–68, 66
  external, 227
    ala, 227
    general morphology, 227
    root, 227
  internal, 228–233
  muscles of, 158
  skeleton, 227–228
  venous drainage of, 232
Notch(es), 17, 325
  mandibular, 105
  mastoid, 100
  superior, 110

thyroid, 113
  superior, 257
  vertebral, 110
  inferior, 110
Nucleus (nuclei), 25, 325
  cuneatus, 274
  gracilis, 274

Obex, 274
Oblique muscle
  inferior, 180
  superior, 180
Obliquus capitis
  inferior, 126
  superior, 126
Occipital artery, 144, 195, 196
  branches of, 144
Occipital nerve
  greater, 116
  lesser, 116
  third, 116
Occipital sinus, 171
Occipital triangle, 131, 325
Occipital vein, 145, 333
Occipitofrontalis muscle. *See* Epicranius muscle
Oculomotor nerve, 173, 182, 282, 284–285, 325
Odontogenesis, 44
Olfactory bulb, 101, 271, 280, 325
Olfactory nerve, 101, 173, 280, *281*, 282, 325
Olfactory tract, 173, 271, 280
Olive, 274
Omohyoid muscle, 133, 141
Opthalmic artery, 185, 276, 328
  branches of, 164, 328
  ethmoidal branches, 232, 328
Ophthalmic nerve, 286–287
Ophthalmic veins
  inferior, 185, 334
  superior, 185, 334
Optic chiasma, 280, 325

Optic nerve, 173, 179, 182, 280, *281*, 282, 325
Oral cavity, 31–48
  proper, 326
Oral fissure, 31
Ora serrata, 179
Orb anatomy, 177, *178*, 179
Orbicularis oculi, 158
Orbicularis oris, 159
Orbit, 74–75, 175
  anterior anatomy, 175–177, *178*
  apex of, 75
  bones of, 176
  bony, 175, *176*
  communications of, 177
  and ear, 175–189
  floor of, 75
  lateral wall, 75
  medial wall of, 75
  muscles surrounding, 158
  nerves of, 182–185
  roof of, 75
  vascular supply of, *181*, 185
Orbital fissure
  inferior, 75
  superior, 75
Orbital plate, 75
Organ, defined, 9
Origin, defined, 326
Oropharyngeal isthmus, 31, 36, 252, 326
Oropharynx, 50, 56, 326
Ossicles of ear, 326
Osteoblasts, 19
Osteoclasts, 20
Osteocytes, 20
Osteoid, 19
Osteology, 73–112
Osteomyelitis, 164
  frontal bone, 234
Otis media, 189, 326
Otosclerosis, 189

Palate, 40, *41*, *42*, 55–56, 245–250
  and associated area, *92*, *93*
  congenital defects of, 262

development, 65–68
  hard, 40, 97, 245, *246*
  muscles of, 248
  soft, 49, 245, *246*
  muscles of, 245
  vascular supply of, *246*, 249
  venous drainage, 249
Palatine artery
  ascending, 144
  lesser, 225, 249, 327
  greater, 225, 249, 327
Palatine foramina
  greater, 98, 225
  lesser, 225, 226
Palatine fovea, 40
Palatine glands, 40
Palatine nerve, greater, 226
Palatine processes, 66
Palatine raphe, 40
Palatine rugae, 40
Palatine tonsil, *246*, 249–250
Palatine torus(i), 55, *56*, 262, 326
Palatine velum, 40
Palatoglossal arch, 36
Palatoglossal fold, 245
Palatoglossus, 247
Palatopharyngeal fold, 50, 245
Palatopharyngeal sphincter, 253–254
Palatopharyngeus, 249
Paleocerebellum, 271
Palbebral fissure, 177, 326
Panniculus adiposus, 10, 326
Papilla
  incisive, 40
  interdental, 36
  parotid, 34, 326
  retrocuspid, 55
  retromolar, 36
Paranasal sinus, 229, 230, *231*, 232–234, 326
  nerve supply of, 232–233
  vascular supply of, 232
  venous drainage of, 232
Parasympathetic nervous system, 326

Parathyroid glands, 146
  inferior, 146
  superior, 146
Parietal operculum, 270
Parotid bed, 191–199
  structures deep to, *196*, 197–199
  arteries and nerves, 198–199
  muscles and ligament, 197–198
  superficial anatomy and boundaries, 191, *192*
Parotid duct, 191
  calculus accumulations in, 199
Parotid fascia, 119, 326
Parotid gland, 191, *192*, *193*, 194
  tumors, of, 199
  vascularization, lymphatics, and innervation, 193, 195
Parotid papilla, 326
Passavant's bar, 56, 326
Peduncles
  cerebellar, 274
  inferior, 274
  middle, 274
  superior, 274
  cerebral, 274
Pericranium, 153
Perikaryon, 25
Perilymph, 188
Perimysium, 13
Periodontal ligament, 44
Periorbita, 175
Periosteal bud, 20
Periosteum, 20, 175
Peripheral nervous system, 326
Petrosal nerve
  deep, 296
  greater, 296–297
    facial canal, hiatus of, 296
  lesser, 300
Petrosal sinus
  inferior, 172
  superior, 172
Petrosquamous sinus, 171

Phagocytic cells, 20
Pharyngeal, defined, 58
Pharyngeal (branchial)
        arch(es), 58, 326
    derivatives, 59
    first, 59
    fourth, 62
    second, 59
    sixth, 62
    third, 61–62
Pharyngeal artery
    ascending, 143, 195,
        249, 320
        branches of, 143, 320
Pharyngeal canal, 226
Pharyngeal clefts, 58, 326
Pharyngeal constrictor
    middle, 48
    superior, 48
Pharyngeal groove
    first, 62
    and pouches, late
        development of, *61*
Pharyngeal isthmus, 250
Pharyngeal nerve, 147,
        226, 300
Pharyngeal plexus, 255,
        326
Pharyngeal pouch(es), 58,
        326
    derivatives, 62–63
    fifth, 63
    first, 62
    fourth, 63
    second, 62
    third, 63
Pharyngeal raphe, 253
Pharyngeal recess, 50,
        250
Pharyngeal vein, 145
Pharyngeal tonsil, 252
Pharyngeal wall, 253–254
Pharyngobasilar fascia,
        253
Pharynx, 48–51, 250, *252*
    floor of, 63–65
    laryngeal, 50, 252
    muscles of, *49, 247,
        248, 251, 252,* 253
        pharyngeal
            constrictor,
            253–254
        salpingopharyngeus,
            254
        stylopharyngeus, 254

nasal, 250–251
oral, *51,* 252
and the pharyngeal
        pouch, derivatives
        of, *65*
regional divisions of,
        50
vascular and nerve
        supply, 254–255
venous drainage, 255
Philtrum, 31
Phrenic nerve, 137
Pia mater, 28, 266, 326
Pigment, red, 12
Pineal body, 272
Pit(s), 17
    nasal, 65
    preauricular, 68
Pituitary gland. *See*
        Hypophysis
Placodes, nasal, 65
Planes
    comparative, 6
    coronal, 7, 320
    frontal, 7, 322
    horizontal, 7, 322
    median, 7, 324
    midsagittal, 7, 325
    sagittal, 7
    transverse, 7
Plasma, 22
Platysma, 114, 159
Pleurisy, 150
Plexus
    basilar, 172
    brachial, 116, 134–135
    cervical, 116, 135–137
    choroid, 266, 275
    parotid, 197, 298
        buccal branch, 298
        cervical branch, 298
        mandibular branch,
            298
        temporal branch, 298
        zygomatic branch,
            298
    pharyngeal, 145, 255,
        300, 326
    pterygoid, 213
    venous, 205
    subtrapezial, 132
    tympanic, 187, 299
Plica fimbriata, 38
Plica sublingualis, 38
Pons, 274

Pontine arteries, 276
Posterior, defined, 5, 326
Posterior auricular nerve,
        297
    auricular branch, 297
    occipital branch, 297
Posterior median raphe,
        48
Postganglionic, 30, 326
Pouch defects, 69
Preganglionic, 30, 327
Premolars, 42
Preoccipital notch, 270
Primary ossification
        center, 20
Process(es), 17
    articular
        inferior, 110
        superior, 110
    clinoid
        anterior, 101
        middle, 102
        posterior, 102
    condylar, 105
    coronoid, 105
    mastoid, 96, 99
    spinous, 110
    styloid, 96, 99
    transverse, 110
    vaginal, 98
Prominence, laryngeal, 257
Protrusion, 327
    osseous, 162
Protuberance
    mental, 77, 103
    occipital
        external, 96
        internal, 103
Proximal, 6, 327
Pterygoid canal
    artery of, 226, 326
    nerve of, 296
Pterygoid muscle
    lateral, 105, *207,* 208,
        209, 210, 211
    medial, *204,* 207, 208,
        209, 210
Pterygoid nerve, lateral,
        293
Pterygomandibular raphe,
        160
Pterygopalatine fossa,
        225, 327
Pterygopalatine nerves,
        226, 290

Pulmonary arteries, left, 22
Pulmonary circuit, 22
Pulmonary trunk, 22
Pulmonary veins, 22
Pulvinar, 273
Puncta, 177
Pupil, 179, 327
Pyramidal decussations, 274
Pyramids, 274
Pyriform recess, 253
Pythagoras, 1

Ranvier, nodes of, 25
Raphe,
        pterygomandibular,
        51
Rathke's pouch, 58, 327
Recti muscles, 180
Rectus capitis anterior,
    144, 150
Rectus capitis lateralis,
    149, 150
Rectus capitis posterior
    major, 126
    minor, 127
Red blood cells
    (erythrocytes), 22
Reflex arc, 28, 327
Refractive media, of eye,
    180
Retina, 175, 179, 180
    detached, 185
Retraction, 327
Retromandibular vein,
    114, 164, 192, 333,
    334
Retromolar pad, 52
Retromolar triangle, 51
Rhinorrhea,
    cerebrospinal, 234
Ridges, 17
Rima, glottidis, 260
Risorius muscle, 159
Rivinus, ducts of, 240
Rods, 327
Rods and cones, 179
Rostral, 327
Rotation, 327
Rotatores spinae, 126
Rotatory motion, 327

Sacral outflow, 30, 327
Sagittal sinus
    inferior, 171
    superior, 171

Salivary glands, 238, 240
    accessory, 37, 38
Scalene(s)
    anterior, 134
    middle, 134
    posterior, 134
Schlemm, canal of, 179
Scalp, 153–155
    bleeding in, 164
    danger zone of, 164
    muscles of, 154–155,
        156
    nerve supply of, 155,
        158
    vascular supply to,
        155, *158*
Sclera, 179, 327
Schwann cells, 25
Sebum, 12
Sellae turcica, 101
Semispinalis capitis, 125
Semispinalis cervicis,
    125
Septal branches,
    posterior, 232
Septum (septa)
    dorsal median, 277
    interdental, 97, 105
    nasal, 76, 228, 234, 325
    pellucidum, 275
Sharpey's fibers, 167
Sheath(s)
    carotid, 117, 120–121
    neurilemma, 25
Sialography, 199, 327
Sigmoid sinus, 172
Sinus(es)
    accessory, 229
    carotid, 24
    cavernous, 165, 172
    confluence of, 171, 320
    ethmoidal, 231
    frontal, 100, 231
    headaches, 234
    intercavernous, 172
    maxillary, 76, 231
    paranasal, 229, 230,
        231, 232–234, 326
    openings of, 231
    venous drainage of,
        232
    petrosal, 172
    inferior, 102
    superior, 102
    petrosquamous, 171

sagittal
    inferior, 171
    superior, groove for,
        103
    sigmoid, groove for,
        103
    sphenoidal, 232
    sphenoparietal, 101,
        172
    transverse, 171
Sinusitis, 234, 327
Skeletal muscle, *13*
Skeletal system, 16–21
Skeleton, 16–17
    appendicular, 16, 17,
        318
    axial, 16, 17, 318
Skin, 9–12
    color, 10
    layers, 10
    keratohyalin, 10
    stratum corneum, 10
    stratum germinativum,
        10
    structure, *11*
Skull, 17, 73–109
    anterior portion, 97–98
    anterior view, 73–74,
        80, 81
    base of, *90,* 91
    bones of, 74
    external aspect of,
        73–77, *78–93,*
        94–100
    foramina of, 106–109
    frontal view of, *78, 79*
    inferior view, 97
    internal aspect of,
        100–103
    internal base of, *94,*
        100–101
    lateral view, 77, *86, 87*
    lateroinferior view of,
        88, 89
    median section of
        with median nasal
            septum intact, *82,*
            83
        with median nasal
            septum removed,
            84, 85
    middle portion, 98–99
    posterior portion, 99–100
    posterior view, 96–97
    superior view, 97

Sling
  mandibular, 208
  pterygomasseteric, 208
Somatic fibers
  afferent
    general, 279
    special, 27, 280
  efferent, general, 279
Sphenoethmoidal recess,
    229
Sphenoidal sinus, 229
Sphenopalatine artery,
    226
Sphenopalatine foramen,
    226
Sphenoparietal sinus, 172
Sphincter,
    palatopharyngeal,
    253–254
Sphincter pupillae
    muscles, 182
Spinal accessory nerve,
    132, 174, 328
Spinal cord, 277
  brain and, 265–277
  dorsal horn of, 27
Spinalis capitis, 125
Spinalis cervicis, 125
Spine(s)
  defined, 17
  mandibular
    inferior, 105
    superior, 105
  nasal
    anterior, 75
    posterior, 75, 98
Splenius capitis, 121
Splenius cervicis, 121
Stapedius muscle, 186
  nerve to, 297
Stapes, 186
Stenson's duct, 34, 191,
    328
Sternocleidomastoid
    artery, 143, 144,
    320, 323
Sternocleidomastoid
    muscle, 113, 128
Sternohyoid muscle, 140
Sternothyroid muscle,
    140
Stomodeum, 58
Straight sinus, 171
Stria medullaris, 272

Styloglossus muscle, 198,
    239
Stylohoid muscle, 198, 236
  nerve to, 298
Stylomandibular
    ligament, 119
Stylomastoid artery, 196,
    324
Stylopharyngeus muscle,
    198
  nerve to, 30
Subarachnoid space, 28,
    266, 328
Subclavian artery(ies),
    137–139, 146, 330
Subclavian triangle, 129,
    131, 328
Subclavian vein, 115, 139
Subclavius muscle, 139
Subcortical nuclei, 270
Subdural space, 28, 265,
    328
Sublingual artery, 242,
    321
  injury to, 244
Sublingual caruncula, 40,
    240, 328
Sublingual duct, 240
  large, 38
  small, 38
Sublingual gland,
    240–241
  autonomic innervation,
    241
Sublingual sulcus, 36
Submandibular duct, 38,
    240
Submandibular gland, 240
  autonomic innervation,
    241
Submandibular nodes,
    243
Submandibular triangle,
    131, 328
Submental artery, 144,
    243, 322
Submental triangle, 131,
    328
Suboccipital nerve, 126,
    128
Suboccipital triangle,
    126, 127–128, 328
  boundaries and
    contents of, 128

Subthalamus, 273
Sulcus, 328
  anterior lateral, 274
  calcarine, 271
  lateral, 270
  median lingual, 324
  olfactory, 271
  parietooccipital, 270
  precentral, 270
  sagittal, 100
  terminal, 64
Sulcus terminalis, 37, 328
Superficial, defined, 5,
    328
Superior, defined, 5
Supraclavicular nerves,
    117
Suprahyoid artery, 242,
    321
Suprahyoid muscles, 236,
    237
  group actions of, 238
Supraorbital artery, 164,
    328
Supraorbital nerve, 161,
    184, 288
Suprascapular artery,
    138, 331
Suprascapular vein, 115,
    334
Suprasternal space, 119
Supratrochlear artery,
    164, 329
Supratrochlear nerve,
    161, 184
Suture, 328
  coronal, 74, 77, 320
  cruciform, 97
  lambdoidal, 77, 96
  metopic frontal, 74
  occiptomastoid, 77
  sagittal, 74, 96, 327
  sphenoparietal, 77
  sphenosquamosal, 77
  squamosal, 77
  temporo-occipital, 100
Swelling, lateral nasal, 65
Sympathectomy, 150
Sympathetic nerve, 185
Sympathetic trunk, 30,
    329
Symphysis, 329
  mandibular, 103
  mental, 77, 103, 324

Synapse, 27, 329
Synovial fluid, 14, 329
Synovial sheath, 14, 329
Systemic circuit, 22
Systems, defined, 9

Tarsal gland, 175
Tear gland. *See* Lacrimal
    gland
Tectum, 274
Tegmentum, 274
Tegmen tympani, 102
Temple, 210
Temporal artery
    maxillary, 144–145,
        326
    superficial, 144, 163,
        196, 324
Temporalis, *204*, 205,
    206
Temporal nerves
    deep, 292
    superficial, 294
Temporal vein,
    superficial, 164,
    193, 333
Temporomandibular
    joint (TMJ),
    213–214, 217–223
    anatomy of, 217–221
    dysfunction syndrome,
        223
    innervation and
        vascularization,
        220
    muscles acting on, 223
    portion of, *19*
    types of movement,
        221–223
        ginglymus (hinge),
            221
        lateral rotation, 222
        translatory (gliding),
            222
Temporoparietalis, 155
Tendon, 14
Tensor tympani, 186
Tensor veli palatini,
    246–247
Tensor tympani, nerve
    to, 213
Tentorium cerebelli,
    167–168, 329
Thalamus, 272, 329

Thoracic duct, 24, 139,
    329
Thoracic spinal cord
    segment and
    nerve, *28*
Thoracolumbar outflow,
    30, 329
Thrombosis, 164, 165
Thyrocervical trunk,
    138–139
Thyroglossal duct, 37,
    69, 145, 329
Thyrohyoid muscle, 141
Thyroid, 69
    aberrant, 69
    accessory, 69
    cartilage, 113
    lingual, 53, 69
Thyroid artery
    inferior, 139, 146, 255,
        261, 331
        ascending branch,
            146
    superior, 146, 254, 261,
        320
        anterior branch, 146
        posterior branch, 146
Thyroidectomy, 152
Thyroid gland, 145
    venous drainage of, 146
Thyroid notch, 113
Thyroid storm, 152
Thyroid vein
    inferior, 146, 335
    middle, 146, 335
    superior, 146, 335
Tic douloureux. *See*
    Neuralgia,
    trigeminal
Tissues, 9
    areolar tissue, loose, 10
    connective tissue
        (hypodermis),
        subcutaneous, 10
    fascia, superficial, 10
TMS. *See*
    Temporamandibular
    joint
Tomography, computed,
    319
Tongue, 36–40, 53,
    63–64, 69
    crenated, 53, 320
    development, *64*

fissured, 53, 321
forms, *54*
muscles, 238–239
    extrinsic, 239
    group actions of,
        239–240
    innervation and
        vascularization,
        239
    intrinsic, 238–239
    principal lymph node
        of, 243, 314, 327
    ventral surface of, *39*
Tonsil(s)
    lingual, 37
    nasopharyngeal, 50,
        325
    palatine, *246*, 249–250
    pharyngeal, 252
Tonsillar artery, 144,
    254, 322
Tonsillar circle, 250
Tonsillar nerve, 300
Tonsillitis, 263
Tooth (teeth), 40–48
    deciduous, 42
    dentin, 44
    development, 44, *48*
    enamel, 44
    eruption, 44
    permanent, 42
    radiographs of, *45*
Torticollis, 149–150
Torus tubarium, 250
Trachea, *256*, 261
Tracheotomy, 263, 329
Transverse cervical
    artery, 138, 139,
    331
Transverse sinus, 171
Trapezius muscle, 113
    paralysis of, 150
Triangle(s)
    anterior, 317
    carotid, 131
    cervical, boundaries of,
        130
    of neck, 128–131
        anterior, 139
        muscles associated
            with posterior,
            132, 133
        posterior, 131–139
    occipital, 325

Triangles (*continued*)
posterior, 326
retromolar, 105
Trigeminal cave, 170
Trigeminal ganglion, 174
Trigeminal nerve, 173,
174, 184, 193, 226,
241, 282, 285, *286,*
289, 329
branches of, 161
mandibular division,
161–162, 213–215
meningeal branch,
213
maxillary division,
161, 184, 215
opthalmic division,
161, 184
Trochlear fovea, 75, 180
Trochlear nerve, 282,
285, 287–288, 329
Tuber cinereum, 273
Tubercle(s), 17
alveolar, 97
articular, 218
genial, 105
mental, 103
pharyngeal, 98
posterior, 112
post-glenoid, 96
Tuberculum, cinereum,
274
Tuberculum cuneatus,
274
Tuberculum gracilis, 274
Tuberculum impar, 63
Tuberculum sellae, 101,
102
Tuberosities, 17
maxillary, 97
Tunics, *178,* 179–180
internal, 179
Tympanic artery,
anterior, 196, 325
Tympanic cavity. *See*
Ear, middle
Tympanic nerve, 299–300
Tympanum, 186, 329

Upper limb
arterial insufficiency
of, 150
uncontrollable bleeding
in, 151
Uvula, 40

Vagus nerve, 146–147,
174, 300–303, 329
auricular branch, 302
cardiac branches,
superior, 303
external laryngeal
branch, 147
inferior ganglion, 302
internal branch, 147
meningeal branch, 302
pharyngeal branches,
302
recurrent laryngeal
branches, 148
superior ganglion, 302
Vallate papillae, 37, 330
Valleculae, 50
epiglottic, 258
Valve
bicuspid, 22
left atrioventricular,
22
right atrioventricular,
22
tricuspid, 22
Vein(s)
angular, 332, 334
auricular
anterior, 333
posterior, 114, 164,
333, 334
brachiocephalic, 139
cerebellar
inferior, 276
superior, 276
cerebral, 276
cervical
deep, 335
transverse, 334
ciliary, 334
in cranial cavity. *See*
Sinus(es), venous
diploic, 172, 173
emissary, 173, 333
facial, 164, 332
common, 243
deep, 332
transverse, 164, 333
frontal, 332
great cerebral, 276
infraorbital, 164
jugular
anterior, 115, 334,
336
arch, 116

external, 114, 193,
333, 334, 336
internal, 145, 171,
335
posterior external,
115, 334
lingual, 243, 335
maxillary, 213, 333
nasofrontal, 334
occipital, 333
ophthalmic, 164
inferior, 185, 334
superior, 185, 334
palatine
greater, 249, 333
lesser, 249, 333
pharyngeal plexus, 145,
255
pterygoid plexus, 164,
213, 333
retromandibular, 114,
164, 192, 333, 334
subclavian, 115, 139,
334, 335
supraorbital, 164, 332
suprascapular, 115, 334
supratrochlear, 164, 332
temporal
middle, 333
superficial, 164, 193,
333
thyroid, 146, 335
tonsillar, 249, 333
transverse cervical,
115, 334
transverse facial, 164,
333
vertebral
anterior, 335
Veli palatini
levator, 246
tensor, 246–247
Vena cava(ae), 22
inferior, 22
superior, 22
Ventral, defined, 5, 330
Ventral horn (motor), 27,
330
Ventral root, 27, 330
Ventricles, 275
fourth, 275
lateral, 271, 275
left, 22
right, 22
third, 275

Vermilion
  border, 31
  zone, 31, 330
Vermis, 271
Vertebra(ae), cervical, 73, 109–112
  body, 110
  typical, 110, *111*
Vertebral artery, 137–138, 276, 330
Vertebral column, 17
Vesalius, Andreas, 2
Vestibular nerve, 298
Vestibule, 33–36, 51–53, 229, 330
  buccal, *52*
Vibrissa(ae), 227
Vidian nerve, 296, 330
Visceral nervous system, 28

Visceral afferent
  general, 279
  special, 27, 280, 328
Visceral efferent
  general, 279
  special, 27, 280, 328
Vomer, 73, 76
Vocal folds, movements of, 260–261
Vocalization, inability to, 263
Voice box. *See* Larynx

Waldeyer, lymphatic ring of, 56.
  See also Tonsillar circle
Wharton's duct. *See* Submandibular duct

White blood cells (leucocytes), 22
White rami communicantes, 30, 330
Willis, circle of, 276
Wisdom tooth, 42
Wolff's Law, 20

Zygoma, 73, 96
  maxillary process of, 76
Zygomatic nerve, 226, 290
Zygomaticofacial artery, 164
Zygomaticofacial nerve, 161, 290
Zygomaticotemporal nerves, 161, 290
Zygomaticus major, 160
Zygomaticus minor, 160